The Prognosis of Metastatic Gastrointestinal Cancer

Survival of patients with metastatic cancer has increased over the past two decades as a result of a progressive improvement of regional and systemic therapies. However, oncologists' estimates of patients' predicted overall survival in metastatic cancer are imprecise. The purpose of this book is to systematize the evidence regarding the prognostic factors of metastatic gastrointestinal tumors, separating the findings with the highest level of evidence among those available for each disease by selecting studies with the highest scientific evidence level.

The Prognosis of Metastatic
Gastrointestinal Cancer

Giuseppe A. Colloca and Antonella Venturino

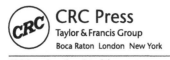

CRC Press
Taylor & Francis Group
Boca Raton London New York

CRC Press is an imprint of the
Taylor & Francis Group, an **informa** business

Designed cover image: Authors

First edition published 2025
by CRC Press
2385 NW Executive Center Drive, Suite 320, Boca Raton FL 33431

and by CRC Press
4 Park Square, Milton Park, Abingdon, Oxon, OX14 4RN

CRC Press is an imprint of Taylor & Francis Group, LLC

© 2025 Giuseppe Colloca and Antonella Venturino

ISBN: 9781032703343 (hbk)
ISBN: 9781032699714 (pbk)
ISBN: 9781032703350 (ebk)

DOI: 10.1201/9781032703350

Typeset in Times
by Deanta Global Publishing Services, Chennai, India

Contents

Introduction

Survival of patients with metastatic cancer has increased over the past two decades as a result of a progressive improvement of regional and systemic therapies. This improvement has been remarkable in some diseases due to immunotherapy, whereas in the area of gastrointestinal (GI) oncology, the improvement was related to the optimization of the integration of regional and systemic treatments in oligometastatic disease (OMD), as well as to new drugs. Some examples are the change in prognosis of patients with metastatic GI stromal tumors after the introduction of imatinib, the median overall survival (OS) of more than 5 years for metastatic neuroendocrine tumors, or that of more than 3 years for metastatic colorectal cancer patients. In this context, therefore, it becomes increasingly important for each of the practitioners involved in the management of patients with metastatic GI tumors to be able to perform a comprehensive evaluation of all prognostic and predictive variables to propose an appropriate therapeutic plan.

Oncologists' estimates of patients' predicted OS in metastatic cancer are imprecise. In one study it was too optimistic in 35% of cases and too pessimistic in 39% [1], although according to another study it was independently associated with observed survival [2]. Improving this prediction is necessary to define appropriate treatment plans.

A prognostic factor (PF) is any variable, usually tumor- or patient-related, that can influence the outcome. The importance of PFs lies in the fact that they can modulate and support therapeutic decisions, aggressive or conservative, relying on the expected clinical evolution. In addition, PFs are essential for research because they enable sample stratification in clinical trials. Unlike predictive factor (PREF), which predicts the efficacy of a specific treatment in a patient population, PF predicts survival independently of treatments and other variables.

Thus, while the evaluation and study of PREFs are closely linked to a specific treatment, PFs are not linked to treatments but only to the host and the disease. Unfortunately, however, their evaluation and analysis are seldom considered in prospective randomized clinical trials (RCTs). Consequently, the lack of evidence-based results of PFs puts the variables included in RCTs at risk and the confounding sometimes necessitates the use of expert opinion to redefine the relevant variables [3]. Ultimately, while RCTs have provided high levels of evidence on the treatment variable, they have not provided equally unambiguous conclusions on PFs. For this reason, in some situations, only retrospective studies have investigated prognostic variables and defined cut-offs and standardizations.

The standardization of prognostic variables remains one of the most critical issues. These variables vary widely among RCTs, and many PFs are questionable because they were identified in uncontrolled studies with inadequate case numbers and statistical power. Since phase III RCTs remain the most objective method for evaluating the efficacy of antineoplastic treatments, they are also an important and reliable source of information on PFs. Indeed, in RCTs, evaluation of all variables that influence survival is essential to support study conclusions, but the PFs analyses are not always appropriate nor homogeneous over time, whenever reported.

The purpose of this book is to systematize the evidence regarding PFs of metastatic GI tumors, separating the findings with the highest level of evidence among those available for each disease by selecting studies with the highest scientific evidence level. This aim is achieved by separately evaluating PFs within a limited number of trials, whose evidence level differed by tumor site (Table S1). A systematic search of two databases (PubMed and Web of Science) enabled the selection of clinical trials related to patients with metastatic disease. Only studies published in English during the period 1970–2022 were considered. These selected studies represented each variable with the highest level of evidence. To avoid confusion the authors restricted the analysis to the exclusive disease setting of unresectable/metastatic disease in the early metastatic timing, before any upfront treatment, and evaluated only the relationship of the PFs with OS.

TABLE S1
Selected studies reporting evaluation of prognostic variables in metastatic gastrointestinal tumors

	Phase III	Phase II	Retrospective	Total
Esophageal cancer	3	3	–	6
Gastric cancer	8	–	–	8
Small bowel adenocarcinoma	–	3	6	9
Pancreatic adenocarcinoma	25	–	–	25
Hepatocellular carcinoma	6	5	–	11
Biliary tree tumors	1	15	–	16
Neuroendocrine neoplasms	6	10	–	16
Gastrointestinal stromal tumors	3	1	–	4
Colorectal cancer	39	–	–	39
Anal cancer	–	–	3	3

To overcome the selection bias of RCTs and include other study samples more similar to current clinical practice, but also to evaluate some PFs when RCTs did not report sufficient information, for each PF, the results of population-based and retrospective/observational studies were separately reported in the text.

To systematize and provide the reader with a systematic treatment of the topics, a distinction has been made between patient-related PFs (performance status, demographic, anthropometric, clinic, and laboratory variables) and tumor-related PFs (tumor burden, primary tumor location, timing of metastasis, site of metastasis, pathology, previous treatments). Although this distinction has often been reported in the literature, we realize that it is a distortion of reality. Indeed, even for seemingly host-related variables such as performance status (PS), it is not possible to separate them from the presence of the tumor, especially in metastatic disease. Therefore, the subdivision of PFs into patient-related and tumor-related is only intended to simplify consultation of the text.

On purpose, composite indices, scores, and nomograms have been avoided as much as possible in the evaluation of variables, since they are not widely accepted and used in the clinic and often confuse the evaluation of individual variables, which are themselves often interconnected and difficult to evaluate separately. Furthermore, although questionnaire scores related to health-related quality of life (HRQoL) have been shown to play a prognostic role, it was decided to exclude them from the analysis, as well as health services related variables.

Whenever at least three studies reporting the same effect size measure were available, in our case hazard ratio, PFs were also evaluated by meta-analysis, performed according to the random-effects model, to give an overall estimate of the overall effect size and heterogeneity of the studies, and forest plots were reported by publication year for all variables that had been evaluated in at least five studies. The results by PFs of the selected studies were summarized in the first table, in each chapter. Subsequent tables listed the findings of the reviewed studies for each prognostic variable.

After the synthesis of the various evidence-level reports for patient- and tumor-related variables, a further paragraph summarizes the PFs reliability in the decision-making in the upfront setting and after progression. This discussion is largely theoretical, and does not take into account the multifaceted and practical aspects of decision-making, such as toxicity profiles, patient's conditions, multidisciplinary treatment plans, available therapeutic procedures and drugs, institution experience, patient preferences, etc.

Finally, at the end of each chapter, a table summarises the conclusions of the PFs analysis based on the selected studies but taking into account all the other findings from the literature, with the indication about the suggested prognostic variables and those needing further study or appropriate standardization.

The procedure followed for reading the available evidence on PFs in prospective studies of upfront metastatic disease has limitations. The most notable of them is the very limited reporting of the results of analyses of PFs, which are mostly used to perform subgroup analyses to better define the effects of treatment on various sub-populations of patients. This tendency to not report the direct effect of PFs on OS appears particularly evident in the last ten years. Another important limitation of the studies is the lack of standardization of many PFs and, within each, the absence of clear cut-offs or methods of assessment (e.g., as a continuous variable or around a clinically relevant cut-off). The unevenness of results across studies often led to reporting the data in tables with the various cut-offs (e.g., PS 2/more vs. PS 0–1, PS 1 vs. PS 0, continuum, etc.). Other critical issues encountered are the variability of the PFs included in the individual studies and the reporting. Some studies report univariate and not multivariate analyses, and this in itself exposes an overestimation of the effect size of the variable. In this book, we have preferred to include the result of the multivariate analysis whenever it was available. Sometimes, in addition to the data from the univariate analysis or obtained by means of other statistical procedures, the results of post-hoc or limited sample analyses presenting the results of the variable under study have been published.

On the other hand, it is necessary to reiterate the strength of the analysis reported in this book, i.e., the attempt to differentiate the quality of the evidence by giving more prominence to selected studies, which in most cases are those reporting prospective and controlled evaluations.

REFERENCES

1. Stockler MR, Tattersall MHN, Boyer MJ, et al. Disarming the guarded prognosis: Predicting survival in newly referred patients with incurable cancer. *Br J Cancer* 2006;94:208–12.
2. Kiely BE, Martin AJ, Tattersall MHN, et al. The median informs the message: Accuracy of individualized scenarios for survival time based on oncologists' estimates. *J Clin Oncol* 2013;31:3565–71.
3. ter Veer E, van Rijssen LB, Besselink MG, et al. Consensus statement on mandatory measurements in pancreatic cancer trials (COMM-PACT) for systemic treatment of unresectable disease. *Lancet Oncol* 2018;19(3):e151–60.

1 Esophageal cancer

1.1 INTRODUCTION

The histological distinction between esophageal squamous cell carcinoma (ESCC) and esophageal adenocarcinoma (EAC) identifies two different diseases rather than two subgroups of esophageal cancer (EC), with the first accounting for 85% of total ECs. In this chapter, the focus is on ESCC, leaving the discussion of EAC for the most part to the second chapter.

1.1.1 EPIDEMIOLOGY

A GLOBOCAN database report estimated 604,000 new cases and 544,100 deaths from EC for 2020, with incidence and mortality of 6.3 and 5.6 per 100,000, respectively [1]. In 2022, in China, the expected new cases were 346,663, with related deaths 323,600, while in the US the estimated new cases were 19,042 with 16,916 deaths [2]. In 2022, in Europe, the age-adjusted standardized incidence rate (ASR) was 6.7/100,000, with 29,825 new cases, and similar rates of mortality with an ASR of 5.8/100,000 and 26,015 cancer deaths. The tumor was more prevalent among males with an incidence ASR of 10.5 vs. 2.6/100,000, and a mortality ASR of 9.3 vs. 2.2/100,000 [3].

The highest registered EC incidences were in Eastern Asia and Southern and Eastern Africa, and the lowest in Western Africa and Central America [1]. An Indian study documented that EC was the most common malignancy of the gastrointestinal tract [4].

The 2019 Global Burden of Disease Study evaluated the time course of EC in high-incidence areas such as China and Japan over 30 years and reported a decline in the mortality ASR. This reduction has stopped among young people [5], but GLOBOCAN data and Chinese National Cancer Centers registries documented that declines in incidence and mortality continued in 2022 [1]. Also in the United States, a Surveillance Epidemiology End Results (SEER) database analysis showed reductions in incidence and mortality [6], and the National Cancer Database (NCDB) documented a reduction in early onset ECs [7]. If rates remain stable 957,000 new cases and 880,000 deaths are expected by 2040 worldwide [1], and an increasing incidence in Europe with an additional 17.8% for males and 17.6% for females [3].

Gender distribution by geographic area, particularly in Europe [8], was highly variable, although EC remains prevalent among males. A worldwide analysis of 171 registries in 54 countries reported that the male-to-female incidence rate ratio increased from young ages with a peak at 60–64, then decreased [9].

1.1.2 STAGING OF METASTATIC DISEASE

It is important to tailor the diagnostic workout and staging to the patient's conditions, thus also considering diet and correction of nutritional status. For diagnosis, flexible endoscopy with biopsy is always indicated [10]. Esophagoscopy allows direct visualization and samples for diagnosis, histological classification, and molecular typization.

Histopathologic and molecular diagnosis requires at least 6–8 endoscopic biopsies. The pathology report must define the diagnosis according to the WHO criteria [11], including any immunohistochemistry (IHC) in undifferentiated tumors to clearly distinguish between ESCC and EAC. In the case of ESCC, PD-L1 must be determined, through clones currently validated in diagnostics

DOI: 10.1201/9781032703350-1

(22C3, 28.8), and expressed as tumor proportion scale (TPS) or combined positive score (CPS). For the EAC of the junction, the same assessments as for gastric cancer must be considered.

A thoraco-abdominal CT is necessary to evaluate the invasion of adjacent structures, lymph nodes, and distant metastases. Any cervical-cephalic tumor, occurring in 6.7% of ESCC patients, should be diagnosed early in consideration of the poor prognosis of ESCC patients in the presence of a second cervical-cephalic district malignancy [12].

Iron deficiency anemia, renal and liver function, weight loss (WL), and inflammation and nutrition-related variables [13, 14] should be assessed, as well as cardio-pulmonary reserve before multimodal therapy.

Other imaging, such as EUS, FDG-PET, and laparoscopy are not indicated in metastatic or locally advanced unresectable esophageal cancer (mEC).

The reference staging is that proposed by the American Joint Committee on Cancer (AJCC) according to the TNM Classification (AJCC 8th edition 2017) [15].

1.1.3 PROGNOSIS OF METASTATIC DISEASE

Survival rates are dismal. Despite treatment improvements, the overall survival (OS) of mEC remains poor, with a 5-year survival rate of 5.7% [1]. About 40% of these patients have rapidly progressive disease at diagnosis, leading to death within three months [16]. Among European people in 2000–2007, 5-year survival rates of 10.3% for males and 14.3% for females were reported [3], and of 20.6% from SEER database in the US from 2012 to 2018 [17].

The poor mEC outcomes are confirmed by median OS, which however has changed over time from 3.5 months in 1980 [18] to 5.7–8.9 months in 1997 [19] until 9.8–12.4 months in 2021 [20].

1.2 ANALYSIS OF PROGNOSTIC VARIABLES IN EARLY METASTATIC DISEASE

A systematic review of prospective trials that studied upfront therapies in patients with mEC resulted in the selection of 36 studies (9 phase III, 27 phase II) published from 1980 to 2022. In six trials an analysis of prognostic variables was done, and in five a multivariate analysis was performed, whose results were partly reported in the articles [18, 19, 21–24]. Table S1 summarizes all prognostic factors (PFs) that have been reported in at least one of the six studies, and the number of studies that found or did not find a relationship between the candidate PFs and OS.

In the present analysis, adenocarcinomas of the cardia are considered as gastric cancers (GC), but some studies of mECs have been included in the analysis although they enrolled a proportion of patients with GC. This has been necessary because of the limited number of mEC trials. Thus, patients with cardial and gastric adenocarcinomas were enrolled in some of the studies, and in three of them, ECs were only a part of the study cohort (48%, 56%, and 70%, respectively) [21, 22, 24].

1.3 PATIENT-RELATED PROGNOSTIC FACTORS

1.3.1 PERFORMANCE STATUS

Despite comparisons between various categories of performance status (PS), two prospective studies documented a significant association between good PS and long survival [25, 26], but in two other studies, the differences were not significant [27, 28]. Except one trial that compared an ECOG PS 0 vs. 1 in patients with oligometastatic disease (OMD) [29], four retrospective experiences consistently found a favorable prognostic role for good PS [30–33].

1.3.1.1 Selected trials

Six studies investigated the PS and included 1,265 patients. Their results are listed in Table 1.1. Patients with PS ≥2 were included in 3 studies and accounted for 22% of all patients. In two studies

TABLE S1
Prognostic factors analyzed in selected clinical trials of patients with unresectable or metastatic esophageal cancer receiving upfront treatment

Variable	No. trials	Prognostic relationship	No prognostic relationship
Patient-related			
Performance status	6	2	4
Demographic			
Age	1	0	1
Sex	1	0	1
Anthropometric			
Clinic			
Weight loss	1	0	1
Lab			
Albumin	2	1	1
Bilirubin	1	1	0
Alkalyne phosphatase	1	1	0
Sodium	1	1	0
Tumor-related			
Tumor burden			
Disease status	4	4	0
Regional infiltration	1	1	0
Primary tumor location	1	0	1
Timing of metastasis			
Site of metastasis			
Liver metastases	1	1	0
Pathology			
DNA ploidy	1	0	1
Previous treatments			
Previous radiotherapy	1	0	1

TABLE 1.1
Prognostic relationships of performance status in selected studies of patients with unresectable or metastatic esophageal cancer receiving upfront treatment

Study [ref]	Phase	No. pts	Scale	Comparison	Prognostic relationship	Effect size
ECOG 1980 [18]	II	63	ECOG	PS 2–3 vs. PS 0–1	No	NR
Ohio SU 1996 [23]	II	27	SWOG	PS 2 vs. PS 0–1	No	NR
British 1997 [19]	III	256	ECOG	PS ≥2 vs. PS 0–1	Yes	HR 1.76 (1.26–2.45)
British 2002 [21]	III	250	ECOG	NR	No	NR
MRC 2002 [22]	III	574	ECOG	NR	No	NR
MDACC 2010 [24]	II	95	ECOG	PS 2 vs. PS 0–1	Yes	HR 2.88 (1.51–5.51)

Legend: ECOG, Eastern Cooperative Oncology Group. HR, hazard ratio. NR, not reported. PS, performance status. SWOG, South Western Oncology Group.

PS was associated with poor prognosis on multivariate analysis [19, 24], and in another study, if albuminemia was excluded from the Cox model, PS returned to predict OS [22].

1.3.2   DEMOGRAPHIC

1.3.2.1   Age

Two SEER database analyses documented poor outcomes for ages >65–70 [16, 34], while other authors did not find significant differences in terms of long-term survivors (>24 months) [35]. The poor outcome of elderly people seems particularly pronounced in patients with multiple sites of metastasis [36] and could be a consequence of a disparity of multimodal treatments [37].

One study of a cohort of patients with mEC and OMD undergoing treatment documented a worse prognosis with increasing age [28], while four prospective cohorts did not find OS differences [25–27, 38]. One retrospective study confirmed reduced survival of patients >50 years [31], while five others reported no difference by age [29, 30, 32, 39, 40], or on the contrary better outcomes for patients >65 years old [33].

1.3.2.2   Sex

Eleven studies of mEC patients did not show OS differences by sex [16, 25, 27, 30, 31–33, 35, 36, 39, 40]. An evaluation of the SEER database found better OS for females [34], with further analyses suggesting that the favorable prognosis was prominent in 46–55-year-old patients [41]. A study from Shandong Cancer Hospital detected only a favorable OS trend for females [29], while another Chinese series documented better outcomes for the male sex [30].

1.3.2.3   Other demographic variables

According to a South African study, residence in metropolitan areas vs. rural areas confers better prognosis for mEC patients [26].

Only one [42] of four SEER database analyses on patients with mEC found a poor prognosis for Whites vs. Blacks in the US population [16, 35, 36].

The three studies from the SEER database that investigated the effect of marital status reported among married patients significantly increased OS [34], lower early death [16], and a higher percentage of patients with OS >24 months [35].

1.3.2.4   Selected trials

Only one randomized phase III trial (RCT) evaluated the prognostic role of age, finding no significant relationship [21].

The same trial examined sex as a PF without reporting an effect on OS [21].

1.3.3   ANTHROPOMETRIC

An Asian pooled analysis of 18 cohort studies [43] and another of two North American cohorts [44] documented increased EC mortality for body mass index (BMI) <18.5 kg/m2 or >25–35 kg/m^2.

In the 384 mEC patients at Grey's Hospital in South Africa who had received palliative treatment, the probability of being alive after 3 months was higher for a baseline BMI >18.5 [26], while two retrospective studies did not find differences at cut-offs of 25 [30] and 18.8 [39].

1.3.4   CLINIC

Among 350 patients enrolled in six prospective studies of cisplatin-based chemotherapy, a WL >5% in the last 3 months was associated with an OS reduction from 12 to 9 months [25], with a similar conclusion at a cut-off of 10% [32]. Other studies suggest that WL and cachexia are early symptoms [45] frequently concomitant to systemic inflammatory response (SIR) activation [46].

On the other hand, dysphagia at onset and its severity did not affect prognosis [26, 27, 32], nor did diabetes mellitus, pulmonary obstructive disease [30], or a previous malignancy [34].

The presence of tracheoesophageal fistula, a complication that is associated with more aggressive ECs and reduced regional treatment options, shortened the median OS of mEC patients with oligometastatic disease (OMD) [29], but produced only a negative trend in another study [32].

Neither the Charlson Comorbidity Index (CCI) [28] nor smoking habit or history of alcohol consumption showed correlations with the outcome [29, 30].

1.3.4.1 Selected trials

A small study of mEC patients receiving chemotherapy documented a median WL of 15%, but a baseline WL >10% did not affect OS [23].

1.3.5 LABORATORY

One study documented a relationship between hemoglobin >11.2 g/dL and better prognosis [32], while others did not [25, 33], similar to platelet count [32, 33]. Leukocyte count >10,000/mcL correlated with poor prognosis in a retrospective analysis [33], but not in a similar study at a cut-off of 8,630/mcL [32]. Lymphocyte [47] and monocyte counts [48] need further confirmation in mEC, as the CD4/CD8 ratio [49]. Similarly, a meta-analysis that included four studies with mEC patients did not report a prognostic effect of neutrophil-to-lymphocyte ratio (NLR) [50], while prognostic effect was reported for the ratio of platelet count to mean platelet volume [51].

Some SIR-related parameters [30, 39, 40] and albuminemia [26, 32] could have an effect on the outcome of mEC. While altered liver function parameters did not seem as relevant [32], analysis of data from six prospective studies reports worse OS for elevated alkaline phosphatase (ALP) or lactic dehydrogenase (LDH) [25].

Few studies have evaluated oncologic markers, with no significant prognostic effect for carcino-embryonic antigen (CEA) [40].

1.3.5.1 Selected trials

Two studies have evaluated the relationship between serum albumin and OS, with one documenting better OS with increasing albumin [21] and the other not [22].

One study included bilirubinemia as a continuous variable and found poor OS with increasing bilirubin [22]. A modest but significant OS reduction was documented for elevated ALP [21].

1.4 TUMOR-RELATED PROGNOSTIC FACTORS

1.4.1 TUMOR BURDEN

Most of the studies that analyzed the prognostic role of T-stage in mEC are negative [27, 28, 30, 36]. While only one study documented that mEC patients with a T3–T4 tumor had lower OS than those with a T1–T2 [31], a similar conclusion from the comparison of T4 vs. T3 was found by the SEER database [35].

No prognostic relationships resulted from studies investigating tumor length along the esophagus [26, 29], nor for N-stage [16, 27–30, 35, 36].

The presence of metastatic vs. unresectable locally advanced disease was a negative PF in two studies [27, 30], but not in others [39, 40].

Some tumor burden (TB)-related variables, such as the diameter of lung metastases, did not show relationships with OS [38], while patients with "extensive dissemination", those with more than 4 metastases, or high metabolic tumor volume had a poor prognosis [25, 29, 52].

Multiple vs. single sites of metastasis usually presented shorter survival [25, 29, 31, 35], except in one study that evaluated patients with resected lung metastases [38].

1.4.1.1 Selected trials

Four studies evaluated the prognostic effect of locally advanced vs. metastatic disease, reporting a poor prognosis of patients with metastatic disease [19, 21–23]. The results of the four studies are summarized in Table 1.2. Pooling data of three of these studies the global ES was significant (HR 1.47, CI 1.22–1.78; Q = 0.65, p-value = 0.7227; I^2 = 0%).

A study published in 1980 reported adjacent organ involvement as an independent variable that correlated with reduced OS [18].

1.4.2 PRIMARY TUMOR LOCATION

A retrospective analysis of a series of 90 mECs from Mansoura University documented improved survival rates proceeding from the lower to the upper third of the esophagus [31], while other authors did not detect different outcomes depending on EC location [16, 27, 29, 30, 32, 34–36].

The 2022 Kyoto Consensus redefined the gastro-esophageal junctional zone and proposed a pathophysiologic classification of GC [53]. In addition, ICD-11 distinguished EAC from junctional adenocarcinomas [54]. Adenocarcinomas of the cardia are increasingly evaluated as GC though they express etiologic characteristics of similarity with both ESCC and non-cardial GC [52].

1.4.2.1 Selected trials

Only one study analyzed mEC location (esophagus vs. junction vs. stomach), finding no effect on OS after multivariate regression [21].

1.4.3 TIMING OF METASTASIS

The outcome of patients with synchronous vs. metachronous metastases was compared in a limited number of studies, with negative results [29, 33].

In metachronous OMD [28] and in patients with resectable lung metastases [38], a disease-free interval (DFI) >12 months appeared to be predictive of longer OS [28, 38], and in a prospective database metachronous recurrence with a median time-to-recurrence (TTR) of 19 months or more was a favorable PF [28].

1.4.4 SITES OF METASTASIS

The lymph node localization of distant metastases predicts a more indolent disease course, with a 1-year survival rate of 53% vs. 11–19% of other sites [31], and this was particularly true for lymph node-limited disease [33] and those involving only one anatomic nodal group [29]. In the context of metastatic lymph node disease, however, other variables might exert an unfavorable prognostic effect, such as high NLR, volume of recurrence [55], and DFI [56].

TABLE 1.2

Prognostic relationships of disease status in selected studies of patients with unresectable or metastatic esophageal cancer receiving upfront treatment

Study [ref]	Phase	No. pts	Variable	Prognostic relationship	Effect size
Ohio SU 1996 [23]	II	27	Metastatic vs. LA	Yes	NR
British 1997 [19]	III	256	Metastatic vs. LA	Yes	HR 1.61 (1.17–2.20)
British 2002 [21]	III	250	Metastatic vs. LA	Yes	HR 1.55 (1.10–2.18)
MRC 2002 [22]	III	508	Metastatic vs. LA	Yes	HR 1.40 (1.15–1.70)

Legend: HR, hazard ratio. LA, locally advanced. NR, not reported.

After the occurrence of liver metastases (LMs), some authors suggest a reduced OS [16, 25, 35], which is not confirmed by others [29, 32, 36]. An analysis of 1,197 mEC patients with LMs from the SEER suggested that some characteristics might contribute to reduced OS, such as male sex, advanced age, ESCC histotype, and multiple extra-hepatic metastases [57].

Excepting one study that reports an increase in early deaths for patients with lung metastases [16], lung metastases do not seem to alter outcome [29, 32, 35], but in the case of lung-limited disease survival could be longer [36]. Moreover, in the context of lung-limited disease, the results of SBRT [58] and surgery [59] seem considerable.

The occurrence of bone disease has been related to shorter OS [16, 31, 35], although not in all studies [29, 32]. Some authors have reported longer OS in patients with EAC, T2 stage, absence of extra-osseous metastases, and previous chemoradiation [60].

Except in a SEER study evaluating mEC early death [16], it remains doubtful that the presence of brain metastases could change the outcome [35, 36], although the prognosis remains poor [61–63]. A possible favorable role of a low number of metastases, good PS, and treatment modality needs further confirmation, while a score based on ECOG PS, number of vertebrae involved, and presence of visceral metastases could estimate the 6-month survival of ESCC patients with secondary epidural spinal cord compression [64].

1.4.4.1 Selected trials

A relationship between the presence of LMs and OS was evaluated in one study, which showed a significant prognostic role, although details of the regression model were not reported [18].

1.4.5 PATHOLOGY

1.4.5.1 Histology

Many studies have compared ESCC with EAC, usually without documenting differences in OS [25, 27–29, 31, 35], while the SEER database suggested increased early deaths for patients with ESCC compared with EAC [16]. Excluding neuroendocrine carcinomas, which will be discussed in Chapter 7, the other histotypes are very uncommon. One study evaluated 29 patients with small cell carcinoma of the esophagus (SCC) and 30 with basaloid squamous cell carcinoma, describing a more advanced stage and poor prognosis for patients with SCC, which improved after systemic therapy [65].

1.4.5.2 Tumor grade

Of four studies that assessed tumor grade, three found OS reduction with increasing grade [16, 31, 35] and one did not [36]. In contrast, differentiation grade correlated with OS in one SEER database analysis [34], but not in the other four studies [25, 28, 32, 39].

1.4.5.3 Other immunopathologic variables

Among ESCC patients cancer-specific survival was longer in patients with tumor-infiltrating lymphocytes (TILs), which were independent PF [66].

It is doubtful that high PD-L1 expression correlates with prognosis in patients with stage III–IV or lymph node metastasis [67].

1.4.5.4 Molecular biology

Molecular and clustering analysis, while not clearly distinguishing EC from GC at the cardial level, captured important differences. EACs of the cardia are almost exclusively represented by one of the four molecular subgroups of GC, the CIN-activated, and the closer EACs were to the stomach, the more intense CIN was, hypermethylation becoming more pronounced and directed toward some genetic profiles, such as to silencing of CDKN2A, MGMT, and CHFR, but never MLH1, with minor activation of the Wnt/beta-catenin pathway. Therefore, in some cases, molecular biology could be a valuable support to characterize the origin of adenocarcinoma in the cardial region.

Microbiota dysbiosis promotes the occurrence and development of ESCC [68, 69]. This microbiota varies with alcohol consumption [70] and is associated with OS [71], but also with various other variables.

1.4.5.5   Selected trials

None of the selected studies evaluated the role of histotype and tumor grading, but a study excluded a possible prognostic relevance for DNA ploidy (aneuploid vs. diploid) [23].

1.4.6   Previous treatments

1.4.6.1   Surgery

Studies do not allow definitive conclusions regarding the prognostic relevance of a previous primary tumor resection (PTR) in mEC patients. Some population studies have documented an improvement in the outcome of patients who previously received a PTR [35, 72, 73], while others have not [74]. In the favorable studies, however, a possible effect on patient selection from PS and TB cannot be excluded [73].

Among 2,981 mEC patients from the SEER database, prior surgery of primary and metastases was more frequent among patients with OS >2 years [35], and other analyses from the same database concluded that having included surgery in the treatment plan was associated with better OS [34], at least in the young [36]. A retrospective cohort also confirmed the better prognosis of patients with prior PTR [32], while no OS improvement was associated with prior stent/PEG placement [27, 32]. Furthermore, after univariate analysis of OMD, surgical or local treatment affected OS if it involved all metastases and not only a part of them [29].

1.4.6.2   Radiotherapy

Some analyses, which assessed the risk of the early death of mEC patients, suggested that previous radiotherapy, chemoradiation, or chemotherapy had a favorable prognostic effect in patients with mEC [16], and radiotherapy in the upfront treatment plan increased 2-year survival rates [75]. Even though radiotherapy is active in treating primary tumors in association with other regional treatments of metastases in OMD [29], few data are available about the treatment of metastases, except SBRT for oligometastatic lung disease [58].

1.4.6.3   Selected trials

A small study did not find any relationship between previous radiotherapy and OS [18].

1.5   PROGNOSTIC FACTORS IN DECISION-MAKING

All patients should be offered early palliative care and nutritional support, but ESCC patients ineligible for local treatments with poor general condition (PS ECOG ≥2) should not receive any antineoplastic treatment. Anyway, for locally advanced or metastatic ESCC that cannot receive definitive CRT (mESCC), prognosis is poor, with a median OS of 9–10 months [76].

Of the eight larger phase III RCTs that have been published in the last years and have changed clinical practice, only two included EAC among the enrolled patients, so overall EAC represented a minority of the examined mEC patients (11%, 428/3866). Therefore, the reported suggestions, which are resumed in Table 1.3, apply mostly to patients with mESCC.

1.5.1   Upfront treatment

In the first-line setting, the association of immunotherapy plus chemotherapy was compared both with chemotherapy alone [20, 77] and with immunotherapy alone [78, 79], with the combination reporting a significant OS improvement in both cases. Therefore, for patients with an ECOG PS

TABLE 1.3

Prognostic and predictive variables in clinical decision-making in metastatic esophageal cancer

A. Upfront systemic treatment

1   PD-L1

CPS ≥10: ICI+CHT favored (PEMB+CHT is better than CHT)

CPS ≥1: ICI+CHT favored (NIVO+CHT is better than CHT)

TPS ≥1%: ICI+CHT favored (CAMR+CHT or TORI+CHT better than CHT or TORI)

2   Disease status

Metastatic: ICI+CHT favored (NIVO+CHT is better than CHT; CAMR+CHT is better than CHT; TORI+CHT is better than TORI)

Multiple sites of metastasis: ICI+CHT favored (CAMR+CHT is better than CHT)

3   Age

≥65 years old: ICI+CHT favored (PEMB+CHT, NIVO+CHT or NIVO+IPIL are better than CHT)

4   Geographic origin

Asian: ICI+CHT favored (PEMB+CHT or NIVO+CHT are better than CHT)

B. Treatment of refractory disease

1   PD-L1

CPS ≥ 110: ICI favored (PEMB is better than CHT),

PD-L1 >1%: ICI favored (NIVO or CAMR are better than CHT)

TAP ≥10%: ICI favored (TISL is better than CHT)

PD-L1 any: ICI favored (NIVO is better than CHT)

2   Smoking

Active smokers: ICI favored (NIVO or TISL are better than CHT)

Legend: CAMR, camrelizumab. CHT, chemotherapy. CPS, combined positive score. ICI, immune checkpoint inhibitor. IPIL, ipilimumab. NIVO, nivolumab. PD-L1, programmed death ligand 1. PEMB, pembrolizumab. TAP, tumor area positive score. TISL, tislelizumab. TORI, toripalimab. TPS, tumor proportion score.

0–1, pembrolizumab+chemotherapy containing platinum and fluoropyrimidine has become the standard of care, with more consistent results in PD-L1 CPS ≥10 tumors [20, 80], but without any improvement in the CPS <10 subgroups [20]. Nivolumab+fluoropyrimidine/platinum-based chemotherapy is recommended in PD-L1 CPS≥1% [77]. Although the association was confirmed to be more effective among patients with high PD-L1 expression, the difficulty remains in conclusions about some subgroups, such as the under-represented female patients (17.3% in studies comparing chemotherapy, 13.5% in studies comparing immunotherapy). Differently from chemotherapy alone, the association appeared to significantly increase OS among the elderly, in patients of Asian origin, and in metastatic vs. loco-regional EC. On the contrary, compared to immunotherapy alone, OS after chemo-immunotherapy seemed to increase significantly in patients with metastatic disease and in one study also in patients with multiple metastatic sites [78]. The ESCORT-1st trial also reported a significant OS benefit from the combination compared to immunotherapy alone even in patients with BMI >20 kg/m^2 and weight >60 kg, former smokers, and those with previous high alcohol consumption [78], results that should be confirmed in future trials.

The only study that compared a combination of nivolumab+ipilimumab vs. front-line chemotherapy has documented better outcomes for the immunotherapy doublet, in particular in some subgroups, such as ECOG PS 0, age ≥65, males, non-Asian, smokers, PDL1 CPS>1, and metastatic vs. locally advanced [77]. These results also need confirmation, as the evaluation of the regimen in females, who made up only 18% of the enrolled patients [77].

1.5.2 TREATMENT OF REFRACTORY DISEASE

Four studies evaluated immunotherapy vs. chemotherapy, comparing anti-PD-L1 vs. taxane or taxane/irinotecan. Nivolumab is recommended after platinum+fluoropyrimidine, achieving higher OS than taxane-based chemotherapy regardless of PD-L1 [81]. Similar results were reported for tislelizumab [82]. All trials have documented a benefit for immunotherapy, except one [80]. However, when patients with EAC were excluded, pembrolizumab was superior to chemotherapy in mESCCs with CPS≥10 [80].

If no subgroup showed better outcomes for the chemotherapy arm, this arm appeared inferior when irinotecan and not taxane were used [78, 82]. In addition to documenting a significant benefit in patients of Asian and Malaysian origin, in tumors with increased PD-L1, and an absence of efficacy of immunotherapy in non-smokers, also in these trials female patients remain poorly represented (13.3%).

1.6 CONCLUSION

In mEC some evidence suggests that the opportunity for a more aggressive multimodal treatment should be evaluated in prospective trials in well-identified subgroups of patients. A retrospective evaluation of 96 patients suggested selecting patients to receive a multimodal regimen by young age, lack of anorexia and fatigue, exclusive dissemination to distant lymph-node, and radiographic response to upfront chemotherapy [83], but other variables such as PS [84, 85], modified Glasgow prognostic score (mGPS), or serum total proteins [84, 85], histotype [85] have been proposed.

From the current analysis, a summary of possible updated recommendations of the examined PFs is already possible, as shown in Table 1.4. It emerges as a large number of PFs need further confirmation, possibly in prospective studies of mESCC patients. On the other hand, a molecular evaluation of EACs is also recommended in future studies to define the true incidence of these forms and the prognostic and molecular differences from GCs.

Moreover, the most recent molecular analyses, in addition to definitively establishing the substantial differences between ESCCs and EACs, have suggested three classes of ESCCs, the clinical and prognostic significance of which must be investigated, in order to identify not only the possible different therapeutic approaches, but also the relative significance of each PF [86].

TABLE 1.4
Prognostic factors evaluated in prospective trials of upfront treatment in patients with unresectable or metastatic esophageal cancer

Suggested	Not suggested	Needing study
Age		Performance status
Esophageal fistula		Sex
		Body mass index
		Neutrophil-to-lymphocyte ratio
		Albumin
		Bilirubin
		Alkaline phosphatase
		Lactic dehydrogenase
Disease status	Primary tumor location	Timing of metastasis
No. sites of metastases		Liver metastases
		Lung-limited metastases
		Tumor grading

REFERENCES

1. Morgan E, Soerjomataram I, Rumgay H, et al. The global landscape of esophageal squamous cell carcinoma and esophageal adenocarcinoma incidence and mortality in 2020 and projections to 2040: New estimates from GLOBOCAN 2020. *Gastroenterol* 2022;163(3):649–58.
2. Xia C, Dong X, Li H, et al. Cancer statistics in China and United States, 2022: Profiles, trends, and determinants. *Chin Med J* 2022;135(5):584–90.
3. ECIS – European Cancer Information System, available at https://ecis.jrc.ec.europa.eu, accessed October 31, 2023.
4. Shakuntala TS, Krishnan SK, Das P, et al. Descriptive epidemiology of gastrointestinal cancers: Results from National Cancer Registry Programme, India. *Asian Pac J Cancer Prev* 2022;23(2):409–18.
5. Li R, Sun J, Wang T, et al. Comparison of secular trends in esophageal cancer mortality in china and Japan during 1990–2019: An age-period-cohort analysis. *Int J Environ Res Public Health* 2022;19:10302.
6. Teglia F, Boffetta P. Association between trends of mortality and incidence, survival and stage at diagnosis for six digestive and respiratory cancers in United States (2009–2013). *Eur J Cancer Prev* 2022;32(2):195–202.
7. Torrejon NV, Deshpande S, Wei W, et al. Proportion of early-onset gastric and esophagus cancers has changed over time with disproportionate impact on Clack and Hispanic patients. *JCO Oncol Pract* 2022;18(5):e759–69.
8. Botterweck AA, Schouten LJ, Volovics A, et al. Trends in incidence of adenocarcinoma of the oesophagus and gastric cardia in ten European countries. *Int J Epidemiol* 2000;29:645–54.
9. Wang S, Zheng R, Arnold M, et al. Global and national trends in the age-specific sex ratio of esophageal cancer and gastric cancer by subtype. *Int J Cancer* 2022;151(9):1447–61.
10. Varghese TK Jr, Hofstetter WL, Rizk NP, et al. The society of thoracic surgeons guidelines on the diagnosis and staging of patients with esophageal cancer. *Ann Thorac Surg* 2013;96(1):346–56.
11. Nagtegaal ID, Odze RD, Klimstra D, et al. The 2019 WHO classification of tumors of the digestive system. *Histopathology* 2020;76(2):182–8.
12. van de Ven S, Bugter O, Hardillo JA, et al. Screening for head and neck second primary tumors in patients with esophageal squamous cell cancer: A systematic review and meta-analysis. *United European Gastroenterol J* 2019;7(10):1304–11.
13. Takeuchi H, Miyata H, Gotoh M, et al. A risk model for esophagectomy using data of 5354 patients included in a Japanese nationwide web-based database. *Ann Surg* 2014;260:259–66.
14. Lu Z-H, Yang L, Yu J-W, et al. Weight loss correlates with macrophage inhibitory cytokine-1 expression and might influence outcome in patients with advanced esophageal squamous cell carcinoma. *Asian Pac J Cancer Prev* 2014;15(15):6047–52.
15. Amin MB, Edge S, Green F, et al. *AJCC Cancer Staging Manual*. 8th Ed. New York; Springer-Verlag, 2017.
16. Shi M, Zhai G-Q. Models for predicting early death in patients with stage IV esophageal cancer: A surveillance, epidemiology, and end results-based cohort study. *Cancer Control* 2022;29:1–11.
17. SEER, available at https://seer.cancer.gov/statfacts/html/stomach.html, accessed January 21, 2023.
18. Ezdinli EZ, Gelber R, Desai DV, et al. Chemotherapy of advanced esophageal carcinoma: Eastern Cooperative Oncology experience. *Cancer* 1980;46:2149–53.
19. Webb A, Cunningham D, Scharffo JH, et al. Randomized trial comparing epirubicin, cisplatin, and fluorouracil versus fluorouracil, doxorubicin, and methotrexate in advanced esophagogastric cancer. *J Clin Oncol* 1997;15:261–7.
20. Sun JM, Shen L, Shah MA, et al. Pembrolizumab plus chemotherapy versus chemotherapy alone for first-line treatment of advanced oesophageal cancer (KEYNOTE-590): A randomised, placebo-controlled, phase 3 study. *Lancet* 2021;398(10302):759–71.
21. Tebbutt NC, Norman A, Cunningham D, et al. A multicentre, randomised phase III trial comparing protracted venous infusion (PVI) 5fluorouracil (5-FU) with PVI 5-FU plus mitomycin C in patients with inoperable oesophago-gastric cancer. *Ann Oncol* 2002;13:1568–75.
22. Ross P, Nicolson M, Cunningham D, et al. Prospective randomized trial comparing mitomycin, cisplatin, and protracted venous-infusion fluorouracil (PVI 5-FU) with epirubicin, cisplatin, and PVI 5-FU in advanced esophagogastric cancer. *J Clin Oncol* 2002;20:1996–2004.
23. Spiridonidis CH, Laufman LR, Jones JJ, et al. A phase II evaluation of high dose cisplatin and etoposide in patients with advanced esophageal adenocarcinoma. *Cancer* 1996;77:2070–7.
24. Overman MJ, Kazmi SM, Jhamb J, et al. Weekly docetaxel, cisplatin, and 5-fluorouracil as initial therapy for patients with advanced gastric and esophageal cancer. *Cancer* 2010;116:1446–53.

25. Polee MB, Hop WCJ, Kok TC, et al. Prognostic factors for survival in patients with advanced oesophageal cancer treated with cisplatin-based combination chemotherapy. *Br J Cancer* 2003;89:2045–50.

26. Ferndale L, Ayeni OA, Chen WC, et al. Development and internal validation of the survival time risk score in patients treated for oesophageal cancer with palliative intent in South Africa. *S Afr J Surg* 2023;61:66–74.

27. Bergquist H, Johnsson A, Hammerlid E, et al. Factors predicting survival in patients with advanced oesophageal cancer: A prospective multicentre evaluation. *Alim Pharmacol Ther* 2008;27:385–95.

28. Ghaly G, Harrison S, Kamel MK, et al. Predictors of survival after treatment of oligometastases after esophagectomy. *Ann Thorac Surg* 2018;105:357–62.

29. Li B, Wang R, Zhang T, et al. Development and validation of a nomogram prognostic model for esophageal cancer patients with oligometastased. *Sci Rep* 2020;10:11259.

30. Cui C, Wu X, Deng L, et al. Modified Glasgow prognostic score predicts the prognosis of patients with advanced esophageal squamous cell carcinoma: A propensity score-matched analysis. *Thorac Cancer* 2022;13:2041–9.

31. Ghazy HF, El-Hadaad HA, Wahba HA, et al. Metastatic esophageal carcinoma: Prognostic factors and survival. *J Gastrointest Cancer* 2022;53(2):446–50.

32. Jung HA, Adenis A, Lee J, et al. Nomogram to predict treatment outcome of fluoropyrimidine/platinum-based chemotherapy in metastatic esophageal squamous cell carcinoma. *Cancer Res Treat* 2013;45(4):285–94.

33. Chen W-W, Lin C-C, Huang T-C, et al. Prognostic factors of metastatic or recurrent esophageal squamous cell carcinoma in patients receiving three-drug combination chemotherapy. *Anticancer Res* 2013;33:4123–8.

34. Saad AM, Al-Husseini MJ, Elgebaly A, et al. Impact of prior malignancy on outcomes of stage IV esophageal carcinoma: SEER based study. *Exp Rev Gastroenterol Hepatol* 2018;12(4):417–23.

35. Liu M, Wang C, Gao L, et al. A nomogram to predict long-time survival for patients with M1 diseases of esophageal cancer. *J Cancer* 2018;9(21):3986–90.

36. Qiu G, Zhang H, Wang F, et al. Patterns of metastasis and prognosis of elderly esophageal squamous cell carcinoma patients in stage IVB: A population-based study. *Transl Cancer Res* 2021;10(11):4591–600.

37. Al-Kaabi A, Baranov NS, van der Post RS, et al. Age-specific incidence, treatment, and survival trends in esophageal cancer: A Dutch population-based cohort study. *Acta Oncol* 2022;61(5):545–52.

38. Shiono S, Kawamura M, Sato T, et al. Disease-free interval length correlates to prognosis of patients who underwent metastasectomy for esophageal lung metastases. *J Thorac Oncol* 2008;3:1046–9.

39. Wu M, Zhu Y, Chen X, et al. Prognostic nutritional index predicts the prognosis of patients with advanced esophageal cancer treated with immune checkpoint inhibitors: A retrospective cohort study. *J Gastrointest Oncol* 2023;14(1):54–63.

40. Kijima T, Arigami T, Uchikado Y, et al. Combined fibrinogen and neutrophil-lymphocyte ratio as a prognostic marker of advanced esophageal squamous cell carcinoma. *Cancer Sci* 2017;108:193–9.

41. Xiang Z-F, Xiong H-C, Hu D-F, et al. Age-related sex disparities in esophageal cancer survival: A population-based study in the United States. *Front Public Health* 2022;10:836914.

42. Li H, Zhang S, Guo J, et al. Hepatic metastasis in newly diagnosed esophageal cancer: A population-based study. *Front Oncol* 2021;11:644880.

43. Lee S, Jang J, Abe SK, et al. Association between body mass index and oesophageal cancer mortality: A pooled analysis of prospective cohort studies with >800000 individuals in the Asia Cohort Consortium. *Int J Epidemiol* 2022;51(4):1190–203.

44. Spreafico A, Coate L, Zhai R, et al. Early adulthood body mass index, cumulative smoking, and esophageal adenocarcinoma survival. *Cancer Epidemiol* 2017;47:28–34.

45. Shen S, Araujo JL, Altorki NK, et al. Variation by stage in the effects of prediagnosis weight loss on mortality in a prospective cohort of esophageal cancer patients. *Dis Esophagus* 2017;30:1–7.

46. Deans DAC, Tan BH, Wigmore SJ, et al. The influence of systemic inflammation, dietary intake and stage of disease on rate of weight loss in patients with gastro-oesophageal cancer. *Br J Cancer* 2009;100:63–9.

47. Zhao Q, Bi Y, Xue J, et al. Prognostic value of absolute lymphocyte count in patients with advanced esophageal cancer treated with immunotherapy: A retrospective analysis. *Ann Transl Med* 2022;10(13):744.

48. Wang X, Zhang B, Chen X, et al. Lactate dehydrogenase and baseline markers associated with clinical outcomes of advanced esophageal squamous cell carcinoma patients treated with camrelizumab (SHR-1210), a novel anti-PD-1 antibody. *Thoracic Cancer* 2019;10:1395–401.

49. Xu S, Zhu Q, Wu L, et al. Association of the CD4+/CD8+ ratio with response to PD-1 inhibitor-based combination therapy and dermatological toxicities in patients with advanced gastric and esophageal cancer. *Int Immunopharmacol* 2023;123:110642.

50. Li B, Xiong F, Yi S, Wang S. Prognostic and clinicopathologic significance of neutrophil-to-lymphocyte ratio in esophageal cancer: An update meta-analysis. *Technol Cancer Res Treat* 2022;21:15330338211070140.

51. Su R, Zhu J, Wu S, et al. Prognostic significance of platelet (PLT) and platelet to mean platelet volume (PLT/MPV) ratio during apatinib second-line or late-line treatment in advanced esophageal squamous cell carcinoma patients. *Tech Cancer Res Treat* 2022;21:1–10.

52. Yu C-W, Chen X-J, Lin Y-H, et al. Prognostic value of 18F-FDG PET/MR imaging biomarkers in oesophageal squamous cell carcinoma. *Eur J Radiol* 2019;120:108671.

53. Sugano K, Spechler SJ, El-Omar EM, et al. Kyoto international consensus report on anatomy, pathophysiology and clinical significance of the gastro-oesophageal junction. *Gut* 2022;71:1488–514.

54. ICD, available at https://icd.who.int/ct11/icd11_mms/en/release, accessed January 21, 2023.

55. Zhou S-B, Guo X-W, Gu L, et al. Influential factor on radiotherapy efficacy and prognosis in patients with secondary lymph node metastasis after esophagectomy of thoracic esophageal squamous cell carcinoma. *Cancer Manage Res* 2018;10:217–25.

56. Yamashita H, Jingu K, Niibe Y, et al. Definitive salvage radiation therapy and chemoradiation therapy for lymph node oligo-recurrence of esophageal cancer: A Japanese multi-institutional study of 237 patients. *Radiat Oncol* 2017;12:38.

57. Li H, Zhang S, Guo J, et al. Hepatic metastasis in newly diagnosed esophageal cancer: A population-based study. *Front Oncol* 2021;11:644880.

58. Yamamoto T, Niibe Y, Matsumoto Y, et al. Stereotactic body radiotherapy for pulmonary oligometastases from esophageal cancer: Results and prognostic factors. *Anticancer Res* 2020;40(4):2065–72.

59. Kozu Y, Sato H, Tsubosa Y, et al. Surgical treatment for pulmonary metastases from esophageal carcinoma after definitive chemoradiothrapy: Experience from a single institution. *J Cardiothorac Surg* 2011;6:135.

60. Wang R-C, Liu X-L, Qi C, et al. Bone metastasis of esophageal carcinoma diagnosed as a first primary tumor: A population-based study. *Trends Cancer Res* 2022;11(1):113–23.

61. Song Z, Lin B, Shao L, et al. Brain metastases from esophageal cancer: Clinical review of 26 cases. *World Neurosurg* 2014;81(1):131–5.

62. Kothary N, Mellon E, Hoffe SE, et al. Outcomes in patients with brain metastasis from esophageal carcinoma. *J Gastrointest Oncol* 2016;7(4):562–9.

63. Ogawa K, Toita T, Sueyama H, et al. Brain metastases from esophageal carcinoma. *Cancer* 2002;94:759–64.

64. Rades D, Huttenlocher S, Bajrovic A, et al. A new instrument for estimating the survival of patients with metastatic epidural spinal cord compression from esophageal cancer. *Radiol Oncol* 2015;49(1):86–90.

65. Ishida H, Kasajima A, Onodera Y, et al. A comparative analysis of clinicopathological factors between esophageal small cell and basaloid squamous cell carcinoma. *Medicine* 2019;98:8.

66. Sudo T, Nishida R, Kawahara A, et al. Clinical impact of tumor-infiltrating lymphocytes in esophageal squamous cell carcinoma. *Ann Surg Oncol* 2017;24(12):3763–70.

67. Jiang D, Song Q, Wang H, et al. Independent prognostic role of PD-L1 expression in patients with esophageal squamous cell carcinoma. *Oncotarget* 2017;8(5):8315–29.

68. Yang L, Lu X, Nossa CW, et al. Inflammation and intestinal metaplasia of the distal esophagus are associated with alterations in the microbiome. *Gastroenterology* 2009;137(2):588–97.

69. Liu N, Ando T, Ishiguro K, et al. Characterization of bacterial biota in the distal esophagus of Japanese patients with reflux esophagitis and Barrett's esophagus. *BMC Infect Dis* 2013;13:130.

70. Rao W, Lin Z, Liu S, et al. Association between alcohol consumption and oesophageal microbiota in oesophageal squamous cell carcinoma. *BMC Microbiol* 2021;21(1):73.

71. Liu Y, Lin Z, Lin Y, et al. Streptococcus and Prevotella are associated with the prognosis of oesophageal squamous cell carcinoma. *J Med Microbiol* 2018;67(8):1058–68.

72. Cai W, Ge W, Yuan Y, et al. A 10-year population-based study of the differences between NECs and carcinomas of the esophagus in terms of clinicopathology and Survival. *J Cancer* 2019;10(6):1520–7.

73. Zhang R, Zou J, Li P, et al. Surgery to the primary tumor is associated with improved survival of patients with metastatic esophageal cancer: Propensity score-matched analyses of a large retrospective cohort. *Dis Esophagus* 2020;33(3):doz051.

74. Coffey MR, Bachman KC, Worrell SG, et al. Palliative surgery outcomes for patients with esophageal cancer: An National Cancer Database analysis. *J Surg Res* 2021;267:229–34.

75. Li X, Zhang H, Jia X, et al. Survival benefit of radiotherapy in metastatic esophageal cancer: A population-based study. *Transl Cancer Res* 2019;8(4):1974–85.
76. Moehler M, Maderer A, Thuss-Patience PC, et al. Cisplatin and 5-fluorouracil with or without epidermal growth factor receptor inhibition panitumumab for patients with non-resectable, advanced or metastatic oesophageal squamous cell cancer: A prospective, open-label, randomised phase III AIO/EORTC trial (POWER). *Ann Oncol* 2020;31(2):228–35.
77. Doki Y, Ajani JA, Kato K, et al. Nivolumab combination therapy in advanced esophageal squamous-cell carcinoma. *N Engl J Med* 2022;386(5):449–62.
78. Luo H, Lu J, Bai Y, et al. Effect of camrelizumab vs placebo added to chemotherapy on survival and progression-free survival in patients with advanced or metastatic esophageal squamous cell carcinoma: The ESCORT-1st randomized clinical trial. *JAMA* 2021;326(10):916–25.
79. Wang ZX, Cui C, Yao J, et al. Toripalimab plus chemotherapy in treatment-naïve, advanced esophageal squamous cell carcinoma (JUPITER-06): A multi-center phase 3 trial. *Cancer Cell* 2022;40(3):277–288.e3.
80. Kojima T, Shah MA, Muro K, et al. Randomized phase III KEYNOTE-181 study of pembrolizumab versus chemotherapy in advanced esophageal cancer. *J Clin Oncol* 2020;38(35):4138–48.
81. Kato K, Cho BC, Takahashi M, et al. Nivolumab versus chemotherapy in patients with advanced oesophageal squamous cell carcinoma refractory or intolerant to previous chemotherapy (ATTRACTION-3): A multicentre, randomised, open-label, phase 3 trial. *Lancet Oncol* 2019;20(11):1506–17.
82. Shen L, Kato K, Kim SB, et al. Tislelizumab versus chemotherapy as second-line treatment for advanced or metastatic esophageal squamous cell carcinoma (RATIONALE-302): A randomized phase III study. *J Clin Oncol* 2022;40(26):3065–76.
83. Wang J, Suri JS, Allen PK, et al. Factors predictive of improved outcomes with multimodality local therapy after palliative chemotherapy for stage IV esophageal cancer. *Am J Clin Oncol* 2016;39(3):228–35.
84. Park JH, Woodley N, McMillan DC, Glen P. Palliative stenting for oesophagogastric cancer: Tumour and host factors and prognosis. *BMJ Support Palliat Care* 2019;9(3):332–9.
85. Qin J, Zhu HD, Guo JH, et al. Factors associated with overall survival and relief of dysphagia in advanced esophageal cancer patients after 125I seed-loaded stent placement: A multicenter retrospective analysis. *Dis Esophagus* 2019;32(12):doz012.
86. CGARN 2017 Cancer Genome Atlas Research Network. Integrated genomic characterization of oesophageal carcinoma. *Nature* 2017;541(7636):169–75.

2 Gastric cancer

2.1 INTRODUCTION

In 2022, an international consensus report modified the endoscopic definition of gastro-esophageal junction (GOJ) and introduced the concept of the GOJ zone, which would be the transitional area 1 cm upstream and 1 cm downstream of GOJ. A redefinition of adenocarcinomas of the cardia, renamed GOJ zone adenocarcinoma, was proposed, to identify tumors arising within 1 cm of the cardia, distinct in pathophysiologic classification [1].

For this chapter, we consider GOJ zone adenocarcinomas as gastric tumors, thus reserving the esophageal site only for adenocarcinomas proximal to the anatomic cardia, according to the distinction made by the ICD-11 classification [2].

2.1.1 EPIDEMIOLOGY

A GLOBOCAN database report for 2020 estimated worldwide 1.1 million new cases and 770,000 deaths from gastric cancer (GC), with age-standardized incidence rates (ASR) of 15.8 vs. 7.0 in males vs. females, and mortality of 11.0 vs. 4.9/100,000 [3]. The ASR for GC in Europe in 2022 was 16.7/100,000, with 74,580 new cases, and the ASR for mortality of 11.6/100,000 with 51,781 cancer deaths, with a male prevalence [4].

The highest incidences were in Eastern Asia, and the lowest in Africa. The highest mortality rates were in Eastern Asia and the lowest in very high human development index countries.

Worldwide, the annual burden is predicted to increase by 2040 [3], and an increasing trend is expected also in Europe, with an additional 23.61% for males and 22.69% for females [4]. However, the analysis of 22 Chinese cancer registries documented a decline in the incidence of GC from 2000 to 2015 and predicted a further 15% reduction by 2030 [5]. In the US, a reduction in noncardial GC in elderly subjects has been documented, but also an increase in young <50 years among non-Hispanic Whites, particularly among women [6].

2.1.2 STAGING OF METASTATIC DISEASE

Clinical examination is recommended in the initial workup and should include an assessment of nutritional status.

Laboratory tests are indicated to rule out iron deficit with/without anemia, determine peripheric leukocyte and platelet counts, and evaluate renal and liver function.

EGDS+biopsy is the gold standard for diagnosis. Sometimes endoscopic mucosal resection and endoscopic submucosal dissection are employed as diagnostic and therapeutic maneuvers. To ensure adequate tumor representation, especially in the presence of ulcerated lesions, at least 5–8 endoscopic biopsies are recommended [7, 8].

Pathologic report should contain the histologic diagnosis by WHO criteria.

Molecular characterization requires the determination of HER2, PD-L1, and mismatch repair (MMR) system status.

Chest-abdomen CT is the imaging of choice for staging. It can evidentiate local or distant lymphoadenomegaly, distant metastasis, and ascites, but the sensitivity for lymph node metastases is variable from 62.5% to 91.9% [9] and there is no consensus on diagnostic criteria for lymph nodes.

TABLE S1

Prognostic factors analyzed in selected clinical trials of patients with unresectable or metastatic gastric cancer receiving upfront treatment

Variable	No. trials	Prognostic relationship	No prognostic relationship
Patient-related			
Performance status	11	10	1
Demographic			
Age	10	3	7
Sex	8	2	6
Geographic area	1	1	0
Ethnicity	1	0	1
Anthropometric			
Body mass index	1	0	1
Clinic			
Ascites	1	1	0
Sufficient ingestion	1	1	0
Lab			
Hemoglobin	2	0	2
Leukocyte count	1	1	0
Neutrophil-lymphocyte ratio	1	1	0
Albumin	1	0	1
Alkalyne phosphatase	5	3	2
Aspartate transaminase	2	1	1
Alanine transaminase	2	0	2
Lactic dehydrogenase	1	1	0
Reactive C-protein	1	1	0
Other	5	0	5
Tumor-related			
Tumor burden			
Sum of tumor diameters	1	1	0
Disease status	4	3	1
No. sites metastases	3	2	1
Measurable disease	5	4	1
Primary tumor location	2	1	1
Timing of metastasis	4	2	2
Site of metastasis	3	0	3
Liver metastases	2	2	0
Peritoneal metastases	3	1	2
Nodal metastases	1	1	0
Lung metastases	1	0	1
Bone metastases	1	1	0
Pathology			
Macroscopic	2	0	2
Histotype	7	3	4
Differentiation grade	1	1	0
Previous treatments			
Previous surgery	4	3	1
Time from diagnosis to chemotherapy	1	0	1

In the metastatic setting, many investigations often used in localized disease, are not routinely recommended, such as EUS, FDG-PET, which can be falsely negative in diffuse or mucinous carcinomas [10], and laparoscopy.

The reference staging system is TNM Classification (AJCC 8th edition 2017) [11].

2.1.3 PROGNOSIS OF METASTATIC DISEASE

Among European registries in 2020, a 5-year survival of 18.7% for males was reported, and 23.4% for females [4]. From data of Surveillance, Epidemiology, and End Results (SEER) the 5-year relative survival was 33.3% [12].

In clinical practice, the prognosis of metastatic or inoperable disease is poor [13], despite in clinical trials median overall survival (OS) increased over time from 5.2 months in 1987 [14], to 9.2 in 2006 [15], up to 17.5 in 2022 [16].

Prognostic models have been proposed over time, but none is extensively used, and many studies attempted to better define the prognosis of the individual patient [17–20].

Overall, TNM 8th stage IV GC is associated with a 5-year survival rate of <5% [21].

2.2 ANALYSIS OF PROGNOSTIC VARIABLES OF EARLY METASTATIC DISEASE

A systematic review of phase III randomized clinical trials (RCTs) that studied upfront therapies in patients with unresectable or metastatic gastric cancer (mGC) resulted in the selection of 56 studies, published from 1985 to 2022. In 14 an analysis of prognostic factors (PFs) was done [14, 22–34], and in 11 a multivariate analysis was performed. The results of the review are summarized in Table S1. It lists all PFs that have been reported in at least one study and the number of studies that found or did not a relationship between the PFs and OS.

2.3 PATIENT-RELATED PROGNOSTIC FACTORS

2.3.1 PERFORMANCE STATUS

Four prospective cohort studies [19, 35–37] and nine retrospective studies [17, 18, 38–44] revealed an unfavorable prognostic role of deteriorated PS in mGC, while in other analyses the relationship was not significant [20, 45–47].

Other authors analyzed 310 Chinese patients in the setting of first-line chemotherapy, comparing the role of other possible PFs in the subgroups with a good PS. ECOG PS 0 patients reported longer OS when they had undergone primary tumor resection (PTR), had a low number of metastatic sites without liver or bone metastases, and low neutrophil-to-lymphocyte ratio (NLR) [48]. A similar evaluation by the same authors on a retrospective cohort of 309 mGC patients with good PS documented as independent PFs, in addition to the number of metastatic sites, the value of carbohydrate antigen 19-9 (CA 19-9), and fibrinogen [49]. Furtherly, patients with baseline ECOG PS 0–1 had a higher likelihood of receiving second-line therapy and better disease control [50].

2.3.1.1 Selected trials

Ten of the eleven studies that evaluated the relationship of PS with OS reported a significant prognostic relationship of PS, as summarized in Table 2.1. Despite the various reported comparisons between PS categories, for the present analysis, the comparison between PS 1–2 vs. PS 0 was evaluated [28]. Eight RCTs, enrolling 3,891 patients, reported an effect size (ES). The meta-analysis confirmed the prognostic relationship (HR 1.43, CI 1.18–1.73; Q = 96.43, p-value <0.0001; I^2 = 92.7%) (Figure 2.1).

TABLE 2.1

Prognostic relationships of performance status in selected studies of patients with unresectable or metastatic gastric cancer receiving upfront treatment

Study [ref]	Phase	No. pts	Scale	Comparison	Prognostic relationship	Effect size
EORTC 1987 [14]	III	189	KPS	continuous	Yes	NR
GITSG 1998 [22]	III	249	ECOG	PS 2–3 vs. PS 0–1	Yes	NR (p <0.01)
Korean 1993 [23]	III	295	ECOG	PS 2–3 vs. PS 0–1	Yes	32.8 m vs. 22.7 m
Swedish 1994 [24]	III	61	KPS	continuous	Yes	HR 0.96 (0.93–0.98)
British 1997 [25]	III	274	NR	PS 2–3 vs. PS 0–1	Yes	HR 1.76 (1.26–2.45)
REAL-2 2008 [27]	III	908	WHO	PS 2–3 vs. PS 0–1	Yes	HR 1.92 (1.54–2.39)
JCOG-9912 2009 [28]	III	642	ECOG	PS 1 vs. PS 0	Yes	HR 1.52 (1.29–1.80)
		425		PS 2 vs. PS 0	No	HR 1.32 (0.63–2.79)
		650		PS 1–2 vs. PS 0	Yes	HR 1.51 (1.28–1.79)
		650		PS 2 vs. PS 0–1	No	HR 1.16 (0.55–2.46)
GC0301 2011 [29]	III	315	ECOG	PS 1–2 vs. PS 0	Yes	HR 1.35 (1.08–1.69)
EXPAND 2013 [30]	III	761	ECOG	PS 1 vs. PS 0	Yes	HR 1.55 (1.32–1.82)
JCOG-0106 2013 [31]	III	237	ECOG	PS 1–2 vs. PS 0	No	HR 1.02 (0.76–1.38)
Japanese 2015 [32]	III	685	ECOG	PS 1–2 vs. PS 0	Yes	HR 1.60 (1.33–1.94)

Legend: ECOG, Eastern Cooperative Oncology Group. HR, hazard ratio. KPS, Karnofsky performance status. m, months. NR, not reported. PS, performance status. WHO, World Health Organization.

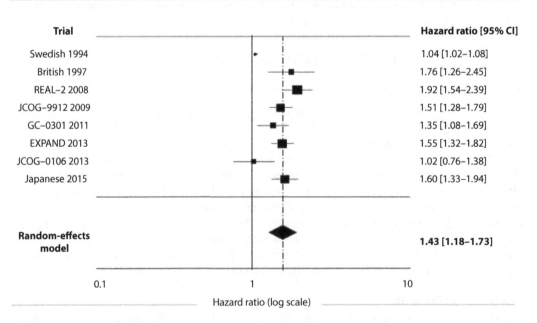

FIGURE 2.1   Forest plot of meta-analysis of performance status in prospective trials of patients with unresectable or metastatic gastric cancer

2.3.2 DEMOGRAPHIC

2.3.2.1 Age

Some population-based analyses, from the SEER database [51–53] and the Ontario Cancer Registry (OCR) [54], found a significant relationship between advanced age and reduced OS, but other studies did not [55, 56]. No evidence of a relationship emerged from other studies on both prospective cohorts and retrospective series, with age cut-offs varying between 54–75 [17, 35–40, 42, 44, 46, 57], in which only one study documented OS reduction in the elderly [45].

Some studies on GC patients at any stage have documented that age of onset <20–30 was more common among females [58, 59] and was associated with poor outcomes [60] and more advanced stages [58, 59, 61, 62]. In contrast, other studies for age at onset <45 reported higher 5-year survival rates [63] or no changes [64].

Other authors focused on elderly patients with GC at any stage, mostly finding poor outcomes in patients with deteriorated PS [65, 66] or frailty and functional decline [67].

2.3.2.2 Sex

Some reports from the SEER [51, 55] and OCR [54] documented better OS for females, while the relationship between sex and survival disappeared in another SEER analysis [56], three prospective cohort studies [19, 35, 36], and 11 retrospective studies [17, 38–46, 57].

The AGAMENON-SEOM registry suggested that in females some characteristics were different, such as lower frequency of HER2-positive, well-differentiated mGCs, peritoneal and liver metastases (LMs), with an increase of diffuse and signet ring cell carcinoma (SRCC) histotypes. Even though women reported more side effects from systemic chemotherapy, such as neutropenia, anemia, and diarrhea, no difference with males in progression-free survival (PFS) and OS was reported [37].

A propensity score-matched analysis of patients with GC at any stage documented that sex was independent PF, with increased rates of recurrences and LMs among males [68].

2.3.2.3 Other demographic variables

Many differences in GC outcomes between the Eastern and Western series have been explained with different characteristics [69] and high rates of advanced stage at diagnosis in the Western (60% vs. 30%). In the AVAGAST trial, an RCT of upfront chemotherapy, the area of origin was related to different mGC characteristics and prognosis [70]. Some biological differences have been documented in the angiogenic response [70], but also regional differences in the healthcare environment [71]. Within Europe, the EUROCARE study showed, after adjustment for age, sex, and PTR, a persisting excessive risk of death in some areas, such as Granada and Yorkshire [72], and similar findings have been reported for some high-incidence areas in Italy [73]. In the analysis of the 1,433 mGC patients of the OCR, even the geographic region of residence was related to the outcome, with poor survival for patients living in rural vs. urban areas [54].

Many studies have evaluated ethnicity, without documenting differences in the US between African-Americans and Whites [51, 55] or differences of other ethnicities vs. Whites [51, 56]. Controversial reports about the comparison of Asians vs. non-Asians have been published [42, 74, 75], but characteristics of patients and stage at diagnosis are frequently unbalanced. In particular, studies in localized GC from SEER and NCDB case series have found that differences by ethnicity are also associated with a better outcome for Asian-American patients [76–78], and differences within different Asian ethnicities have also been reported [79]. These differences were explained by a more frequent diagnosis of oligometastatic disease (OMD) and stage migration [69, 80]. However, in mGC increased use of second-line chemotherapy [81] and different drug toxicity profiles by race [82, 83] have been reported.

Finally, married patients more rarely than nonmarried experienced early death within three months of diagnosis [48].

2.3.2.4 Selected trials

Ten studies analyzed age as a PF, but only in five a measure of the ES was available [27, 28, 30–32], as resumed in Table 2.2. The cut-off ranged between 50 and 70 years. Three studies found better prognosis in younger subjects [27, 30, 33]. Five trials reported ES by evaluating 3,241 patients, and their pooled analysis did not show a significant relationship with OS (HR 0.96, CI 0.89–1.05; Q = 5.55, p-value = 0.2352; I^2 = 27.9%).

TABLE 2.2

Prognostic relationships of age in selected studies of patients with unresectable or metastatic gastric cancer receiving upfront treatment

Study [ref]	Phase	No. pts	Comparison	Prognostic relationship	Effect size
EORTC 1987 [14]	III	189	NR	No	NR
Korean 1993 [23]	III	295	> vs. ≤60	No	37.4 vs. 29.4 m
Swedish 1997 [24]	III	61	continuous	No	NR
REAL-2 2008 [27]	III	908	≥ vs. <60	Yes	HR 0.85 (0.74–0.98)
JCOG-9912 2009 [28]	III	650	≥ vs. <65	No	HR 0.99 (0.85–1.17)
GC0301 2011 [29]	III	315	NR	No	NR
EXPAND 2013 [30]	III	761	≥ vs. <65	Yes	HR 0.98 (0.97–0.99)
JCOG-0106 2013 [31]	III	237	≥ vs. <65	No	HR 1.16 (0.86–1.57)
Japanese 2015 [32]	III	685	≥ vs. <70	No	HR 0.92 (0.76–1.12)
TRIO-LOGiC 2015 [33]	III	487	≥ vs. <60	Yes	NR

Legend: HR, hazard ratio. m, months. NR, not reported.

TABLE 2.3

Prognostic relationships of sex in selected studies of patients with unresectable or metastatic gastric cancer receiving upfront treatment

Study [ref]	Phase	No. pts	Comparison	Prognostic relationship	Effect size
EORTC 1987 [14]	III	189	M vs. F	No	NR
Korean 1993 [23]	III	295	M vs. F	No	OS 31.9 vs. 28.2 m
Swedish 1994 [24]	III	61	M vs. F	Yes	HR 2.13 (1.09–3.85)
JCOG-9912 2009 [28]	III	650	M vs. F	Yes	HR 0.83 (0.68–0.99)
GC0301 2011 [29]	III	315	M vs. F	No	NR
EXPAND 2013 [30]	III	761	M vs. F	No	HR 0.93 (0.74–1.17)
JCOG-0106 2013 [31]	III	237	M vs. F	No	HR 0.83 (0.62–1.12)
Japanese 2015 [32]	III	685	M vs. F	No	HR 1.11 (0.90–1.36)

Legend: F, female. HR, hazard ratio. M, male. m, months. NR, not reported. OS, overall survival.

Eight studies investigated the prognostic role of sex, and HR was available in five, including 2,394 patients, as listed in Table 2.3. Only two studies documented an effect of sex on OS [24, 28], with one study reporting a favorable prognostic effect for female sex [24] and the other for males [28]. The pooled analysis did not report a significant ES (HR 0.98, CI 0.70–1.37; Q = 11.30, p-value = 0.0234; I^2 = 64.6%).

One study evaluated the relationship between geographic areas (North America, Asia, rest of the world) and found a statistically significant effect of the region, favoring Asian patients [33]. On the other hand, a trend favoring non-Asian patients was reported in a Japanese trial [30].

2.3.3 ANTHROPOMETRIC

A retrospective study of 518 mGC patients with peritoneal carcinomatosis reported a better prognosis of the subgroup with body mass index (BMI) >23 kg/m² [84]. In other studies, BMI was unable to predict the outcome of mGC patients [41], even at a cut-off <18.5–20 [36, 42, 57].

Among the nutritional status-related variables in mGC patients, the reduced third lumbar vertebra level skeletal muscle index (L3-SMI) was associated with reduced OS [43, 57, 85], as were other nutritional scores [42, 86] confirming the unfavorable effect on the outcome of poor nutritional status [86].

2.3.3.1 Selected trials

An evaluation of the EXPAND study allowed analysis of body composition-related variables in 761 patients, evaluating muscle and fat parameters, and only mean muscle attenuation clustered with fat parameters and was independent PF [30].

2.3.4 CLINIC

Some authors investigated symptoms at diagnosis in mGC patients, with few mGC-related symptoms showing prognostic significance, such as dysphagia and weight loss (WL) [87, 88]. WL occurs in 72% of mGC patients, with various symptoms coexisting, such as dysphagia, anorexia, early satiety, emesis, and pain [89].

With all the limitations related to patient-reported measurements, WL of 5–10% in the three months preceding diagnosis was associated with a reduction in OS in two studies [39, 45], and in another study, the association was significant only after univariate analysis [41]. Some studies that evaluated WL after the start of upfront chemotherapy also documented its close relationship with the outcome [90–92].

The presence of ascites showed a poor prognostic role in two studies of mGC patients [17, 39].

The occurrence of venous thromboembolic events (VTE) could affect 0.5–24.4% of GC patients [93], especially mGC [94]. However, VTE is rarely reported in mGC, and the size of the negative effect on OS is unknown, as an analysis of 612 GC patients with VTE from the RIETE registry reported a 6-month mortality rate of 44% and VTE recurrence in 6.5% of cases [95].

In contrast, pain [45], other comorbidities such as diabetes and hypertension [39] or a high comorbidity index [54] did not influence the outcome.

2.3.4.1 Selected trials

The JCOG-0106 trial reported that ascites were associated with a poor OS, while patients maintaining a sufficient ingestion had longer survival [31].

2.3.5 LABORATORY

2.3.5.1 Hematology

Some authors have reported a relationship of anemia with poor outcomes, with hemoglobin cut-offs 9–10.6 g/dL [39, 46], with a similar effect for the need for blood transfusions [45]. Other studies, however, did not find relationships between hemoglobin levels and prognosis [17–19].

Increasing leukocyte count >9,000/mcL presented an inverse relationship with OS in one study [36], but not in others [17–19, 39, 41]. Despite the unfavorable prognostic trend of an increase in neutrophil count or a reduction in peripheral lymphocytes [36, 41], they did not affect OS. However, other authors have reported a negative effect on OS by increasing NLR [37, 41, 44]. A meta-analysis of 10 studies, enrolling 2,952 patients, evaluated baseline NLR and concluded that it was an independent PF at any stage, including the subgroup of III/IV TNM stage [96], with another study defining a value of 2.5 as an appropriate cut-off for mGC patients [36]. However, higher values between 3.1 and 4 were also effective [44, 97, 98].

No role emerged for platelet count, but the analyzed cut-offs were low [17–19, 39, 46]. Conversely, a meta-analysis of 13 studies that included 6,280 patients with GC, of whom 683 mGC, documented that a platelet-to-lymphocyte ratio (PLR) >160 was associated with poor outcomes [99].

2.3.5.2 Chemistry

Of five studies investigating serum albumin, two reported an inverse relationship with OS [17, 57] and three only after univariate analysis [19, 41, 45]. In addition to the effect on the outcome of the numerous albumin-related indexes and scores, some studies have suggested a prognostic role of inflammation-related variables [41], except for C-reactive protein [41, 45]. Although the increase in liver enzymes is not associated with the outcome in mGC [17, 18, 39], some studies have highlighted an unfavorable prognostic effect of serum bilirubin >0.5 mg/dL [17, 18], even in the absence of LMs, confirming that biliary obstruction could aggravate mGC outcome. On the other hand, the increase of serum alkaline phosphatase (ALP) levels, which seems to be related more to tumor burden (TB) than LMs [19], was associated with reduced OS [17, 44], but not in others [18, 39], while sometimes the efficacy as PF varied depending on the cut-off [19]. In the first-line setting only two [45, 46] of four retrospective studies [18, 39] documented a negative effect on OS by lactic dehydrogenase (LDH) >225 U/L, and a possible predictive role of LDH concerning immunotherapy was described [100]. In particular, the negative effect of LDH on the outcome is a continuum and was reported even within the normal range values, as suggested in a study of 365 mGC patients, that noted a poor prognosis for patients with a serum LDH 158–245 U/L vs. LDH <157 U/L [101]. See Figure 2.2.

2.3.5.3 Tumor markers

Traditional oncological markers are controversial PFs. Besides studies favoring a negative prognostic effect by high carcino-embryonic antigen (CEA) level [46, 57, 102] and for CA 19–9 [46, 97, 103, 104], there are other negative studies [39, 45]. Although CEA is expressed more often than CA 19-9 [105], a predictive role for CA 19–9 has been hypothesized in patients receiving chemotherapy [104].

2.3.5.4 Selected trials

Three studies analyzed hematological laboratory parameters. Two studies evaluated hemoglobin, without reporting a relationship with OS [24, 28], while a leukocyte count >4,000/mcL was inversely associated with OS [28], as in another RCT was NLR >3 [27].

ALP was evaluated in five studies, of which three documented a prognostic effect. The four studies reporting the ES were pooled in a meta-analysis, including 2,497 patients, that documented for high serum ALP levels a non-significant negative trend to poor OS (HR 1.15, CI 0.92–1.44; Q = 18.70, p-value = 0.0003; I^2 = 84.0%) [26–28, 32]. Two studies investigated aspartate transaminase (AST) and alanine transaminase (ALT), with mixed results, without affecting OS in one [24], and with an inverse relationship with OS for AST in the other [28]. Finally, one trial explored the

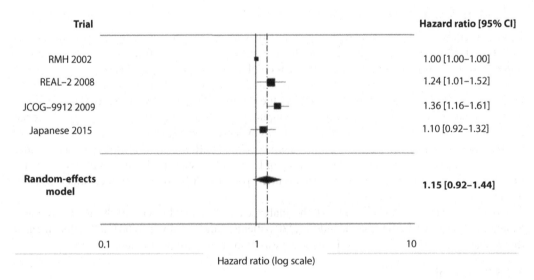

FIGURE 2.2   Forest plot of meta-analysis of alkaline phosphatase in prospective trials of patients with unresectable or metastatic gastric cancer

TABLE 2.4

Prognostic relationships of laboratory variables in selected studies of patients with unresectable or metastatic gastric cancer receiving upfront treatment

Study [ref]	Phase	No. pts	Variable	Cut-off	Prognostic relationship	Effect size
GITSG profile						
GITSG 1988 [22]	III	249	Multiple	NR	Yes	NR
Red blood cells						
Swedish 1994 [24]	III	61	Hb	NR	No	NR
JCOG-9912 2009 [28]	III	650	Hb	11 g/L	No	HR 1.06 (0.90–1.26)
White blood cells						
JCOG-9912 2009 [28]	III	650	WBCC	4000/mcL	Yes	HR 0.68 (0.47–0.98)
NLR						
REAL-2 2008 [27]	III	908	NLR	3	Yes	HR 1.67 (1.45–1.93)
Liver function						
Swedish 1994 [24]	III	61	AST	NR	No	NR
			ALT	NR	No	NR
			ALP	NR	No	NR
RMH 2002 [26]	III	254	ALP	NR	Yes	HR 1.001 (1.00–1.002)
REAL-2 2008 [27]	III	908	ALP	ULN	Yes	HR 1.24 (1.01–1.52)
JCOG-9912 2009 [28]	III	650	Albumin	ULN	No	HR 1.11 (0.95–1.31)
			Bilirubin	ULN	No	HR 0.78 (0.55–1.10)
			AST	ULN	Yes	HR 1.33 (1.10–1.60)
			ALT	ULN	No	HR 1.14 (0.93–1.39)
			ALP	ULN	Yes	HR 1.36 (1.16–1.61)
Japanese 2015 [32]	III	685	ALP	258 IU/L	No	HR 1.10 (0.92–1.32)

Legend: ALP, alkaline phosphatase. ALT, alanine aminotransferase. AST, aspartate aminotransferase. Hb, hemoglobin. HR, hazard ratio. NLR, neutrophil-to-lymphocyte ratio. NR, not reported. WBCC, white blood cells count.

possible prognostic role of high serum LDH [28], which was uninfluent after multivariate analysis. The results of the studies are reported in Table 2.4.

2.4 TUMOR-RELATED PROGNOSTIC FACTORS

2.4.1 TUMOR BURDEN

For mGC patients a consensus conference characterized OMD as a condition of tumor spread limited to one organ with three metastases or one extra-regional lymph node station [106], but OMD was not evaluated as PF.

2.4.1.1 Tumor size

Studies of mGC patients are contradictory regarding the prognostic effect of primary tumor size [53, 56], but also of T-stage, with favorable [53, 56] and negative results [43, 55], N-stage, which is prognostic in one [56] but not in other studies [52, 55], and the presence of measurable disease [17, 57].

2.4.1.2 Disease status

Disease status did not affect prognosis when comparing metastatic disease vs. locally advanced [19, 39], while when resected disease vs. recurrent vs. initially metastatic were compared, a better outcome for resected disease was documented [38, 40].

2.4.1.3   Number of metastatic sites

Though the number of metastatic sites may be a surrogate for TB, the results of studies in mGC patients are variable. The number of sites of metastasis resulted in an evaluable PF in three studies [18, 35, 54] but was not associated with the outcome in the other four [38, 40, 44, 46].

2.4.1.4   Other variables

An analysis of the AGAMENON-SEOM database evaluated patients with mGC based on a categorization of TB into five groups, relying on the number of involved organs, the number of metastases, the sum of diameters of the metastases, presence of ascites, and liver involvement >50%, and concluded for a progressive reduction of OS with the increasing class of TB [37]. Another retrospective Korean study evaluated TB as low in patients with a resected metastatic or recurrent disease and high in the initially metastatic group and concluded that TB was independently associated with OS [17].

2.4.1.5   Selected trials

Various trials have addressed TB using various approaches. One of the most recent studies used the sum of tumor diameter around the median of 76.5 mm to define TB [32]. Four studies evaluated disease status, comparing the prognosis of patients with locally advanced vs. metastatic cancer and reporting mixed results, with one negative trial [27] and three showing a poor prognosis for metastatic disease [14, 25, 26]. A pooled analysis of the three RCTs reporting an ES, including 1,436 patients, resulted in an overall trend of reduced OS for patients with metastatic tumors (HR 1.40, CI 0.97–2.04; Q = 2.41, p-value = 0.2996; I^2 = 17.0%). The number of metastatic sites also correlated with OS in two trials [28, 30], but not in a third [31]. Five studies evaluated the measurability of disease [14, 22, 23, 28, 29], of which only two quantifying the ES, and four RCTs suggested a negative prognostic role for the occurrence of measurable disease [14, 22, 28, 29].

2.4.2   PRIMARY TUMOR LOCATION

Most of the studies that have investigated the role of the site of origin of the mGC within the stomach have not reported OS differences [17, 19, 37, 38, 44, 45, 51, 54, 56, 57], with exception of SEER analyses documenting poor OS for distal tumors [53, 55]. On the contrary, an old series of patients with GC at any stage suggested worse outcomes for proximal tumors [107, 108]. One explanation could be the different genetic composition in terms of molecular subgroups, since CINs would be more frequent in proximal locations, EBV-related in the distal.

Proximal GCs have been well characterized, and some population-based studies investigated specific PFs for mGC of the cardia [109, 110].

A pathophysiologic classification into type Ia, Ib, and II has been proposed, distinguishing GERD-related GCs of the cardia (Ia) from HP-associated tumors such as gastric antral GCs (Ib), while GCs with atrophic gastritis and absence of GERD, which are often HP-related (II), are separate [1]. However, the prognostic relevance was not investigated.

2.4.2.1   Selected trials

Conflicting results come from two RCTs that evaluated tumor location. One study did not highlight any difference in OS between GOJ and stomach in a post-hoc analysis [27]. On the contrary, another study reported that tumors not involving pylorus presented longer OS and PFS [33].

2.4.3   TIMING OF METASTASIS

In a Japanese study metastatic disease at diagnosis compared to recurrent disease was associated with poor OS [111], but also in metachronous disease a reduced time to relapse predicted shorter OS [52, 112]. On the other hand, other studies have not found OS differences in synchronous vs. metachronous metastases [44, 57].

Among mGC, there is a substantial number of patients with interval metastases, for whom the diagnosis of mGC occurs during surgery and in any case after diagnosis and initiation of therapy for localized disease, that have specific biologic characteristics, such as lymph node and peritoneal metastases, frequently undergoing extensive resection, for whom rates of MSI-H were around 8% [113].

2.4.3.1 Selected trials

In contrast to two studies that documented no differences between the advanced vs. recurrent subgroups [29, 31], the other two reported a significant relationship with poor OS for patients with unresectable vs. recurrent disease [28, 32]. The pooled analysis of three Japanese studies reporting an ES [28, 31, 32] suggested a non-significant unfavorable prognostic trend for synchronous metastases (HR 1.30, CI 0.51–3.32; Q = 10.24, p-value = 0.0060; I^2 = 80.5%).

2.4.4 SITE OF METASTASIS

2.4.4.1 Liver metastases

LMs are prevalently metachronous (37% vs. 3–14%) [114, 115], and associated with extensive dissemination, since even within patients with liver-limited disease only 26% have limited TB that fits the definition of OMD [106]. If the risk of early death increases with LMs occurrence [55], the results of the studies are not in agreement on the relationship between LMs and poor prognosis, which is significant in some studies [19, 36, 45, 52, 53, 116] but not in others [17, 38–40, 43, 44, 46, 54]. However, several studies have attempted to define PFs in the subgroup of patients with LMs from mGC [57, 104, 117, 118].

2.4.4.2 Lung metastases

A SEER database analysis reported that lung metastases occur in 11% of mGC patients [53]. Their prognostic significance is unclear. While reports from the SEER database support a negative prognostic role [46, 52, 53, 119, 120], other authors, mostly after retrospective studies, have not confirmed the relationship [19, 39, 40, 43–45, 54].

2.4.4.3 Peritoneal metastases

NCDB reported that 43% of mGC patients had peritoneal metastases, 26% LMs, 20% lymph node, and 11% metastases at other sites. Peritoneal metastases were more frequent with antral location, SRCC histotype, and poor differentiation [121], but rates of peritoneal metastases were affected by diagnostic methods [122].

If three studies are excluded [38, 40, 43], most of the authors reported worse outcomes for peritoneal metastases [18, 19, 39, 44–46, 54], but the extent of peritoneal involvement appears more important than the peritoneal site itself [123–125].

2.4.4.4 Bone metastases

Autopsy series documented a 10-fold higher frequency of bone metastasis than clinical studies [126], with population-based studies reporting incidences around 2–4% [127, 128], until 14% of a SEER database analysis, which suggested more bone metastases among cardial tumors and SRCC histotype [129].

With some exceptions [39, 45], studies are quite in agreement on the poor prognosis in the presence of bone metastases [17, 18, 40, 43, 52–56, 130]. Even though mGC patients with bone metastases represent an extremely heterogeneous subgroup [131], their poor prognosis has been associated with various concomitant characteristics, such as deteriorated PS [131, 132], synchronous timing [133], increased LDH, CEA and CA 19-9 levels [132].

2.4.4.5   Other sites

Except for a SEER database report suggesting longer OS for patients with lymph node metastases [56], most authors agree that the occurrence of lymph node metastases does not affect the prognosis [38, 40, 43–45, 54].

No relationship with prognosis has been highlighted for ovarian metastases [17, 44, 45, 54], even though, according to some authors, peritoneum surgery was more likely to be successful in cases of only metachronous ovarian localization [134].

Few studies have investigated brain metastases, reporting divergent results on the outcome [43, 55].

2.4.4.6   Selected trials

Three old studies analyzed the site of metastatic disease and found no significant differences of median OS [14, 23, 24]. Further, researchers have focused on specific sites of metastasis. Three studies evaluated peritoneal metastases [27, 28, 32], of which only one showed a correlation with poor OS [27]. It should be considered, however, that none of the three studies included surgical staging and that in one case, patients with "severe peritoneal disease" were not eligible [28]. A pooled analysis of the three studies yielded a non-significant relationship (HR 1.17, CI 0.86–1.59; Q = 3.70, p-value = 0.1571; I^2 = 46%). Concordant were the results of the two studies that evaluated the presence of LMs, which had a negative relationship with OS [27, 28]. Only a Japanese trial evaluated a possible prognostic role for other sites of metastasis [28], evidencing poor outcomes for patients with lymph node and bone localizations, but not for those with lung metastases.

2.4.5   PATHOLOGY

2.4.5.1   Histology

Even though the WHO 2019 classification distinguishes 14 morphological GC histotypes [135], most studies report the comparison between intestinal and diffuse. Intestinal-type GCs include papillary, tubular, and mucinous adenocarcinoma; diffuse-type are the SRCC and the poorly cohesive carcinoma [136]. Diffuse histotypes have been associated with a worse prognosis than intestinal types, especially in mGC patients [137]. However, it is unclear whether the poor OS of SRCCs is limited to early or advanced stages [138–141]. In the US, SRCC and poorly cohesive cell carcinoma account for 25% of GCs, are often distal, and affect female sex and early age, with synchronous metastases in 50% [138].

The comparison between intestinal vs. diffuse mGCs did not produce homogeneous results, with some studies documenting better prognosis for patients with intestinal histotypes [37, 44], while others did not detect differences [17, 35, 57]. Analogous is the uncertainty that comes from the studies comparing adenocarcinoma to SRCC, sometimes reporting better prognosis for adenocarcinomas [39], sometimes no difference [38, 43, 51, 55].

2.4.5.2   Tumor grade

Various analyses of the SEER database concluded that poorly differentiated mGCs had a significantly poor prognosis compared to well/moderately differentiated tumors [51–53, 55, 56]. Four retrospective studies did not document any difference in survival by tumor differentiation [17, 39, 46, 98]. Tumor grade was found to be a PF in the analysis of the AGAMENON database [37] and in one retrospective study [45], but not in the other two [43, 57].

2.4.5.3   Molecolar biology

The Cancer Genome Atlas (TCGA) research network proposed a genomic classification in four subtypes: genomically stable GC (GS, 20%), that prevailed among patients with diffuse histotype; GC with chromosomal instability (CIN, 50%), that represented 65% of proximal or junctional tumors;

GCs with microsatellite instability (MSI, 22%); Epstein-Barr virus-associated GC (EBV-related, 9%), which accounted for 62% of body-antrum GCs [142].

The currently necessary molecular characterization requires the determination of HER2, PD-L1, and MMR status, as they are predictive markers of drug response. Other determinations, such as TMB and EBV, are increasingly used.

HER2 is overexpressed in 10–30% of GCs, and is more frequent in males, proximal tumors, intestinal-type, and Asians [143–145]. Although reported as a negative PF, this role has not been confirmed [146]. In the HER2-positive mGC poor PS and multiple sites of metastasis have been associated with poor outcomes [147], as well as HER IHC 3+ vs. 0–1 [37].

MSI-H in GCs appears more prevalent in localized GC, female sex, and older age, with the primary tumor localizing in the gastric antrum [142, 148]. Although the prognosis of patients with MSI-H vs. MSS is better [112], the most consolidated role for MSI-H is to be a predictive variable of immunotherapy activity. An analysis of 5 RCTs that had enrolled 2,264 mGC patients showed that immune checkpoint inhibitors (ICIs) were associated with significantly improved OS in patients with MSI-H [149].

EBV-positive GC is more frequent in men and is characterized by specific genetic, epigenetic, and histological molecular features [142, 145, 150]. EBV-positive GC subtype also has amplifications of PD-L1 [142], and PIK3CA mutations [142], with impressive response rates to immunotherapy [151].

2.4.5.4 Selected trials

Among the heterogeneous comparisons between GC histologies, seven studies evaluated the prognosis of intestinal vs. diffuse mGCs, with a significant association with OS in three, as resumed in Table 2.5. Four studies, comparing outcomes of 1,923 patients, calculated an ES and were included in a meta-analysis [28, 29, 31, 32], that resulted in an overall non-significant trend to poor prognosis for diffuse histotypes (HR 1.23, CI 0.81–1.86; Q = 14.66, p-value = 0.0021; I^2 = 79.5%).

Grading was explored as a PF in one trial, that reported reduced OS of patients with poorly differentiated mGC [31]. See also Figure 2.3.

2.4.6 PREVIOUS TREATMENTS

Of the studies evaluating PTR, some documented a relationship with improved prognosis [17, 44, 45, 51, 52, 54, 55], while others did not [35, 53].

TABLE 2.5
Prognostic relationships of histotype in selected studies of patients with unresectable or metastatic gastric cancer receiving upfront treatment

Study [ref]	Phase	No. pts	Variable	Prognostic relationship	Effect size
Korean 1993 [14]	III	295	Intestinal vs. diffuse	No	OS 28 vs. 33 weeks
REAL-2 2008 [27]	III	888	Adenocarcinoma vs. SCC	No	NR
JCOG-9912 2009 [28]	III	650	Intestinal vs. diffuse	No	HR 0.94 (0.81–1.11)
GC0301 2011 [29]	III	315	Intestinal vs. diffuse	Yes	HR 1.72 (1.16–2.55)
JCOG-0106 2013 [31]	III	273	Intestinal vs. diffuse	No	HR 1.12 (0.78–1.62)
Japanese 2015 [32]	III	685	Intestinal vs. diffuse	Yes	HR 0.72 (0.61–0.87)
TRIO-LOGiC 2015 [33]	III	487	Intestinal vs. diffuse	Yes	NR

Legend: HR, hazard ratio. NR, not reported. OS, overall survival. SCC, squamous cell carcinoma.

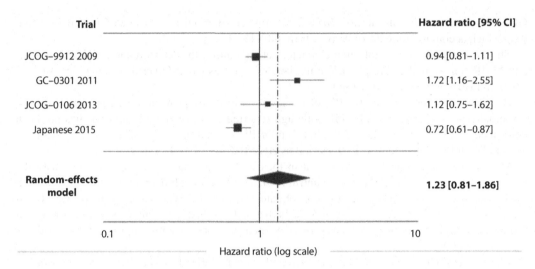

FIGURE 2.3   Forest plot of meta-analysis of histologic tumor type in prospective trials of patients with unresectable or metastatic gastric cancer

Prior radiotherapy was associated with better outcome in SEER database [51] and OCR analyses [54], while only one study evaluated the role of previous adjuvant chemotherapy, which was associated with longer OS only after univariate analysis [57].

2.4.6.1   Primary tumor resection

In addition to the favorable results of some population-based studies [51, 52, 54, 55, 152–154], many studies that evaluated prior PTR documented a relationship with a better prognosis [17, 44, 45, 97], that was not confirmed by other authors [35, 39, 41, 53]. However, in most studies it was not palliative PTR, therefore the favorable effect of PTR could be a bias related to a metachronous relapsing disease. On the other hand, a systematic review of 19 studies identified 2,911 mGC patients who underwent palliative gastrectomy, that was associated with increased 1-year survival rates compared with both other conservative procedures and no resection [155].

A RCT assigned 175 mGC patients to chemotherapy alone or gastrectomy followed by chemotherapy, and did not document any OS improvement from PTR [156]. Therefore, palliative PTR is currently reserved for treating symptoms related to the primary tumor. In the opinion of some authors, the benefit from PTR was limited to patients with CEA and CA 19–9 in the normal range [157] or symptomatic [158]. Other authors suggested that palliative PTR improved OS/PFS after subsequent chemotherapy [159], or after response to chemotherapy and in patients with good PS [160], such that despite the negative RCT, nomograms were defined to select candidates for palliative gastrectomy [161].

2.4.6.2   Extensive surgery

Few studies have explored the role of extensive surgery in GC. Although they are generally favoring surgery [97, 152, 162], they should be considered with caution [163]. Two meta-analyses [164, 165] and several retrospective series [117, 166, 167] have reported a possible benefit of LMs surgery, but a selection bias is probable.

2.4.6.3   Selected trials

Of the four studies that evaluated the relationship of PTR with OS, three documented a significant correlation. In particular, an Asian study found longer OS for patients with previous PTR (44.9 vs. 28.4 weeks) [23], while a small Swedish trial had ruled out an independent effect on OS for PTR

[24]. Finally, other two RCTs documented the poor prognosis of patients who had not undergone gastrectomy [14, 28].

2.5 PROGNOSTIC FACTORS IN DECISION-MAKING

In the setting of mGC the prognosis remains severe, but the introduction of targeted therapy and immunotherapy in combination with chemotherapy has improved outcomes [168, 169], and some PFs could support clinical management of mGC patients (Table 2.6).

Currently, in mGC patients a gastrectomy is not recommended unless palliation of symptoms is necessary [170, 171]. Notably, a RCT excluded a benefit from palliative PTR on OS [156], but was closed early. No subgroup recorded a significant benefit from gastrectomy, and in particular patients with upper third mGC and those with clinical stage cN0–1 had a significant increase in post-operative mortality.

Resection of metastases is still being studied and cannot be advised, but it could be considered in carefully selected OMD patients, who are responsive to chemotherapy [172, 173]. HIPEC in limited peritoneal disease is a safe procedure but studies are insufficient [174, 175].

Early palliative care and nutritional support, including nasogastric tube or PEG in order to contain WL [176], should be part of the management of patients with mGC, as documented in a RCT that showed a benefit from early interdisciplinary supportive care, particularly pronounced in young male patients [177].

2.5.1 UPFRONT TREATMENT

2.5.1.1 Untargetable tumors

After early studies documented an OS benefit from chemotherapy [24, 178, 179], four trials have reported further OS improvement from two-drug vs. single-drug regimens [23, 28, 180, 181], particularly among patients with good PS and low TB (not measurable disease), with synchronous metastases and/or without PTR. Therefore, currently the recommended upfront chemotherapy is a two-drug regimen of platinum+fluoropyrimidine. While S-1 is more commonly used in Asia, in Europe oxaliplatin is the preferred platinum, especially in the elderly, due its safety profile [182]. A recent trial of elderly patients confirmed the usefulness of reduced doses of doublets [183].

Various attempts to improve outcomes of the upfront platinum-fluoropyrimidine doublet adding a third drug, ended in negative studies for many drugs (bevacizumab, cetuximab, panitumumab, ornatuzumab, rilotumumab, ramucirumab). On the other hand, a triplet including docetaxel has been evaluated in four RCTs, including two with increased OS but at the cost of prohibitive toxicity, which prevented the triplet from becoming an accepted new standard of care [15, 34, 184, 185]. However, docetaxel-based triplets significantly improved outcomes in patients with good PS, early onset, distal tumors, and increased TB (with LMs, without PTR).

In contrast, a three-drug regimen including an ICI showed favorable results in two trials [186, 187], even though limited to the mGC patients with PD-L1 CPS>10 for pembrolizumab [186] and CPS >5 for nivolumab [187]. The ICI-based regimens appeared most effective in the subgroups with high TB (tumor size above median; multiple sites of metastasis) [186, 187], in young patients with diffuse histotype [193], and in those with ECOG PS 1, males, with distal tumors [187].

Two studies also reported a direct comparison of an immunotherapy arm with chemotherapy, concluding that the immunotherapy arm was more active in patients with a low TB, while the profile of the young patient with diffuse histotype and distal gastric origin was confirmed as the most ICI-responsive [186].

TABLE 2.6

Prognostic and predictive variables in clinical decision-making in metastatic gastric cancer (HER2-negative/MSS)

A. Upfront systemic treatment

1   PD-L1
- Positive (CPS >5-10): ICI+CHT or ICI alone favored (PEMB+CHT or PEMB is better than CHT [CPS >10]; NIVO+CHT is better than CHT [CPS >5])
- Negative: CHT favored (triplet is better than doublet; doublet is better than mono)

2   Tumor burden
- High (PD-L1 positive): ICI+CHT favored (PEMB+CHT is better than CHT [CPS >1]; NIVO+CHT is better than CHT [CPS >5])
- High (PD-L1 negative): docetaxel-containing triplet favored (triplet is better than doublet)
- Low (PD-L1 positive): ICI favored (PEMB is better than CHT in CPS >10)

3   Age
- <65 years old: ICI+CHT or ICI favored (PEMB+CHT or PEMB [CPS >10] are better than CHT)
- <70 years old: docetaxel-containing triplet favored (triplet is better than doublet)

4   Location
- Distal tumors: ICI+CHT or ICI favored (PEMB+CHT is better than CHT [CPS >10]; NIVO+CHT is better than CHT [CPS >5])

B. Treatment of refractory disease

1   Performance status
- Good: RAMU+PACL or CHT or PEMB favored (RAMU+PACL is better than PACL; CHT with taxane or irinotecan is better than placebo; PEMB is better than PACL [CPS >1])
- Poor: RAMU favored (RAMU is better than placebo, particularly when weight loss does not occur)

2   Age
- <70 years old: doublet favored (doublet is better than mono)
- >65 years old: ICI favored (NIVO is better than placebo)

3   Location
- Proximal tumors: RAMU+PACL, ICI or CHT favored (RAMU+PACL is better than PACL; PEMB is better than PACL [CPS >1]; docetaxel is better than placebo)

4   Treatment line
- Second line: RAMU+PACL, docetaxel, or RAMU favored (RAMU+PACL is better than PACL; docetaxel or RAMU are better than placebo)
- Third or later lines: TAS-102, NIVO or APA favored (TAS-102, NIVO or APA are better than placebo; TAS-102 is better than placebo after previous taxane)

5   Tumor burden
- Multiple sites of metastasis: ICI favored (NIVO is better than placebo)
- Low tumor burden: RAMU+PACL, CHT and APA favored (RAMU+PACL or APA are better than PACL in <3 sites of metastasis; CHT with irinotecan or taxane is better than placebo in non-measurable disease)

Legend: APA, apatinib. CHT, chemotherapy. CPS, combined positive score. HER2, Human epidermal growth factor receptor 2. ICI, immune checkpoint inhibitor. MSS, microsatellite stability. NIVO, nivolumab. PACL, paclitaxel. PD-L1, programmed death ligand 1. PEMB, pembrolizumab. RAMU, ramucirumab. TAS-102, trifluridine/tipiracil.

2.5.1.2   Targetable tumors

As mentioned above, HER2 status predicts activity of HER2-directed drugs. In mGC patients with HER2 over-expressed, only one of four studies reported longer OS for the combination of trastuzumab with chemotherapy vs. chemotherapy [188]. Subgroups documented a significant advantage in patients with ECOG PS 0–1, elderly, with intestinal histotype, and with increased TB (measurable disease, >4 metastases; >2 metastatic sites, visceral organ involvement, no previous PTR).

More recently, based on results of protocol-specified first interim analysis of Keynote-811, pembrolizumab in combination with trastuzumab, fluoropyrimidine, and platinum-containing chemotherapy, has been approved as upfront treatment of HER2-positive unresectable locally advanced or metastatic adenocarcinoma of the stomach or GOJ expressing PD-L1 with a CPS $\geq$ 1 [189].

2.5.2 TREATMENT OF REFRACTORY DISEASE

2.5.2.1 Untargetable tumors

Combination therapy of ramucirumab with paclitaxel or as monotherapy, and chemotherapy are recommended options. Four of five RCTs reported improved OS after monochemotherapy or ramucirumab therapy in comparison to best supportive care (BSC) [190–193]. Chemotherapy was more active in patients with ECOG PS 0, elderly, males, proximal tumors and limited TB, whereas ramucirumab was more effective in those with a poor PS, diffuse histotype, without WL.

Pembrolizumab did not improve OS in comparison with paclitaxel, but was active in mGC with a PD-L1 CPS >1%. Within the study sample, it reported better results in patients with cardia location and ECOG PS 0 [194].

2.5.2.2 Targetable tumors

In the setting of refractory disease, HER2-directed therapy failed to improve the outcome, either by lapatinib [195] or TDM1 [196]. However, a RCT documented better ORR and OS for trastuzumab-deruxtecan, that was more pronounced among patients with a previous PTR and having received at least two previous systemic regimens, diffuse histotype, IHC 3+, advanced age [197].

Besides HER2, another target for predicting immunotherapy efficacy is MSI-H. To date, immunotherapy alone with pembrolizumab as the treatment of choice is frequently limited to the second-line setting [194, 198, 199]. Although there is no dedicated study for MSI-H mGCs, the pooled analysis of three trials indicates that MSI-H status may be a biomarker for pembrolizumab therapy, regardless of the line of therapy in which it was received, and suggests that early introduction of pembrolizumab appears beneficial in patients with this molecular subtype [198].

Three drugs were evaluated in subsequent lines, each reporting longer OS over BSC [200–202], but with different activity by patients subgroups. Apatinib was more effective in patients with low TB and in earlier lines, whereas nivolumab was more active with high TB and in more advanced lines, but also in male and elderly patients, without hepatic or peritoneal involvement. Finally, trifluridine/tipiracil was more active in patients who previously received taxane-based chemotherapy but not irinotecan.

2.6 CONCLUSION

Apart from the pattern of metastases, with worse prognosis in liver or bone metastases, none of the other variables appear to predict reliably the outcome of mGC patients, as resumed in Table 2.7. Peritoneal metastases themselves also do not associate significantly with OS, but it is clear that their staging remains suboptimal in mGC, since peritoneal carcinomatosis index (PCI) determination and surgical staging do not always appear appropriate. Good PS itself does not always predict better OS but is affected by other variables such as PTR and NLR.

Consequently, an evaluation of the prognostic role of more easily reproducible TB-related variables, such as the recent definition of OMD and TB according to AGAMENON-SEOM, is needed.

At the same time, understanding the microenvironment of liver metastasis and changes after vtreatment response, such as clarifying the effect on OS of myeloid-derived tumor-associated macrophages at the tumor invasive margin, could allow better characterization of the prognostic effect of NLR and PLR, that of primary tumor and timing of metastasis.

TABLE 2.7

Prognostic factors evaluated in prospective trials of upfront treatment in patients with unresectable or metastatic gastric cancer

Suggested	Not suggested	Needing study
Performance status	Age	Sex
Geographic area		Body mass index
		Weight loss
		Neutrophil-to-lymphocyte ratio
		Platelet-to-lymphocyte ratio
		Albumin
		Lactic dehydrogenase
Liver metastases	Primary tumor location	Disease status
Bone metastases	Lung metastases	Peritoneal metastases and PCI
		Histotype
		Tumor grade
		Primary tumor resection

REFERENCES

1. Sugano K, Spechler SJ, El-Omar EM, et al. Kyoto international consensus report on anatomy, pathophysiology and clinical significance of the gastro-oesophageal junction. *Gut* 2022;71(8):1488–1514.
2. ICD-11 Classification, available at: https://icd.who.int/ct11/icd11_mms/en/release, accessed January 21, 2023.
3. Morgan E, Arnold M, Camargo MC, et al. The current and future incidence and mortality of gastric cancer in 185 countries, 2020–40: A population-based modelling study. *EClinicalMedicine* 2022;47:101404.
4. ECIS – European Cancer Information System, available at: https://ecis.jrc.ec.europa.eu, accessed October 31, 2023.
5. Zhou J, Zheng R, Zhang S, et al. Gastric and esophageal cancer in China 2000 to 2030: Recent trends and short-term predictions of the future burden. *Cancer Med* 2022;11:1902–12.
6. Anderson WF, Rabkin CS, Turner N, et al. The changing face of noncardia gastric cancer incidence among US non-hispanic whites. *J Natl Cancer Inst* 2018;110(6):608–615.
7. Gullo I, Grillo F, Molinaro L, et al. Minimum biopsy set for HER2 evaluation in gastric and gastroesophageal junction cancer. *Endosc Int Open* 2015;3(2):E165–70.
8. Tominaga N, Gotoda T, Hara M, et al. Five biopsy specimens from the proximal part of the tumor reliably determine HER2 protein expression status in gastric cancer. *Gastric Cancer* 2016;19(2):553–560.
9. Kwee RM, Kwee TC. Imaging in local staging of gastric cancer: A systematic review. *J Clin Oncol* 2007;25(15):2107–16.
10. Gertsen EC, Brenkman HJF, van Hillegersberg R, et al. 18F-Fludeoxyglucose-positron emission tomography/computed tomography and laparoscopy for staging of locally advanced gastric cancer: A multicenter prospective dutch cohort study (PLASTIC). *JAMA Surg* 2021;156(12):e215340.
11. Amin MB, Edge S, Green F, et al. *AJCC Cancer Staging Manual.* 8th Ed. New York; Springer-Verlag, 2017.
12. NIH SEER Programme, available at: https://seer.cancer.gov/statfacts/html/stomach.html, accessed January 21, 2023.
13. Pape M, Kuijper SC, Vissers PAJ, et al. Beyond median overall survival: Estimating trends for multiple survival scenarios in patients with metastatic esophagogastric cancer. *J Natl Compr Cancer Netw* 2022;20(12):1321–9.
14. Lacave A, Wils J, Bleiberg H, et al. An EORTC gastrointestinal group phase III evaluation of combinations of methyl-CCNU, 5-fluorouracil, and adriamycin in advanced gastric cancer. *J Clin Oncol* 1987;5:1387–93.
15. Van Cutsem E, Moiseyenko VM, Tjulandin S, et al; V325 Study Group. Phase III study of docetaxel and cisplatin plus fluorouracil compared with cisplatin and fluorouracil as first-line therapy for advanced gastric cancer: A report of the V325 Study Group. *J Clin Oncol* 2006;24(31):4991–7.

16. Kang YK, Chen LT, Ryu MH, et al. Nivolumab plus chemotherapy versus placebo plus chemotherapy in patients with HER2-negative, untreated, unresectable advanced or recurrent gastric or gastro-oesophageal junction cancer (ATTRACTION-4): A randomised, multicentre, double-blind, placebo-controlled, phase 3 trial. *Lancet Oncol* 2022;23(2):234–47.

17. Lee J, Lim T, Uhm JE, et al. Prognostic model to predict survival following first-line chemotherapy in patients with metastatic gastric adenocarcinoma. *Ann Oncol* 2007;18(5):886–91.

18. Kim JG, Ryoo B-Y, Park YH, et al. Prognostic factors for survival of patients with advanced gastric cancer treated with cisplatin-based chemotherapy. *Cancer Chemother Pharmacol* 2008;61(2):301–7.

19. Chau I, Norman AR, Cunningham D, et al. Multivariate prognostic factor analysis in locally advanced and metastatic esophago-gastric cancer – Pooled analysis from three multicenter, randomized, controlled trials using individual patient data. *J Clin Oncol* 2004;22(12):2395–403.

20. Kanagavel D, Pokataev IA, Fedyanin MY, et al. A prognostic model in patients treated for metastatic gastric cancer with second-line chemotherapy. *Ann Oncol* 2010;21:1779–85.

21. Graziosi L, Marino E, Donini A. Survival comparison in gastric cancer patients between 7th and 8th edition of the AJCC TNM staging system: The first western single center experience. *Eur J Surg Oncol* 2019;45(6):1105–8.

22. Gastrointestinal Tumor Study Group. Triazinate and platinum efficacy in combination with 5-fluorouracil and doxorubicin: Results of a three-arm randomized trial in metastatic gastric cancer. *J Natl Cancer Inst* 1988;80:1011–5.

23. Kim NK, Park YS, Heo DS, et al. A phase III randomized study of 5-fluorouracil and cisplatin versus 5-fluorouracil, doxorubicin, and mitomycin C versus 5-fluorouracil alone in the treatment of advanced gastric cancer. *Cancer* 1993;71:3813–8.

24. Glimelius B, Ekstrom K, Hoffman K, et al. Randomized comparison between chemotherapy plus supportive care with best supportive care in advanced gastric cancer. *Ann Oncol* 1997;8:163–8.

25. Webb A, Cunningham D, Scarffe JH, et al. Randomized trial comparing epirubicin, cicplatin, and fluorouracil versus fluorouracil, doxorubicin, and methotrexate in advanced esophagogastric cancer. *J Clin Oncol* 1997;15:261–7.

26. Tebbutt NC, Norman A, Cunningham D, et al. A multicentre, randomised phase III trial comparing protracted venous infusion (PVI) 5-fluorouracil (5-FU) with PVI 5-FU plus mitomycin C in patients with inoperable oesophago-gastric cancer. *Ann Oncol* 2002;13:1568–75.

27. Grenader T, Waddell T, Peckitt C, et al. Prognostic value of neutrophil-to-lymphocyte ratio in advanced oesophago-gastric cancer: Exploratory analysis of the REAL-2 trial. *Ann Oncol* 2016;27:687–92.

28. Takahari D, Boku N, Mizusawa J, et al. Determination of prognostic factors in Japanese patients with advanced gastric cancer using the data from a randomized controlled trial, Japan Clinical Oncology Group 9912. *Oncologist* 2014;19:358–66.

29. Narahara H, Iishi H, Imamura H, et al. Randomized phase III study comparing the efficacy and safety of irinotecan plus S-1 with S-1 alone as first-line treatment for advanced gastric cancer (study GC0301/TOP-002). *Gastric Cancer* 2011;14:72–80.

30. Hacker UT, Hasenclever D, Linder N, et al. Prognostic role of body composition parameters in gastric/gastroesophageal junction cancer patients from the EXPAND trial. *J Cachexia Sarcop Muscle* 2020;11:135–44.

31. Shirao K, Boku N, Yamada Y, et al. Randomized phase III study of 5-fluorouracil continuous infusion vs. sequential methotrexate and fluorouracil therapy in far advanced gastric cancer with peritoneal metastasis (JCOG0106). *Jpn J Clin Oncol* 2013;43(10):972–80.

32. Yamada Y, Higuchi K, Nishikawa K, et al. Phase III study comparing oxaliplatin plus S-1 with cisplatin plus S-1 in chemotherapy-naive patients with advanced gastric cancer. *Ann Oncol* 2015;26:141–8.

33. Hecht JR, Bang Y-J, Qin SK, et al. Lapatinib in combination with capecitabine plus oxaliplatin in human epidermal growth factor receptor 2-positive advanced or metastatic gastric, esophageal, or gastroesophageal adenocarcinoma: TRIO-013/LOGiC-a randomized phase III trial. *J Clin Oncol* 2016;34:443–51.

34. Yamada Y, Boku N, Mizusawa J, et al. Docetaxel plus cisplatin and S-1 versus cisplatin and S-1 in patients with advanced gastric cancer (JCOG1013): An open-label, phase 3, randomised controlled trial. *Lancet Gastroenterol Hepatol* 2019;4:501–10.

35. Yoshida M, Ohtsu A, Boku N, et al. Long-term survival and prognostic factors in patients with metastatic gastric cancers treated with chemotherapy in the Japan Clinical Oncology Group (JCOG) study. *Jpn J Clin Oncol* 2004;34(11):654–9.

36. Yamanaka T, Matsumoto S, Teramukai S, et al. The baseline ratio of neutrophils to lymphocytes is associated with patient prognosis in advanced gastric cancer. *Oncology* 2007;73:215–20.

37. Gallego Plazas J, Arias-Martinez A, Lecumberri A, et al. Sex and gender disparities in patients with advanced gastroesophageal adenocarcinoma: Data from the AGAMENON-SEOM registry. *ESMO Open* 2022;7(3):100514.
38. Lee SS, Lee J-L, Ryu M-H, et al. Combination chemotherapy with capecitabine (X) and cisplatin (P) as first line treatment in advanced gastric cancer: Experience of 223 patients with prognostic factor analysis. *Jpn J Clin Oncol* 2007;37(1):30–7.
39. Inal A, Kaplan MA, Kicukoner M, et al. Prognostic factors in first-line chemotherapy treated metastatic gastric cancer patients: A retrospective study. *Asia Pac J Cancer Prev* 2012;13:3869–72.
40. Koo DH, Ryu M-H, Ryoo B-Y, et al. Three-week combination chemotherapy with S-1 and cisplatin as first-line treatment in patients with advanced gastric cancer: A retrospective study with 159 patients. *Gastric Cancer* 2012;15:305–12.
41. Demirelli B, Babacan NA, Ercelep O, et al. Modified Glasgow prognostic score, prognostic nutritional index and ECOG performance score predicts survival better than sarcopenia, cachexia and some inflammatory indices in metastatic gastric cancer. *Nutr Cancer* 2021;73(2):230–8.
42. Ma LX, Taylor K, Espin-Garcia O, et al. Prognostic significance of nutritional markers in metastatic gastric and esophageal adenocarcinoma. *Cancer Med* 2021;10:199–207.
43. Hinzpeter R, Mirshahvalad SA, Kulanthaivelu R, et al. Prognostic value of [18F]-FDG PET/CT radiomics combined with sarcopenia status among patients with advanced gastroesophageal cancer. *Cancers* 2022;14:5324.
44. Nakayama I, Takahari D, Shimozaki K, et al. Clinical progress in inoperable or recurrent advanced gastric cancer treatment from 1004 single institute experiences between 2007 and 2018. *Oncologist* 2022;27:e506–17.
45. Sogioultzis S, Syrios J, Xynos ID, et al. Palliative gastrectomy and other factors affecting overall survival in stage IV gastric adenocarcinoma patients receiving chemotherapy: A retrospective analysis. *Eur J Surg Oncol* 2011;37(4):312–8.
46. Zhou Q, Lan X, Li N, et al. Analysis of prognostic factors and design of prognosis model for patients with stage IV gastric cancer following first-line palliative chemotherapy. *Cancer Manage Res* 2020;12:10461–8.
47. Parisi A. Weight loss and body mass index in advanced gastric cancer patients treated with second-line ramucirumab: A real-life multicentre study. *J Cancer Res Cllin Oncol* 2019;145(9):2365–73.
48. Wang J, Qu J, Li Z, et al. A prognostic model in metastatic or recurrent gastric cancer patients with good performance status who received first-line chemotherapy. *Transl Oncol* 2016;9(3):256–61.
49. Wang J, Yang B, Li Z, et al. Nomogram-based prediction of survival in unresectable or metastatic gastric cancer patients with good performance status who received first-line chemotherapy. *Ann Transl Med* 2020;8(6):311.
50. Touchefeu Y, Guimbaud R, Louvet C, et al. Prognostic factors in patients treated with second-line chemotherapy for advanced gastric cancer: Results from the randomized prospective phase III FFCD-0307 trial. *Gastric Cancer* 2019;22(3):577–86.
51. Yang D, Hendifar A, Lenz C, et al. Survival of metastatic gastric cancer: Significance of age, sex and race/ethnicity. *J Gastrointest Oncol* 2011;2(2):77–84.
52. Chen Y, Shou L, Xia Y, et al. Artificial intelligence annotated clinical-pathologic risk model to predict outcomes of advanced gastric cancer. *Front Oncol* 2023;13:1099360.
53. Liu X, Ren Y, Wang F, et al. Development and validation of prognostic nomogram for patients with metastatic gastric adenocarcinoma based on the SEER database. *Medicine* 2023;102(9):e33019.
54. Dixon M, Mahar AL, Helyer LK, et al. Prognostic factors in metastatic gastric cancer: Results of a population-based, retrospective cohort study in Ontario. *Gastric Cancer* 2016;19(1):150–9.
55. Zhu Y, Fang X, Wang L, Zhang T, Yu D. A predictive nomogram for early death of metastatic gastric cancer: A retrospective study in the SEER database and China. *J Cancer* 2020;11(18):5527–35.
56. Ren J, Dai Y, Chao F, et al. A nomogram for predicting the cancer-specific survival of patients with initially diagnosed metastatic gastric cancer. *Clin Med Insights Oncol* 2022;16:11795549221142095.
57. Xiong J, Wu Y, Hu H, et al. Prognostic significance of preoperative sarcopenia in patients with gastric cancer liver metastases receiving hepatectomy. *Front Nutr* 2022;9:878791.
58. Park HJ, Ahn JY, Jung H-Y, et al. Clinical characteristics and outcomes for gastric cancer patients aged 18–30 years. *Gastric Cancer* 2014;17(4):649–60.
59. Zhong N, Yu Y, Chen J, et al. Clinicopathological characteristics, survival outcome and prognostic factors of very young gastric cancer. *Clin Exp Med* 2023;23(2):437–445.
60. Guan WL, Yuan LP, Yan XL, et al. More attention should be paid to adult gastric cancer patients younger than 35 years old: Extremely poor prognosis was found. *J Cancer* 2019;10(2):472–478.

61. Zhou L, Jiang Z, Gu W, Han S. STROBE-clinical characteristics and prognosis factors of gastric cancer in young patients aged ≤30 years. *Medicine* 2021;100(26):e26336.

62. Abele M, Grabner L, Blessing T, et al. Epidemiology and characteristics of gastric carcinoma in childhood-an analysis of data from population-based and clinical cancer registries. *Cancers* 2023;15(1):317.

63. Kong X, Wang JL, Chen HM, Fang JY. Comparison of the clinicopathological characteristics of young and elderly patients with gastric carcinoma: A meta analysis. *J Surg Oncol* 2012;106(3):346–52.

64. Ramos MFKP, Pereira MA, Sagae VMT, et al. Gastric cancer in young adults: A worse prognosis group? *Rev Col Bras Cir* 2019;46(4):e20192256.

65. Lu Z, Lu M, Zhang X, et al. Advanced or metastatic gastric cancer in elderly patients: Clinicopathological, prognostic factors and treatments. *Clin Transl Oncol* 2013;15(5):376–83.

66. Lord SR, Hall PS, McShane P, et al. Factors predicting outcome for advanced gastroesophageal cancer in elderly patients receiving palliative chemotherapy. *Clin Oncol* 2010;22(2):107–13.

67. Loizides S, Papamichael D. Considerations and challenges in the management of the older patients with gastric cancer. *Cancers* 2022;14(6):1587.

68. Hsu L-W, Huang K-H, Chen M-H, et al. Genetic alterations in gastric cancer patients according to sex. *Aging* 2021;13(1):376–388.

69. Yamada T, Yoshikawa T, Taguri M, et al. The survival difference between gastric cancer patients from the UK and Japan remains after weighted propensity score analysis considering all background factors. *Gastric Cancer* 2016;19:479–489.

70. Hacker UT, Escalona-Espinosa L, Consalvo N, et al. Evaluation of Angiopoietin-2 as a biomarker in gastric cancer: Results from the randomised phase III AVAGAST trial. *Br J Cancer* 2016;114(8):855–62.

71. Sawaki A, Yamada Y, Yamaguchi K, et al. Regional differences in advanced gastric cancer: Exploratory analyses of the AVAGAST placebo arm. *Gastric Cancer* 2018;21(3):429–38.

72. Bouvier AM, Sant M, Verdecchia A, et al. What reasons lie behind long-term survival differences for gastric cancer within Europe? *Eur J Cancer* 2010;46(6):1086–92.

73. Marrelli D, Pedrazzani C, Corso G, et al. Different pathological features and prognosis in gastric cancer patients coming from high-risk and low-risk areas of Italy. *Ann Surg* 2009;250(1):43–50.

74. Al-Refaie WB, Tseng JF, Gay G, et al. The impact of ethnicity on the presentation and prognosis of patients with gastric adenocarcinoma. Results from the National Cancer Data Base. *Cancer* 2008;113(3):461–9.

75. Kim J, Sun C-L, Mailey B, et al. Race and ethnicity correlate with survival in patients with gastric adenocarcinoma. *Ann Oncol* 2010;21:152–60.

76. Wang J, Sun Y, Bertagnolli MM. Comparison of gastric cancer survival between Caucasian and Asian patients treated in the United States: Results from the Surveillance Epidemiology and End Results (SEER) database. *Ann Surg Oncol* 2015;22(9):2965–71.

77. Tee MC, Pirozzi N, Brahmbhatt RD, et al. Oncologic and surgical outcomes for gastric cancer patients undergoing gastrectomy differ by race in the United States. *Eur J Surg Oncol* 2020;46(10 Pt A):1941–7.

78. Zhang Y, Lin Y, Duan J, et al. A population-based analysis of distant metastasis in stage IV gastric cancer. *Med Sci Monit* 2020;26:e923867.

79. Kim J, Mailey B, Senthil M, et al. Disparities in gastric cancer outcomes among Asian ethnicities in the USA. *Ann Surg Oncol* 2009;16(9):2433–41.

80. Markar SR, Karthikesalingam A, Jackson D, Hanna GB. Long-term survival after gastrectomy for cancer in randomized, controlled oncological trials: Comparison between West and East. *Ann Surg Oncol* 2013;20(7):2328–38.

81. Takashima A, Iizumi S, Boku N. Survival after failure of first-line chemotherapy in advanced gastric cancer patients: Differences between Japan and the rest of the world. *Jpn J Clin Oncol* 2017;47(7):583–9.

82. Ma Y, Tang L, Wang HX, et al. Capecitabine for the treatment for advanced gastric cancer: Efficacy, safety and ethnicity. *J Clin Pharm Ther* 2012;37(3):266–75.

83. Hsu C, Shen YC, Cheng CC, et al. Geographic difference in safety and efficacy of systemic chemotherapy for advanced gastric or gastroesophagealcarcinoma: A meta-analysis and meta-regression. *Gastric Cancer* 2012;15(3):265–80.

84. Chen S, Nie R-C, OuYang L-Y, et al. Body mass index (BMI) may be a prognostic factor for gastric cancer with peritoneal dissemination. *World J Surg Oncol* 2017;15:52.

85. Park SE, Choi JH, Park JY, et al. Loss of skeletal muscle mass during palliative chemotherapy is a poor prognostic factor in patients with advanced gastric cancer. *Sci Rep* 2020;10(1):17683.

86. Sachlova M, Majek O, Tucek S. Prognostic value of scores based on malnutrition or systemic inflammatory response in patients with metastatic or recurrent gastric cancer. *Nutr Cancer.* 2014;66(8):1362–70.

87. Maconi G, Manes G, Porro GB. Role of symptoms in diagnosis and outcome of gastric cancer. *World J Gastroenterol* 2008;14(8):1149–55.

88. Puhr HC, Pablik E, Berghoff AS, et al. Viennese risk prediction score for Advanced Gastroesophageal carcinoma based on Alarm Symptoms (VAGAS score): Characterisation of alarm symptoms in advanced gastro-oesophageal cancer and its correlation with outcome. *ESMO Open* 2020;5(2):e000623.

89. Takayoshi K, Uchino K, Nakano M, et al. Weight loss during initial chemotherapy predicts survival in patients with advanced gastric cancer. *Nutr Cancer* 2017;69(3):408–15.

90. Ock CY, Oh DY, Lee J, et al. Weight loss at the first month of palliative chemotherapy predicts survival outcomes in patients with advanced gastric cancer. *Gastric Cancer* 2016;19(2):597–606.

91. Namikawa T, Marui A, Yokota K, et al. Frequency and prognostic impact of cachexia during drug treatment for unresectable advanced gastric cancer patients. *Surg Today* 2022;52(11):1560–7.

92. Lu Z, Yang L, Yu J, et al. Change of body weight and macrophage inhibitory cytokine-1 during chemotherapy in advanced gastric cancer: What is their clinical significance? *PLoS One* 2014;9(2):e88553.

93. Lee KW, Bang SM, Kim S, et al. The incidence, risk factors and prognostic implications of venous thromboembolism in patients with gastric cancer. *J Thromb Haemost* 2010;8(3):540–7.

94. Abdel-Razeq H, Mustafa R, Sharaf B, et al. Patterns and predictors of thromboembolic events among patients with gastric cancer. *Sci Rep* 2020;10(1):18516.

95. Majmudar K, Golemi I, Tafur AJ, et al. Outcomes after venous thromboembolism in patients with gastric cancer: Analysis of the RIETE Registry. *Vasc Med* 2020;25(3):210–7.

96. Zhang X, Zhang W, Feng L-J. Prognostic significance of neutrophil lymphocyte ratio in patients with gastric cancer: A meta-analysis. *PLOS ONE* 2014;9(11):e111906.

97. Mohri Y, Tanaka K, Ohi M, et al. Identification of prognostic factors and surgical indications for metastatic gastric cancer. *BMC Cancer* 2014;14:409.

98. Shen H, Wu S, Su R, et al. A nomogram combining neutrophil-to-lymphocyte ratio and D-Dimer predicts chemosensitivity of oxaliplatin-based first-line chemotherapy in patients with unresectable advanced gastric cancer. *Technol Cancer Res Treat* 2022;21:15330338221112741.

99. Gu X, Gao XS, Cui M, et al. Clinicopathological and prognostic significance of platelet to lymphocyte ratio in patients with gastric cancer. *Oncotarget* 2016;7(31):49878–87.

100. Hu J, Yang S, Wang J, et al. Blood alkaline phosphatase predicts prognosis of patients with advanced HER2-negative gastric cancer receiving immunotherapy. *Ann Transl Med* 2021;9(16):1316.

101. Zhao Z, Han F, Yang S, et al. The clinicopathologic importance of serum lactic dehydrogenase in patients with gastric cancer. *Dis Markers* 2014;2014:140913.

102. Wang Q, Yang Y, Zhang Y-P, et al. Prognostic value of carbohydrate tumor markers and inflammation-based markers in metastatic or recurrent gastric cancer. *Med Oncol* 2014;31(12):289.

103. Jo J-C, Ryu M-H, Koo D-H, et al. Serum CA 19–9 as a prognostic factor in patients with metastatic gastric cancer. *Asia Pac J Clin Oncol* 2013;9(4):324–30.

104. Sun Z, Jia J, Du F, et al. Clinical significance of serum tumor markers for advanced gastric cancer with the first-line chemotherapy. *Transl Cancer Res* 2019;8(8):2680–90.

105. Namikawa T, Kawanishi Y, Fujisawa K, et al. Serum carbohydrate antigen 125 is a significant prognostic marker in patients with unresectable advanced or recurrent gastric cancer. *Surg Today* 2018;48(4):388–94.

106. Kroese TE, van Laarhoven HWM, Schoppman SF, et al. Definition, diagnosis and treatment of oligometastatic oesophagogastric cancer: A Delphi consensus study in Europe. *Eur J Cancer* 2023;185:28–39.

107. Wanebo HJ, Kennedy BJ, Chmiel J, et al. Cancer of the stomach. A patient care study by the American College of Surgeons. *Ann Surg* 1993;218(5):583–92.

108. Gill S, Shah A, Le N, et al. Asian ethnicity-related differences in gastric cancer presentation and outcome among patients treated at a Canadian cancer center. *J Clin Oncol* 2003;21(11):2070–6.

109. Chen K, Deng X, Yang Z, et al. Survival nomogram for patients with metastatic siewert type II adenocarcinoma of the esophagogastric junction: A population-based study. *Expert Rev Gastroenterol Hepatol* 2020;14(8):757–64.

110. Custodio A, Carmona-Bayonas A, Jiménez-Fonseca P, et al. Nomogram-based prediction of survival in patients with advanced oesophagogastric adenocarcinoma receiving first-line chemotherapy: A multicenter prospective study in the era of trastuzumab. *Br J Cancer* 2017;116(12):1526–35.

111. Yamanaka T, Matsumoto S, Teramukai S, et al. The baseline ratio of neutrophils to lymphocytes is associated with patient prognosis in advanced gastric cancer. *Oncology* 2007;73:215–20.

112. Apostolidis L, Lang K, Sisic L, et al. Outcome and prognostic factors in patients undergoing salvage therapy for recurrent esophagogastric cancer after multimodal treatment. *J Cancer Res Clin Oncol* 2023;149:1373–82.

113. Polom K, Böger C, Smyth E, et al. Synchronous metastatic gastric cancer-molecular background and clinical implications with special attention to mismatch repair deficiency. *Eur J Surg Oncol* 2018;44(5):626–31.

114. Saiura A, Umekita N, Inoue S, et al. Clinicopathological features and outcome of hepatic resection for liver metastasis from gastric cancer. *Hepatogastroenterology* 2002;49(46):1062–5.

115. Zacherl J, Zacherl M, Scheuba C, et al. Analysis of hepatic resection of metastasis originating from gastric adenocarcinoma. *J Gastrointest Surg* 2002;6(5):682–9.

116. Louvet C, Carrat F, Mal F, et al. Prognostic factor analysis in advanced gastric cancer patients treated with hydroxyurea, leucovorin, 5-fluorouracil, and cisplatin (HLFP regimen). *Cancer Invest* 2003;21(1):14–20.

117. Aurello P, Minervini A, Pace M, et al. The role of surgery in the treatment of metachronous liver metastasis from gastric cancer: A systematic review. *Anticancer Res* 2022;42(1):25–33.

118. Wang Z, Dong Z, Zhao G, et al. Prognostic role of myeloid-derived tumor-associated macrophages at the tumor invasive margin in gastric cancer with liver metastasis (GCLM): A single-center retrospective study. *J Gastrointest Oncol* 2022;13(3):1340–50.

119. Wang X, Espin-Garcia O, Jiang DM, et al. Impact of sites of metastatic dissemination on survival in advanced gastroesophageal adenocarcinoma. *Oncology* 2022;100(8):439–48.

120. Kim HS, Yi SY, Jun HJ, et al. Clinical outcome of gastric cancer patients with bone marrow metastases. *Oncology* 2007;73:192–7.

121. Sirody J, Kaji AH, Hari DM, Chen KT. Patterns of gastric cancer metastasis in the United States. *Am J Surg* 2022;224:445–8.

122. Kienle P, Koch M. Are "micrometastases" of the peritoneum equivalent to distant metastases? *Dig Surg* 2002;19(6):453–8.

123. Ji Z-H, Yu Y, Liu G, et al. Peritoneal cancer index (PCI) based patient selecting strategy for complete cytoreductive surgery plus hyperthermic intraperitoneal chemotherapy in gastric cancer with peritoneal metastasis: A single-center retrospective analysis of 125 patients. *Eur J Surg Oncol* 2021;47:1411–9.

124. Yagi Y, Seshimo A, Kameoka S. Prognostic factors in stage IV gastric cancer: Univariate and multivariate analyses. *Gastric Cancer* 2000;3(2):71–80.

125. Sadeghi B, Arvieux C, Glehen O, et al. Peritoneal carcinomatosis from non-gynecologic malignancies. Results of the EVOCAPE 1 multicentric prospective study. *Cancer* 2000;88(2):358–63.

126. Yoshikawa K, Kitaoka H. Bone metastasis of gastric cancer. *Jpn J Surg* 1983;13(3):173–6.

127. Liang C, Chen H, Yang Z, et al. Risk factors and prognosis of bone metastases in newly diagnosed gastric cancer. *Future Oncol* 2020;16(12):733–48.

128. Qiu MZ, Shi SM, Chen ZH, et al. Frequency and clinicopathological features of metastasis to liver, lung, bone, and brain from gastric cancer: A SEER-based study. *Cancer Med* 2018;7(8):3662–72.

129. Huang L, Zhao Y, Shi Y, et al. Bone metastasis from gastric adenocarcinoma—What are the risk factors and associated survival? A large comprehensive population-based cohort study. *Front Oncol* 2022;12:743873.

130. Xiaobin C, Zhaojun X, Tao L, et al. Analysis of related risk factors and prognostic factors of gastric cancer with bone metastasis: A SEER-based study. *J Immunol Res* 2022;12:3251051.

131. Petrillo A, Giunta EF, Pappalardo A, et al. Bone metastases from gastric cancer: What we know and how to deal with them. *J Clin Med* 2021;10:1777.

132. Turkoz FP, Solak M, Kilickap S, et al. Bone metastasis from gastric cancer: The incidence, clinicopathological features, and influence on survival. *J Gastric Cancer* 2014;14(3):164–72.

133. Kim YJ, Kim SH, Kim JW, et al. Gastric cancer with initial bone metastasis: A distinct group of diseases with poor prognosis. *Eur J Cancer* 2014;50(16):2810–21.

134. Zhang C, Hou W, Huang J, et al. Effects of metastasectomy and other factors on survival of patients with ovarian metastases from gastric cancer: A systematic review and meta-analysis. *J Cell Biochem* 2019;120(9):14486–98.

135. Carneiro F, Fukayama M, Grabsch HI, et al. Gastric adenocarcinoma. In: *WHO Classification of Tumours*, Editorial Board, ed. Digestive System Tumours. 5th ed Lyon, France; International Agency for Research on Cancer, 2019. pp. 85–95.

136. Hu B, El Hajj N, Sittler S, et al. Gastric cancer: Classification, histology and application of molecular pathology. *J Gastrointest Oncol* 2012;3(3):251–61.

137. Park JM, Jang YJ, Kim JH, et al. Gastric cancer histology: Clinicopathologic characteristics and prognostic value. *J Surg Oncol* 2008;98(7):520–5.

138. Taghavi S, Jayarajan SN, Davey A, Willis AI. Prognostic significance of signet ring gastric cancer. *J Clin Oncol* 2012;30(28):3493–8.

139. Zhang C, Liu R, Zhang WH, et al. Difference between signet ring cell gastric cancers and non-signet ring cell gastric cancers: A systematic review and meta-analysis. *Front Oncol* 2021;11:618477.
140. Zhao B, Lv W, Zhang J, et al. Different prognostic significance of signet ring cell histology for early and advanced gastric cancer patients: A systematic review and meta-analysis. *Expert Rev Gastroenterol Hepatol* 2020;14(6):499–509.
141. Tang D, Ni M, Zhu H, et al. Differential prognostic implications of gastric adenocarcinoma based on Lauren's classification: A Surveillance, Epidemiology, and End Results (SEER)-based cohort study. *Ann Transl Med* 2021;9(8):646.
142. Cancer Genome Atlas Research Network. Comprehensive molecular characterization of gastric adenocarcinoma. *Nature* 2014;513(7517):202–9.
143. Lei YY, Huang JY, Zhao QR, et al. The clinicopathological parameters and prognostic significance of HER2 expression in gastric cancer patients: A meta-analysis of literature. *World J Surg Oncol* 2017;15(1):68.
144. Wang HB, Liao XF, Zhang J. Clinicopathological factors associated with HER2-positive gastric cancer: A meta-analysis. *Medicine* 2017;96(44):e8437.
145. Kim M, Seo AN. Molecular pathology of gastric cancer. *J Gastric Cancer* 2022;22(4):273–305.
146. Plum PS, Gebauer F, Krämer M, et al. HER2/neu (ERBB2) expression and gene amplification correlates with better survival in esophageal adenocarcinoma. *BMC Cancer* 2019;19(1):38.
147. Dogan I, Karabulut S, Tastekin D, et al. Evaluation of prognostic factors and trastuzumab-based treatments in HER2/Neu-positive metastatic gastric cancer. *J Coll Physicians Surg Pak* 2022;32(8):1014–9.
148. Shitara K, Van Cutsem E, Bang YJ, et al. Efficacy and safety of pembrolizumab or pembrolizumab plus chemotherapy vs chemotherapy alone for patients with first-line, advanced gastric cancer: The KEYNOTE-062 phase 3 randomized clinical trial. *JAMA Oncol* 2020;6(10):1571–80.
149. Kundel Y, Sternschuss M, Moore A, et al. Efficacy of immune-checkpoint inhibitors in metastatic gastric or gastroesophageal junction adenocarcinoma by patient subgroups: A systematic review and meta-analysis. *Cancer Med* 2020;9:7613–25.
150. Murphy G, Pfeiffer R, Camargo MC, Rabkin CS. Meta-analysis shows that prevalence of Epstein-Barr virus-positive gastric cancer differs based on sex and anatomic location. *Gastroenterol* 2009;137:824–33.
151. Kim ST, Cristescu R, Bass AJ, et al. Comprehensive molecular characterization of clinical responses to PD-1 inhibition in metastatic gastric cancer. *Nat Med* 2018;24(9):1449–58.
152. Yang L-P, Wang Z-X, He M-M, et al. The survival benefit of palliative gastrectomy and/or metastasectomy in gastric cancer patients with synchronous metastasis: A population-based study using propensity score matching and coarsened exact matching. *J Cancer* 2019;10(3):602–10.
153. Warschkow R, Baechtold M, Leung K, et al. Selective survival advantage associated with primary tumor resection for metastatic gastric cancer in a Western population. *Gastric Cancer* 2018;21(2):324–37.
154. Kamarajah SK, Markar SR, Phillips AW, et al. Palliative gastrectomy for metastatic gastric adenocarcinoma: A national population-based cohort study. *Surgery* 2021;170(6):1702–10.
155. Lasithiotakis K, Antoniou SA, Antoniou GA, et al. Gastrectomy for stage IV gastric cancer. a systematic review and meta-analysis. *Anticancer Res* 2014;34(5):2079–85.
156. Fujitani K, Yang HK, Mizusawa J, et al. Gastrectomy plus chemotherapy versus chemotherapy alone for advanced gastric cancer with a single non-curable factor (REGATTA): A phase 3, randomised controlled trial. *Lancet Oncol* 2016;17(3):309–18.
157. Chiu CF, Yang HR, Yang MD, et al. Palliative gastrectomy prolongs survival of metastatic gastric cancer patients with normal preoperative CEA or CA19-9 values: A retrospective cohort study. *Gastroenterol Res Pract* 2016;2016:6846027.
158. Collins A, Hatzaras I, Schmidt C, et al. Gastrectomy in advanced gastric cancer effectively palliates symptoms and may improve survival in select patients. *J Gastrointest Surg* 2014;18(3):491–6.
159. Shin HB, Lee SH, Son YG, et al. Chemoresponse after non-curative gastrectomy for M1 gastric cancer. *World J Surg Oncol* 2015;13:13.
160. Fornaro L, Fanotto V, Musettini G, et al. Selecting patients for gastrectomy in metastaticesophago- gastric cancer: Clinics and pathology are not enough. *Future Oncol* 2017;13(25):2265–75.
161. Li Z, Zheng H, Zhao Z, et al. Identification of optimal primary tumor resection candidates for metastatic gastric cancer: Nomograms based on propensity score matching. *Cancer Med* 2023;12(12):13063–75.
162. Sun J, Nan Q. Survival benefit of surgical resection for stage IV gastric cancer: A SEER-based propensity score-matched analysis. *Front Surg* 2022;9:927030.
163. Tapia Rico G, Townsend AR, Klevansky M, Price TJ. Liver metastases resection for gastric and esophageal tumors: Is there enough evidence to go down this path? *Expert Rev Anticancer Ther* 2016;16(12):1219–25.

164. Granieri S, Altomare M, Bruno F, et al. Surgical treatment of gastric cancer liver metastases: Systematic review and meta-analysis of long-term outcomes and prognostic factors. *Crit Rev Oncol Hematol* 2021;163:103313.

165. Montagnani F, Crivelli F, Aprile G, et al. Long-term survival after liver metastasectomy in gastric cancer: Systematic review and meta-analysis of prognostic factors. *Cancer Treat Rev* 2018;69:11–20.

166. Minciuna C-E, Tudor S, Micu A, et al. Safety and efficacy of simultaneous resection of gastric carcinoma and synchronous liver metastasis—A western center experience. *Medicina* 2022;58:1802.

167. Schmidt T, Alldinger I, Blank S, et al. Surgery in oesophago-gastric cancer with metastatic disease: Treatment, prognosis and preoperative patient selection. *Eur J Surg Oncol* 2015;41(10):1340–7.

168. Wagner AD, Syn NL, Moehler M, et al. Chemotherapy for advanced gastric cancer. *Cochrane Database Syst Rev* 2017;8(8):CD004064.

169. Okines AFC, Norman AR, McCloud P, et al. Meta-analysis of the REAL-2 and ML17032 trials: Evaluating capecitabine-based combination chemotherapy and infused 5-fluorouracil-based combination chemotherapy for the treatment of advanced oesophago-gastric cancer. *Ann Oncol* 2009;20(9):1529–34.

170. Lim S, Muhs BE, Marcus SG, et al. Results following resection for stage IV gastric cancer; are better outcomes observed in selected patient subgroups? *J Surg Oncol* 2007;95(2):118–22.

171. Brar SS, Mahar AL, Helyer LK, et al. Processes of care in the multidisciplinary treatment of gastric cancer: Results of a RAND/UCLA expert panel. *JAMA Surg* 2014;149(1):18–25.

172. Al-Batran SE, Homann N, Pauligk C, et al. Effect of neoadjuvant chemotherapy followed by surgical resection on survival in patients with limited metastatic gastric or gastroesophageal junction cancer: The AIO-FLOT3 Trial. *JAMA Oncol* 2017;3(9):1237–44.

173. Kataoka K, Kinoshita T, Moehler M, et al. Current management of liver metastases from gastric cancer: What is common practice? New challenge of EORTC and JCOG. *Gastric Cancer* 2017;20:904–12.

174. Bonnot PE, Piessen G, Kepenekian V, et al. Cytoreductive surgery with or without hyperthermic intraperitoneal chemotherapy for gastric cancer with peritoneal metastases (CYTO-CHIP study): A propensity score analysis. *J Clin Oncol* 2019;37(23):2028–40.

175. Rau B, Lang H, Konigsrainer A, et al. The effect of hyperthermic intraperitoneal chemotherapy (HIPEC) upon cytoreductive surgery (CRS) in gastric cancer (GC) with synchronous peritoneal metastasis (PM): A randomized multicentre phase III trial (GASTRIPEC-I-trial). *Ann Oncol* 2021;32(S5):S1040.

176. Mansoor W, Roeland EJ, Chaudhry A, et al. Early weight loss as a prognostic factor in patients with advanced gastric cancer: Analyses from REGARD, RAINBOW, and RAINFALL phase III studies. *Oncologist* 2021;26(9):e1538–47.

177. Lu Z, Fang Y, Liu C, et al. Early interdisciplinary supportive care in patients with previously untreated metastatic esophagogastric cancer: A phase III randomized controlled trial. *J Clin Oncol* 2021;39(7):748–56.

178. Murad AM, Santiago FF, Petroianu A, et al. Modified therapy with 5-fluorouracil, doxorubicin, and methotrexate in advanced gastric cancer. *Cancer* 1993;72:37–41.

179. Pyrhonen S, Kuitunen T, Nyandoto P, Kouri M. Randomised comparison of fluorouracil, epidoxorubicin and methotrexate (FEMTX) plus supportive care with supportive care alone in patients with non-resectable gastric cancer. *Br J Cancer* 1995;71:587–91.

180. Koizumi W, Narahara H, Hara T, et al. S-1 plus cisplatin versus S-1 alone for first-line treatment of advanced gastric cancer (SPIRITS trial): A phase III trial. *Lancet Oncol* 2008;9(3):215–21.

181. Koizumi W, Kim YH, Fujii M, et al. Addition of docetaxel to S-1 without platinum prolongs survival of patients with advanced gastric cancer: A randomized study (START). *J Cancer Res Clin Oncol* 2014;140(2):319–28.

182. Al-Batran SE, Hartmann JT, Probst S, et al. Phase III trial in metastatic gastroesophageal adenocarcinoma with fluorouracil, leucovorin plus either oxaliplatin or cisplatin: A study of the Arbeitsgemeinschaft Internistische Onkologie. *J Clin Oncol* 2008;26(9):1435–42.

183. Hall PS, Swinson D, Cairns DA, et al. Efficacy of reduced-intensity chemotherapy with oxaliplatin and capecitabine on quality of life and cancer control among older and frail patients with advanced gastroesophageal cancer: The GO2 phase 3 randomized clinical trial. *JAMA Oncol* 2021;7(6):869–77.

184. Ochenduszko S, Puskulluoglu M, Konopka K, et al. Comparison of efficacy and safety of first-line palliative chemotherapy with EOX and mDCF regimens in patients with locally advanced inoperable or metastatic HER2-negative gastric or gastroesophageal junction adenocarcinoma: A randomized phase 3 trial. *Med Oncol* 2015;32:242.

185. Wang J, Xu R, Li J, et al. Randomized multicenter phase III study of a modified docetaxel and cisplatin plus fluorouracil regimen compared with cisplatin and fluorouracil as first-line therapy for advanced or locally recurrent gastric cancer. *Gastric Cancer* 2016;19:234–44.

186. Shitara K, Van Cutsem E, Bang YJ, et al. Efficacy and safety of pembrolizumab or pembrolizumab plus chemotherapy vs chemotherapy alone for patients with first-line, advanced gastric cancer: The KEYNOTE-062 phase 3 randomized clinical trial. *JAMA Oncol* 2020;6(10):1571–80.

187. Janjigian YY, Shitara K, Moehler M, et al. First-line nivolumab plus chemotherapy versus chemotherapy alone for advanced gastric, gastro-oesophageal junction, and oesophageal adenocarcinoma (CheckMate 649): A randomised, open-label, phase 3 trial. *Lancet* 2021;398(10294):27–40.

188. Bang YJ, Van Cutsem E, Feyereislova A, et al. Trastuzumab in combination with chemotherapy versus chemotherapy alone for treatment of HER2-positive advanced gastric or gastro-oesophageal junction cancer (ToGA): A phase 3, open-label, randomised controlled trial. *Lancet* 2010;376(9742):687–97.

189. Janjigian YY, Kawazoe A, Yañez P, et al. The KEYNOTE-811 trial of dual PD-1 and HER2 blockade in HER2-positive gastric cancer. *Nature* 2021;600(7890):727–30.

190. Thuss-Patience PC, Kretzschmar A, Bichev D, et al. Survival advantage for irinotecan versus best supportive care as second-line chemotherapy in gastric cancer--A randomised phase III study of the Arbeitsgemeinschaft Internistische Onkologie (AIO). *Eur J Cancer* 2011;47(15):2306–14.

191. Kang JH, Lee SI, Lim DH, et al. Salvage chemotherapy for pretreated gastric cancer: A randomized phase III trial comparing chemotherapy plus best supportive care with best supportive care alone. *J Clin Oncol* 2012;30:1513–8.

192. Ford HE, Marshall A, Bridgewater JA, et al. Docetaxel versus active symptom control for refractory oesophagogastric adenocarcinoma (COUGAR-02): An open-label, phase 3 randomised controlled trial. *Lancet Oncol* 2014;15(1):78–86.

193. Fuchs CS, Tomasek J, Yong CJ, et al. Ramucirumab monotherapy for previously treated advanced gastric or gastro-oesophageal junction adenocarcinoma (REGARD): An international, randomised, multicentre, placebo-controlled, phase 3 trial. *Lancet* 2014;383(9911):31–9.

194. Shitara K, Özgüroğlu M, Bang YJ, et al. Pembrolizumab versus paclitaxel for previously treated, advanced gastric or gastro-oesophageal junction cancer (KEYNOTE-061): A randomised, open-label, controlled, phase 3 trial. *Lancet* 2018;392(10142):123–33.

195. Satoh T, Xu RH, Chung HC, et al. Lapatinib plus paclitaxel versus paclitaxel alone in the second-line treatment of HER2-amplified advanced gastric cancer in Asian populations: TyTAN–A randomized, phase III study. *J Clin Oncol* 2014;32(19):2039–49.

196. Thuss-Patience PC, Shah MA, Ohtsu A, et al. Trastuzumab emtansine versus taxane use for previously treated HER2-positive locally advanced or metastatic gastric or gastro-oesophageal junction adenocarcinoma (GATSBY): An international randomised, open-label, adaptive, phase 2/3 study. *Lancet Oncol* 2017;18(5):640–53.

197. Shitara K, Bang YJ, Iwasa S, et al. Trastuzumab Deruxtecan in previously treated HER2-positive gastric cancer. *N Engl J Med* 2020;382(25):2419–30.

198. Chao J, Fuchs CS, Shitara K, et al. Assessment of pembrolizumab therapy for the treatment of microsatellite instability-high gastric or gastroesophageal junction cancer among patients in the KEYNOTE-059, KEYNOTE-061, and KEYNOTE-062 clinical trials. *JAMA Oncol* 2021;7(6):895–902.

199. Marabelle A, Le DT, Ascierto PA, et al. Efficacy of pembrolizumab in patients with noncolorectal high microsatellite instability/mismatch repair-deficient cancer: Results from the phase II KEYNOTE-158 study. *J Clin Oncol* 2020;38(1):1–10.

200. Li J, Qin S, Xu J, et al. Randomized, double-blind, placebo-controlled phase III trial of apatinib in patients with chemotherapy-refractory advanced or metastatic adenocarcinoma of the stomach or gastroesophageal junction. *J Clin Oncol* 2016;34(13):1448–54.

201. Kang YK, Boku N, Satoh T, et al. Nivolumab in patients with advanced gastric or gastro-oesophageal junction cancer refractory to, or intolerant of, at least two previous chemotherapy regimens (ONO-4538-12, ATTRACTION-2): A randomised, double-blind, placebo-controlled, phase 3 trial. *Lancet* 2017;390(10111):2461–71.

202. Shitara K, Doi T, Dvorkin M, et al. Trifluridine/tipiracil versus placebo in patients with heavily pretreated metastatic gastric cancer (TAGS): A randomised, double-blind, placebo-controlled, phase 3 trial. *Lancet Oncol* 2018;19(11):1437–48.

3 Small bowel adenocarcinoma

3.1 INTRODUCTION

3.1.1 EPIDEMIOLOGY

Small bowel adenocarcinomas (SBAs) are 40% of small bowel [1] and 2–4% of gastrointestinal (GI) tumors [2, 3]. From a previous combined analysis of the National Cancer Database (NCDB) and Surveillance, Epidemiology, and End Results (SEER) databases, 37.6% of the small bowel tumors were endocrine neoplasms and 36.9% SBAs [1].

The incidence ranges between 0.12–1.45/100,000 and is higher in Western countries. An analysis by the RARECARE working group documented 3,595 SBAs in 162 million subjects in 21 European countries (1995–2002), with geographic variation [4].

In the US the incidence increased slower than neuroendocrine tumors [1, 5, 6], similar to the Danish Cancer Registry, which specifically showed an increase in duodenal adenocarcinomas [7].

A Chinese series reported a male:female ratio 1.58:1, with male sex prevalence for some locations, such as duodenum, jejunum and duodenal ampulla [8]. SBA remains more frequent in Blacks and slightly more common in males [9], is rare before age 40, and predominates in >60 [10].

3.1.2 STAGING OF METASTATIC DISEASE

SBA is often asymptomatic. Signs of intestinal obstruction or perforation may be found, while jaundice, positive fecal occult blood test, or acute GI bleeding are rare.

Laboratory may detect chronic anemia, elevated serum transaminases, bilirubin, and CEA.

Enteroclysis of the small intestine with double contrast barium enema reported a sensitivity of 95%, but CT is easier to carry out and allows a more precise definition of primary tumor and metastases, sometimes identifying SBAs that are inaccessible to endoscopy [11], than CT is the reference investigation. Sensitivity varies according to tumor location, decreasing from 93% to 60% progressing from duodenum to the ileum [12], but remains higher than endoscopic techniques [13].

Enteroscopy can identify duodenal and proximal jejunal SBAs with sensitivity respectively of 89–92% and 24–30%, allowing diagnostic biopsy [12], but the procedures are rather difficult and require deep sedation. On the other hand, colonoscopy with retrograde ileoscopy may be useful in identifying ileal tumors.

Endoscopic videocapsule is an alternative method to explore the small bowel, with a sensitivity of 50–67% [14], but can be performed only in patients without sub-occlusive symptoms [10].

SBA is staged according to the American Joint Committee on Cancer TNM Classification (AJCC 8th edition 2017) [15].

3.1.3 PROGNOSIS OF METASTATIC DISEASE

A Japanese retrospective study reported metastases at diagnosis in 21% of duodenal tumors and 41% of jejunal-ileal [16]. However, single-institution series describing outcomes of patients with

DOI: 10.1201/9781032703350-3

TABLE S1

Prognostic factors analyzed in selected clinical trials of patients with unresectable or metastatic small bowel adenocarcinoma receiving upfront treatment

Variable	No. comparisons	Prognostic relationship	No prognostic relationship
Patient-related			
Performance status	7	4	3
Demographic			
Age	6	1	5
Sex	5	0	5
Anthropometric			
Ethnia	1	0	1
Clinic			
Crohn's disease	1	0	1
Familial adenomatous polyposis	1	0	1
Lynch syndrome	1	0	1
Lab			
Carcinoembrionic antigen	4	2	2
Carbohydrate antigen 19-9	3	1	2
Tumor-related			
Tumor burden			
Disease status	3	0	3
No. sites metastases	3	1	2
Primary tumor location	8	1	7
Timing of metastasis			
Synchronous vs. metachronous	2	0	2
Site of metastasis			
Liver metastases	3	0	3
Nodal metastases	3	0	3
Lung metastases	2	0	2
Peritoneal metastases	4	1	3
Pathology			
Histotype (mucinous)	1	0	1
Grading	5	1	4
Previous treatments			
Primary tumor resection	4	2	2
Previous adjuvant chemotherapy	4	1	3

unresectable or metastatic small intestine adenocarcinoma (mSBA) are rare. In 2020 in Europe, 5-year survival rates of 40–45% were reported for SBAs at any stage [17].

Over the past three decades early detection did not improve prognosis [18], and the effect of adjuvant chemotherapy remains to be established [1].

3.2 ANALYSIS OF PROGNOSTIC VARIABLES IN EARLY METASTATIC DISEASE

A systematic review of studies including mSBA patients receiving upfront therapies resulted in the selection of 21 studies, published from 1984 to 2022, ten phase II trials and eleven retrospective studies. In nine studies an analysis of prognostic factors (PFs) was done and the results were reported [19–27]. Six of them were retrospective. With the limitations related to the analysis of the PFs and the retrospective data, this review evaluated all PFs that have been reported (Table S1).

3.3 PATIENT-RELATED PROGNOSTIC FACTORS

3.3.1 PERFORMANCE STATUS

The analysis of an Asian database identified 91 mSBA patients and reported a significantly shorter median overall survival (OS) for Eastern Cooperative Oncology Group Performance Status (ECOG PS) 2–3 vs. ECOG PS 0–1 patients, a difference that disappeared after multivariate analysis [28].

Similarly, three retrospective studies showed longer OS for patients with good PS [16, 29, 30], even though only by univariate analysis in one of them [30].

3.3.1.1 Selected studies

Seven studies evaluated PS, and four documented a significant relationship between poor PS and reduced OS. Their results are reported in Table 3.1.

3.3.2 DEMOGRAPHIC

3.3.2.1 Age

SEER database analyses suggested a negative prognostic effect from advanced age. Despite the large sample size of the studies, a low number of mSBA patients was included [31–34]. Similar unfavorable results for advanced age were suggested from two NCDB analyses [35, 36].

Also, three retrospective studies concluded for a poor outcome of elderly SBA patients [8, 16, 37].

3.3.2.2 Sex

The results of two SEER database analyses suggested longer survival for female sex [31, 34].

3.3.2.3 Other demographic variables

A SEER analysis documented that SBAs were more frequent in Blacks vs. Caucasians with a trend to lower 5-year survival rates [38]. In contrast, NCDB suggested a better prognosis for African-Americans vs. Whites [36].

Unmarried SBA patients had worse OS in three analyses of the SEER database [31–33].

3.3.2.4 Selected studies

Six studies evaluated age, four around a cut-off of 65 and one at 50. Only one study reported a negative prognostic role for age >65 years [23] (Table 3.2).

TABLE 3.1

Prognostic relationships of performance status in selected studies of patients with unresectable or metastatic small bowel adenocarcinoma receiving upfront treatment

Study [ref]	Phase	No. pts	Scale	Comparison	Prognostic relationship	Effect size
SKCCC 2005 [19]	II	39	ECOG	PS 2 vs. 1 vs. 0	Yes	NR
BCCA 2007 [20]	R	37	NR	NR	No	NR
AGEO 2010 [22]	R	93	WHO	PS ≥2 vs. PS 0–1	Yes	HR 11.00 (4.22–28.72)
SYUCC 2011 [23]	R	34	ECOG	PS 2 vs. PS 0–1	No	NR
FAHNU 2012 [24]	II	33	ECOG	PS 2 vs. PS 0–1	Yes	HR 6.36 (2.07–19.61)
Japanese 2012 [25]	R	132	ECOG	PS 2 vs. 1 vs. 0	Yes	HR 1.62 (1.11–2.36)
Japanese 2017 [27]	II	24	ECOG	PS 1 vs. PS 0	No	HR 2.60 (0.73–9.28)

Legend: ECOG, Eastern Cooperative Oncology Group. HR, hazard ratio. NR, not reported. PS, performance status. R, retrospective study. WHO, World Health Organization.

TABLE 3.2

Prognostic relationships of age in selected studies of patients with unresectable or metastatic small bowel adenocarcinoma receiving upfront treatment

Study [ref]	Phase	No. pts	Comparison	Prognostic relationship	Effect size
SKCCC 2005 [19]	II	39	<65 vs. ≥65	No	NR
MDACC 2008 [21]	R	80	<50 vs. ≥50	No	NR
AGEO 2010 [22]	R	93	<65 vs. ≥65	No	HR 1.73 (0.98–3.07)
SYUCC 2011 [23]	R	34	<65 vs. ≥65	Yes	NR
Japanese 2012 [25]	R	132	<65 vs. ≥65	No	NR
Japanese 2016 [26]	R	25	<60 vs. ≥60	No	NR

Legend: HR, hazard ratio. NR, not reported. R, retrospective study.

TABLE 3.3

Prognostic relationships of sex in selected studies of patients with unresectable or metastatic small bowel adenocarcinoma receiving upfront treatment

Study [ref]	Phase	No. pts	Comparison	Prognostic relationship	Effect size
SKCCC 2005 [19]	II	39	M vs. F	No	NR
AGEO 2010 [22]	R	93	M vs. F	No	HR 1.17 (0.70–1.96)
SYUCC 2011 [23]	R	34	M vs. F	No	NR
Japanese 2012 [25]	R	132	M vs. F	No	NR
Japanese 2016 [26]	R	25	M vs. F	No	NR

Legend: F, females. HR, hazard ratio. M, males. NR, not reported. R, retrospective study.

Five studies evaluated sex as a PF, without reporting significant relationships, as shown by Table 3.3.

3.3.3 ANTHROPOMETRIC

A retrospective analysis of 28 advanced SBA patients concluded that those with a body mass index (BMI) ≥25 kg/m^2 had longer OS after chemotherapy [39].

3.3.4 CLINIC

Symptoms at diagnosis were associated with poor prognosis, as a retrospective Japanese study demonstrated, reporting symptoms in 62% of patients, prevalently stenosis- and bleeding-related [16].

3.3.4.1 Predisposing conditions

About 12–20% of SBA were diagnosed as a possible consequence of a predisposing condition, such as familial adenomatous polyposis (FAP), Lynch syndrome (HNPCC), Peutz-Jeghers syndrome, Crohn's disease, coeliac disease (CD), cystic fibrosis, peptic ulcer, and ulcerative colitis [40, 41].

A nationwide ARCAD-NADEGE prospective cohort confirmed the consistent prevalence of the predisposing diseases. Notably, Crohn's disease was associated with younger age, poorly differentiated SBAs, and ileal origin. SBAs arising in patients with HNPCC were poorly differentiated and with early onset, but predominantly with duodenal location and early stage [42]. In contrast, another study identified an independent favorable outcome for a diagnosis of CD [43].

Many SBA patients develop additional malignancies, especially of the stomach and colon, and this percentage according to some authors is around 16% [41, 44].

3.3.4.2 Selected studies
One study investigated the relationship between some predisposing conditions to mSBA and OS, without finding any effect of Crohn's disease, FAP, or HNPCC [22].

3.3.5 LABORATORY

3.3.5.1 Hematology
Hemoglobin, neutrophil-to-lymphocyte ratio and platelet count were not associated with the outcome among the 54 mSBA patients of a Japanese study [16].

3.3.5.2 Chemistry
The negative prognostic role of low serum albumin and high lactic dehydrogenase levels was not confirmed in mSBA patients [16].

3.3.5.3 Tumor markers
Carcinoembryonic antigen (CEA) levels >5 ng/mL were associated with poor prognosis [16].

3.3.5.4 Selected studies
Data of laboratory variables are resumed in Table 3.4. The four studies that evaluated the relationship between baseline CEA and OS defined different cut-offs (5 and 10 ng/mL). Two studies reported a significant relationship between elevated CEA and poor outcomes [22, 25], while another showed a non-significant trend [23].

Three of the same studies analyzed carbohydrate antigen 19-9 (CA 19-9) at the cut-off of 37 U/L, and one documented a relationship with OS [22].

TABLE 3.4

Prognostic relationships of tumor markers in selected studies of patients with unresectable or metastatic small bowel adenocarcinoma receiving upfront treatment

Study [ref]	Phase	No. pts	Comparison	Prognostic relationship	Effect size
Carcinoembryonic antigen (ng/mL)					
AGEO 2010 [22]	R	93	≤ vs. > 5	Yes	HR 2.85 (1.19–6.81)
SYUCC 2011 [23]	R	34	≤ vs. > 10	No	NR
Japanese 2012 [25]	R	132	< vs. ≥ 5	Yes	HR 2.21 (1.06–4.78)
Japanese 2017 [27]	II	24	< vs. ≥ 5	No	HR 1.61 (0.43–6.00)
Carbohydrate antigen 19-9 (IU/mL)					
AGEO 2010 [22]	R	93	≤ vs. > 37	Yes	HR 2.26 (1.06–4.78)
SYUCC 2011 [23]	R	34	≤ vs. > 37	No	NR
Japanese 2012 [25]	R	132	< vs. ≥ 37	No	NR

Legend: HR, hazard ratio. NR, not reported. R, retrospective study.

3.4 TUMOR-RELATED PROGNOSTIC FACTORS

3.4.1 TUMOR BURDEN

3.4.1.1 Disease status

An NCDB analysis of 4,995 SBA patients documented a progressive reduction of median OS in patients with local vs. regional vs. distant disease (50.1 vs. 22.2 vs. 8.6 months) [35]. An unfavorable prognostic effect for the advanced stage has been confirmed by the SEER database [34] and retrospective studies [29, 37, 45]. In another analysis of a surgical series local tumor extent, presence of distant metastases, and residual disease after surgery were associated with poor OS [46].

3.4.1.2 Number of metastatic sites

Multiple sites of metastasis correlated with reduced OS in a population-based study [34], but not in a single-centre retrospective analysis [43]. Patients undergoing metastasectomy with curative intent had more often single-site metastases (91% vs. 9%) [43].

3.4.1.3 Selected studies

Three studies compared mSBA patients with those with localized tumors. Locally advanced disease was uncommon and accounted for 8.8–14% in two studies [22, 23], while the third study retrospectively compared patients with localized vs. metastatic tumors [20]. The three studies did not observe any significant difference in OS according to disease status.

An evaluation of the number of metastatic sites was performed in three studies, but only the comparison of single vs. multiple sites displayed a significant survival difference (14.7 vs. 4.1 months; p-value = 0.001) [23] (Table 3.5).

3.4.2 PRIMARY TUMOR LOCATION

SBA originates in duodenum (45–95%), followed by jejunum (3.4–45.5%) and ileum (1.6–26%) [10]. Two of three SEER database analyses documented that jejunal tumors had a better prognosis than duodenal [33, 47], even though the trend was not significant in the third study [34]. A NCDB study evaluating 7,954 SBA patients, of which 57.9% were duodenal, 15.6% jejunal and 10.8% ileal,

---

TABLE 3.5

Prognostic relationships of tumor burden-related variables in selected studies of patients with unresectable or metastatic small bowel adenocarcinoma receiving upfront treatment

Study [ref]	Phase	No. pts	Comparison	Prognostic relationship	Effect size
Disease status					
BCCA 2007 [20]	R	37	Metastatic vs. Loc	No	NR
AGEO 2010 [22]	R	93	Metastatic vs. LA	No	HR 0.56 (0.24–1.30)
SYUCC 2011 [23]	R	34	Metastatic vs. LA	No	OS 14.7 vs. 29.4 m
Number of metastatic sites					
AGEO 2010 [22]	R	93	2 vs. 1	No	HR 1.24 (0.72–2.15)
			>2 vs. 1	No	HR 1.58 (0.74–3.36)
SYUCC 2011 [23]	R	34	>1 vs. 1	Yes	NR
Japanese 2012 [25]	R	132	continuous	No	NR

Legend: HR, hazard ratio. LA, locally advanced. Loc, localized. m, months. NR, not reported. OS, overall survival. R, retrospective study.

---

concluded for a trend to poor outcome of duodenal tumors [36], while the difference was significant in a previous NCDB analysis [35]. The reduced OS of patients with a duodenal primary tumor was significant when compared with jejunal but not ileal cancers [36], and was reported by various studies [28, 45, 48, 49]. Recent case series confirmed the poor prognosis of duodenal tumors [50, 51], both in localized and metastatic disease, which specifically reported median OS of duodenal vs. jejunal vs. ileal mSBAs of 4.2 vs. 11.4 vs. 6.9 months [50]. On the other hand, many other studies did not report any prognostic role for SBA primary tumor location [12, 18, 37, 46, 52].

The possible poor prognosis of duodenal SBAs was attributed to the different natural history, with the diagnosis at a more advanced stage, and to the low rates of patients receiving surgery and adjuvant chemotherapy [12]. This hypothesis is supported by a retrospective Japanese series, that showed that the diagnosis of asymptomatic disease occurred in 43% of duodenal and 16% of jejunal-ileal SBAs [16].

3.4.2.1 Selected studies

Eight studies analyzed SBA locations. Two studies compared three locations [18, 20], while five compared duodenal vs. distal tumors [21–24, 26], and another jejunal vs. non-jejunal [25], but only one study documented a prognostic effect with a poor outcome for duodenal tumors [24] (Table 3.6).

3.4.3 TIMING OF METASTASIS

The MD Anderson Tumor Registry did not show any survival difference according to the timing of metastasis [43], while the other two retrospective series suggested a poor OS for synchronous metastases [29, 30].

3.4.3.1 Selected studies

One study examined the timing of metastasis, and it did not report any effect on OS [20]. Another study investigated the timing from diagnosis to cytoreductive surgery of the peritoneum, not reporting prognostic relationships [26].

3.4.4 SITE OF METASTASIS

The liver is the more frequent site of metastasis, but few data are available on prognosis by site of metastasis. A SEER analysis concluded that the metastasis pattern was independent PF, and was the single variable with the most significant effect on OS. In particular, the occurrence of liver metastases

---

TABLE 3.6
Prognostic relationships of primary tumor location in selected studies of patients with unresectable or metastatic small bowel adenocarcinoma receiving upfront treatment

Study [ref]	Phase	No. pts	Comparison	Prognostic relationship	Effect size
SKCCC 2005 [19]	II	39	Duod vs. jej vs. distal	No	NR
MDACC 2008 [21]	R	80	Duod vs. jej vs. ileum	No	NR
AGEO 2010 [22]	R	93	Duod vs. jej+ileum	No	HR 1.48 (0.88–2.50)
SYUCC 2011 [23]	R	34	Duod vs. jej+ileum	No	NR
FAHNU 2012 [24]	II	33	Duod vs. jej+ileum	No	NR
Japanese 2012 [25]	R	132	Duod vs. jej+ileum	Yes	HR 2.50 (1.67–3.89)
Japanese 2016 [26]	R	25	Jej vs. non-jej	No	NR
Japanese 2017 [27]	II	24	Duod vs. jej	No	HR 2.85 (0.85–9.52)

Legend: Duod, duodenum. HR, hazard ratio. Jej, jejunum. NR, not reported. R, retrospective study.

(LMs) was associated with reduced OS, as was the presence of metastasis in other sites such as bone, brain or lung [34]. Multivariate analysis of a mSBA series showed that LMs and intra-abdominal lymph node metastases were associated with poor survival [28], while another retrospective analysis of patients undergoing metastasectomy did not show any prognostic effect of the site of metastasis [43].

3.4.4.1   Selected studies

One of four studies evaluating peritoneal metastases reported a significantly longer OS of patients with a peritoneal cancer index (PCI) <15 [26]. Three studies investigated LMs, three distant lymph node metastases, and two evaluated lung metastasis, without finding significant results, as summarized in Table 3.7.

3.4.5   PATHOLOGY

3.4.5.1   Histology

Five SBA histologies have been described, such as glandular, diffuse poorly cohesive or signet ring, mixed, medullary-type, and non-medullary solid [53]. A SEER database evaluation of two histologic forms, the signet ring cell small bowel adenocarcinoma (SRCSBA) and the mucinous small bowel adenocarcinoma, suggested a poor prognosis only for SRCSBAs [47]. SRCSBAs were more often associated with poor differentiation, local invasion, and lymphonodal metastasis [47], and tended to be more frequent in association with inflammatory bowel diseases [54].

3.4.5.2   Tumor grade

The WHO classification distinguishes four histological grades. Population-based studies from SEER [31, 34] or NCDB databases [36] support the prognostic role of grade, with G III/IV vs. G I/II being among the unfavorable PFs.

TABLE 3.7

Prognostic relationships of site of metastasis in selected studies of patients with unresectable or metastatic small bowel adenocarcinoma receiving upfront treatment

Study [ref]	Phase	No. pts	Comparison	Prognostic relationship	Effect size
Liver					
MDACC 2008 [21]	R	80	Yes vs. not	No	NR
AGEO 2010 [22]	R	93	Yes vs. not	No	HR 2.70 (0.98–7.69)
SYUCC 2011 [23]	R	34	Yes vs. not	No	NR
Peritoneum					
MDACC 2008 [21]	R	80	Yes vs. not	No	NR
AGEO 2010 [22]	R	93	Yes vs. not	No	HR 1.30 (0.78–2.17)
SYUCC 2011 [23]	R	34	Yes vs. not	No	NR
Japanese 2016 [26]	R	25	Yes vs. not	Yes	NR
Lung					
AGEO 2010 [22]	R	93	Yes vs. not	No	HR 0.79 (0.34–1.85)
SYUCC 2011 [23]	R	34	Yes vs. not	No	NR
Distant lymph nodes					
AGEO 2010 [22]	R	93	Yes vs. not	No	HR 0.78 (0.43–1.43)
SYUCC 2011 [23]	R	34	Yes vs. not	No	NR
Japanese 2016 [26]	R	25	Yes vs. not	No	NR

Legend: HR, hazard ratio. NR, not reported. R, retrospective study.

The other two retrospective studies concluded that poorly differentiated forms had shorter OS [29, 51]. Another tumor registry did not indicate different outcomes by grade, but patients undergoing metastasectomy were more frequently affected by G I/II tumors [43].

3.4.5.3 Molecular biology

The surface area of the small intestine is much larger than that of the large intestine, yet the rate of cancer is approximately 50–100-fold less [55–57]. Although genomic profiles suggest that SBAs are a molecularly unique intestinal entity [58], duodenal adenocarcinomas demonstrated genomic aberrations more typical of upper GI tumors (CDKN2A/B, ERBB2) [58]. From a molecular comparison with colorectal cancer, SBAs had fewer alterations in APC and more in CDKN2A, with similar BRAF mutation rates. When compared with gastric cancer, SBAs had more KRAS, APC and SMAD4 alterations. Another study suggested that MSI-H was associated with localized disease and local recurrences [59].

3.4.5.4 Selected studies

An article reported poor outcomes for patients with GIII vs. GI/GII [26]. However, other four studies investigating tumor grade [21, 23–25] and one investigating mucinous histotype [21] did not demonstrate any relationships with OS (Table 3.8).

3.4.6 Previous treatments

3.4.6.1 Primary tumor resection

At least five SEER database analyses found that previous primary tumor resection (PTR) correlated with better outcomes [31–34, 47], and similar reports came from NCDB [35, 36], which in addition documented that duodenal vs. jejunal tumors more rarely received surgery (50.2% vs. 90.8%) [36]. Retrospective evidence confirmed the poor prognosis of patients without PTR [28, 45].

3.4.6.2 Extensive surgery

Retrospective data documented that patients who underwent metastasectomy were 17.1% and had better prognosis, regardless of the site of metastasis, but more often had a single site of metastases [43].

3.4.6.3 Previous adjuvant chemotherapy

Duodenal vs. jejunal SBAs more rarely received adjuvant chemotherapy, but whenever the patients received adjuvant chemotherapy, OS improved [36]. Some retrospective studies have not documented

---

TABLE 3.8
Prognostic relationships of tumor grade in selected studies of patients with unresectable or metastatic small bowel adenocarcinoma receiving upfront treatment

Study [ref]	Phase	No. pts	Comparison	Prognostic relationship	Effect size
MDACC 2008 [21]	R	80	G III/IV vs. G I/II	No	NR
SYUCC 2011 [23]	R	34	G III/IV vs. G I/II	No	NR
FAHNU 2012 [24]	II	33	G III/IV vs. G I/II	No	HR 0.46 (0.20–1.06)
Japanese 2012 [25]	R	132	Undiffer. vs. differ.	No	NR
Japanese 2016 [26]	R	25	G III vs. GI/II	Yes	NR

Legend: Differ, differentiated. G, grade. HR, hazard ratio. NR, not reported. R, retrospective study. Undiffer, undifferentiated.

TABLE 3.9

Prognostic relationships of previous treatments in selected studies of patients with unresectable or metastatic small bowel adenocarcinoma receiving upfront treatment

Study [ref]	Phase	No. pts	Comparison	Prognostic relationship	Effect size
Primary tumor resection					
MDACC 2008 [21]	R	80	Yes vs. not	Yes	HR 0.53 (0.31–0.90)
SYUCC 2011 [23]	R	34	Yes vs. not	No	NR
Japanese 2012 [25]	R	132	Yes vs. not	No	NR
Japanese 2017 [27]	II	24	Yes vs. not	Yes	HR 0.25 (0.08–0.83)
Adjuvant chemotherapy					
MDACC 2008 [21]	R	80	Yes vs. not	Yes	HR 2.35 (1.01–5.47)
AGEO 2010 [22]	R	93	Yes vs. not	No	HR 1.01 (0.54–1.92)
SYUCC 2011 [23]	R	34	Yes vs. not	No	NR
Japanese 2012 [25]	R	132	Yes vs. not	No	NR

Legend: HR, hazard ratio. NR, not reported. R, retrospective study.

a prognostic role for prior adjuvant chemotherapy [29, 45], while the analysis of a Chinese series reported a favorable prognostic effect [8].

Some studies evaluated the variable of "prior chemotherapy" without specifying the adjuvant or metastatic setting, which was associated with improved outcomes [28, 31, 36, 47].

3.4.6.4 Selected studies

Of the four studies that investigated prior PTR, two documented a longer OS for patients with a previous PTR [21, 27], while in the other there was only a favorable trend [23]. Table 3.9 lists the results of the studies.

A retrospective analysis of 80 mSBA patients receiving upfront chemotherapy, found poor outcomes for patients with previous adjuvant chemotherapy [21].

3.5 PROGNOSTIC FACTORS IN DECISION-MAKING

There are no standard treatment regimens for mSBA. Retrospective data prevails, as there are few prospective dedicated trials. However, some considerations could be made about decision-making by the occurrence of different PFs, as resumed in Table 3.10. Although the role of metastasectomy is not defined, in oligometastatic disease this approach might be considered [43]. Some data also support the association of surgical cytoreduction plus HIPEC in patients with peritoneal disease, detecting PCI <15 and HIPEC as independent predictors of improved survival [26].

3.5.1 UPFRONT TREATMENT

The combination of oxaliplatin+fluoropyrimidine with or without bevacizumab is a commonly used upfront regimen, despite few prospective trials [21, 24, 27, 60]. In a retrospective study of patients receiving oxaliplatin-based treatment, PS 0 and bevacizumab inclusion were significantly favorable PFs [61]. On the other hand, in a monoinstitutional study, bevacizumab was not significantly associated with improved OS, while fluoropyrimidine-based regimens were superior to non-fluoropyrimidine-based [43]. In another retrospective study conducted on 93 patients who received frontline chemotherapy with infusional fluorouracil and leucovorin or combined with irinotecan, either

TABLE 3.10

Prognostic and predictive variables in clinical decision-making in metastatic small bowel adenocarcinoma

A. Upfront systemic treatment

1   Performance status
           • Good: FU-based or OXA+FUP favored
2   Location
           • Jejunum-ileum: OXA+FUP regimen favored
3   Primary tumor resection
           • PTR: OXA+FUP favored
4   Age
           • <65 years old: FUP-based favored

B. Treatment of refractory disease

1   Mismatch repair system
           • MSI-H: ICI favored (PEMB or AVEL)
           • MSI-H: taxane-based favored (retrospective)
2   APC
           • APC wild-type: nab-paclitaxel favored
3   First-line regimen
           • Previous FOLFOX: FOLFIRI favored (retrospective)

Legend: APC, adenomatous polyposis coli gene. AVEL, avelumab. FU, fluoro-uracil. FUP, fluoropyrimidine. MSI-H, microsatellite instability–high. OXA, oxaliplatin. PEMB, pembrolizumab. PTR, primary tumor resection.

platinum regimens, PS and elevated CEA and CA 19-9 levels were independent PFs; after multivariate analysis, FOLFOX was associated with better outcomes than cisplatin+LV5FU2 regimen [22].

Good PS was favorable PF in patients receiving upfront treatment [19, 24]. The jejunal primary tumor location reported better OS, though not significant [24, 27], while confirmation of the favorable outcome of age <65 [19] and previous PTR [27] is lacking.

3.5.2 TREATMENT OF REFRACTORY DISEASE

In refractory disease, studies of nab-paclitaxel [62] and pembrolizumab [63, 64] have been published. They confirm the predictive effect of MSI-H on pembrolizumab efficacy [64] and better performance of taxane-based regimens in MSI-H patients [65] and those with wild-type APC. A possible increased activity of the FOLFIRI regimen after FOLFOX but not after fluorouracil has been hypothesized [22].

3.6 CONCLUSION

Although palliative chemotherapy improved outcomes of mSBA patients, especially after the introduction of irinotecan, oxaliplatin and gemcitabine [29, 49], even in prospective studies the median OS varied greatly [65–67], with little effect of immunotherapy [64, 68].

A synthesis of the final recommendations about the examined PFs is reported in Table 3.11. Beyond the stage at diagnosis and some TB-related variables, other studies of larger cohorts suggested poor outcomes for patients with deteriorated PS, elevated serum CEA and advanced age. It remains unclear whether the outcome is worse in duodenal tumors or better in jejunal mSBAs.

TABLE 3.11

Prognostic factors evaluated in prospective trials of upfront treatment in patients with unresectable or metastatic small bowel adenocarcinoma

Suggested	Not suggested	Needing study
Performance status	Sex	Predisposing conditions
Age	Ethnicity	CA 19-9
CEA		
Primary tumor location	Disease status	Number of sites of metastases
	Histotype	Site of metastasis
	Previous adjuvant chemotherapy	Timing metastasis
		Tumor grade
		Primary tumor resection

Therefore, due to the rarity of the disease, extensive data on the prognostic effect of variables are unlikely in the future. Consequently, a molecular characterization is warranted for patients with MSS metastatic SBA.

REFERENCES

1. Bilimoria KY, Bentrem DJ, Wayne JD, et al. Small bowel cancer in the United States: Changes in epidemiology, treatment, and survival over the last 20 years. *Ann Surg* 2009;249(1):63–71.
2. Locher C, Batumona B, Afchain P, et al. Small bowel adenocarcinoma: French intergroup clinical practice guidelines for diagnosis, treatments and follow-up (SNFGE, FFCD, GERCOR, UNICANCER, SFCD, SFED, SFRO). *Dig Liver Dis* 2018;50(1):15–9.
3. Aparicio T, Zaanan A, Svrcek M, et al. Small bowel adenocarcinoma: Epidemiology, risk factors, diagnosis and treatment. *Dig Liver Dis* 2014;46:97–104.
4. Faivre J, Trama A, De Angelis R, et al. Incidence, prevalence and survival of patients with rare epithelial digestive cancers diagnosed in Europe in 1995–2002. *Eur J Cancer* 2012;48(10):1417–24.
5. Siegel RL, Miller KD, Jemal A. Cancer statistics, 2019. *CA: Cancer J Clin* 2019;69:7–34.
6. Siegel R, Naishadham D, Jemal A. Cancer statistics, 2012. *CA: Cancer J Clin* 2012:62(1):10–29.
7. Bojesen RD, Andersson M, Riis LB, et al. Incidence of, phenotypes of and survival from small bowel cancer in Denmark, 1994–2010: A population-based study. *J Gastroenterol* 2016;51:891–9.
8. Guo X, Mao Z, Su D, et al. The clinical pathological features, diagnosis, treatment and prognosis of small intestine primary malignant tumors. *Med Oncol* 2014;31(4):913.
9. Goodman MT, Matsuno RK, Shvetsov YB. Racial and ethnic variation in the incidence of small-bowel cancer subtypes in the United States, 1995–2008. *Dis Colon Rectum* 2013;56(4):441–8.
10. Lech G, Korcz W, Kowalczyk E, et al. Primary small bowel adenocarcinoma: Current view on clinical features, risk and prognostic factors, treatment and outcome. *Scand J Gastroenterol* 2017;52(11):1194–202.
11. Fernandes DD, Galwa RP, Fasih N, Fraser-Hill M. Cross-sectional imaging of small bowel malignancies. *Can Assoc Radiol J* 2012;63(3):215–21.
12. Wu TJ, Yeh CN, Chao TC, et al. Prognostic factors of primary small bowel adenocarcinoma: Univariate and multivariate analysis. *World J Surg* 2006;30(3):391–8.
13. Neely D, Ong J, Patterson J, et al. Small intestinal adenocarcinoma: Rarely considered, often missed? *Postgrad Med J* 2013;89(1050):197–201.
14. Eliakim R. Wireless capsule video endoscopy: Three years of experience. *World J Gastroenterol* 2004;10(9):1238–9.
15. American Joint Committee on Cancer. *Small Intestine. AJCC Cancer Staging Manual.* 8th Ed. NewYork; Springer, 2017, 221–34.
16. Sakae H, Kanzaki H, Nasu J, et al. The characteristics and outcomes of small bowel adenocarcinoma: A multicentre retrospective observational study. *Br J Cancer* 2017;117:1607–13.

17. ECIS – European Cancer Information System, available at: https://ecis.jrc.ec.europa.eu, accessed October 31, 2023.
18. Colina A, Hwang H, Wang H, et al. Natural history and prognostic factors for localised small bowel adenocarcinoma. *ESMO Open* 2020;5(6):e000960.
19. Gibson MK, Holcroft CA, Kvols LK, Haller D. Phase II study of 5-fluorouracil, doxorubicin, and mitomycin C for metastatic small bowel adenocarcinoma. *Oncologist* 2005;10:132–7.
20. Czaykowski P, Huiy D. Chemotherapy in small bowel adenocarcinoma: 10-year experience of the British Columbia Cancer Agency. *Clin Oncol* 2007;19:143–9.
21. Overman MJ, Kopetz S, Wen S, et al. Chemotherapy with 5-fluorouracil and a platinum compound improves outcomes in metastatic small bowel adenocarcinoma. *Cancer* 2008;113(8):2038–45.
22. Zaanan A, Costes L, Gauthier M, et al. Chemotherapy of advanced small-bowel adenocarcinoma: A multicenter AGEO study. *Ann Oncol* 2010;21(9):1786–93.
23. Zhang L, Wang LY, Deng YM, et al. Efficacy of the FOLFOX/CAPOX regimen for advanced small bowel adenocarcinoma: A three-center study from China. *J BUON* 2011;16(4):689–96.
24. Xiang XJ, Liu YW, Zhang L, et al. A phase II study of modified FOLFOX as first-line chemotherapy in advanced small bowel adenocarcinoma. *Anticancer Drugs* 2012;23(5):561–6.
25. Tsushima T, Taguri M, Honma Y, et al. Multicenter retrospective study of 132 patients with unresectable small bowel adenocarcinoma treated with chemotherapy. *Oncologist* 2012;17(9):1163–70.
26. Liu Y, Ishibashi H, Takeshita K, et al. Cytoreductive surgery and hyperthermic intraperitoneal chemotherapy for peritoneal dissemination from small bowel malignancy: Results from a single specialized center. *Ann Surg Oncol* 2016;23(5):1625–31.
27. Horimatsu T, Nakayama N, Moriwaki T, et al. A phase II study of 5-fluorouracil/L-leucovorin/oxaliplatin (mFOLFOX6) in Japanese patients with metastatic or unresectable small bowel adenocarcinoma. *Int J Clin Oncol* 2017;22(5):905–12.
28. Koo DH, Yun SC, Hong YS, et al. Systemic chemotherapy for treatment of advanced small bowel adenocarcinoma with prognostic factor analysis: Retrospective study. *BMC Cancer* 2011;11:205.
29. Fishman PN, Pond GR, Moore MJ, et al. Natural history and chemotherapy effectiveness for advanced adenocarcinoma of the small bowel: A retrospective review of 113 cases. *Am J Clin Oncol* 2006;29(3):225–31.
30. Aydin D, Sendur MA, Kefeli U, et al. Evaluation of prognostic factors and treatment in advanced small bowel adenocarcinoma: Report of a multi-institutional experience of Anatolian Society of Medical Oncology (ASMO). *J BUON* 2016;21(5):1242–9.
31. Wang N, Yang J, Lyu J, et al. A convenient clinical nomogram for predicting the cancer-specific survival of individual patients with small-intestine adenocarcinoma. *BMC Cancer* 2020;20(1):505.
32. Wang D, Li C, Li Y, et al. Specific survival nomograms based on SEER database for small intestine adenocarcinoma. *Ann Palliat Med* 2021;10(7):7440–57.
33. Zheng Z, Zhou X, Zhang J, et al. Nomograms predict survival of patients with small bowel adenocarcinoma: A SEER-based study. *Int J Clin Oncol* 2021;26(2):387–98.
34. Gu Y, Deng H, Wang D, Li Y. Metastasis pattern and survival analysis in primary small bowel adenocarcinoma: A SEER-based study. *Front Surg* 2021;8:759162.
35. Howe JR, Karnell LH, Menck HR, Scott-Conner C. The American college of surgeons commission on cancer and the American Cancer Society. Adenocarcinoma of the small bowel: Review of the National Cancer Data Base, 1985–1995. *Cancer* 1999;86(12):2693–706.
36. Akce M, Jiang R, Zakka K, et al. Clinical outcomes of small bowel adenocarcinoma. *Clin Colorectal Cancer* 2019;18(4):257–68.
37. Halfdanarson TR, McWilliams RR, Donohue JH, Quevedo JF. A single-institution experience with 491 cases of small bowel adenocarcinoma. *Am J Surg* 2010;199(6):797–803.
38. Qubaiah O, Devesa SS, Platz CE, et al. Small intestinal cancer: A population-based study of incidence and survival patterns in the United States, 1992 to 2006. *Cancer Epidemiol Biomarkers Prev* 2010;19(8):1908–18.
39. Lee D-W, Kyung-Hun Lee K-H, Tae-Yong Kim T-Y, et al. Prognostic role of body mass index in advanced small bowel adenocarcinoma patients receiving palliative chemotherapy. *Nutr Cancer* 2016;68(5):750–5.
40. Ugurlu MM, Asoglu O, Potter DD, et al. Adenocarcinomas of the jejunum and ileum: A 25-year experience. *J Gastrointest Surg* 2005;9(8):1182–8.
41. Chang HK, Yu E, Kim J, et al. Adenocarcinoma of the small intestine: A multi-institutional study of 197 surgically resected cases. *Hum Pathol* 2010;41(8):1087–96.
42. Aparicio T, Henriques J, Manfredi S, et al. Small bowel adenocarcinoma: Results from a nationwide prospective ARCAD-NADEGE cohort study of 347 patients. *Int J Cancer* 2020;147(4):967–77.

43. Bhamidipati D, Colina A, Hwang H, et al. Metastatic small bowel adenocarcinoma: Role of metastasectomy and systemic chemotherapy. *ESMO Open* 2021;6(3):100132.
44. Veyrières M, Baillet P, Hay JM, et al. Factors influencing long-term survival in 100 cases of small intestine primary adenocarcinoma. *Am J Surg* 1997;173(3):237–9.
45. Dabaja BS, Suki D, Pro B, et al. Adenocarcinoma of the small bowel presentation, prognostic factors, and outcome of 217 patients. *Cancer* 2004;101(3):518–26.
46. Agrawal S, McCarron EC, Gibbs JF, et al. Surgical management and outcome in primary adenocarcinoma of the small bowel. *Ann Surg Oncol* 2007;14(8):2263–9.
47. Zhou YW, Xia RL, Chen YY, et al. Clinical features, treatment, and prognosis of different histological types of primary small bowel adenocarcinoma: A propensity score matching analysis based on the SEER database. *Eur J Surg Oncol* 2021;47(8):2108–18.
48. Overman MJ, Hu CY, Wolff RA, Chang GJ. Prognostic value of lymph node evaluation in small bowel adenocarcinoma: Analysis of the surveillance, epidemiology, and end results database. *Cancer* 2010;116(23):5374–82.
49. Moon YW, Rha SY, Shin SJ, et al. Adenocarcinoma of the small bowel at a single Korean institute: Management and prognosticators. *J Cancer Res Clin Oncol* 2010;136:387–94.
50. Yu IS, Al-Hashami Z, Chapani P, et al. Impact of tumor location on patient outcomes in small bowel cancers. *Clin Colorectal Cancer* 2022;21(2):107–13.
51. Zhang S, Yuan W, Zhang J, et al. Clinicopathological features, surgical treatments, and survival outcomes of patients with small bowel adenocarcinoma. *Medicine* 2017;96(31):e7713.
52. Hong SH, Koh YH, Rho SY, et al. Primary adenocarcinoma of the small intestine: Presentation, prognostic factors and clinical outcome. *Jpn J Clin Oncol* 2009;39(1):54–61.
53. Vanoli A, Di Sabatino A, Martino M, et al. Small bowel carcinomas in celiac or Crohn's disease: Distinctive histophenotypic, molecular and histogenetic patterns. *Mod Pathol* 2017;30(10):1453–66.
54. Giuffrida P, Arpa G, Grillo F, et al. PD-L1 in small bowel adenocarcinoma is associated with etiology and tumor-infiltrating lymphocytes, in addition to microsatellite instability. *Mod Pathol* 2020;33(7):1398–409.
55. DeSesso JM, Jacobson CF. Anatomical and physiological parameters affecting gastrointestinal absorption in humans and rats. *Food Chem Toxicol* 2001;39(3):209–28.
56. Haselkorn T, Whittemore AS, Lilienfeld DE. Incidence of small bowel cancer in the United States and worldwide: Geographic, temporal, and racial differences. *Cancer Causes Control* 2005;16(7):781–7.
57. Siegel RL, Miller KD, Jemal A. Cancer statistics, 2016. *CA: Cancer J Clin* 2016;66(1):7–30.
58. Schrock AB, Devoe CE, McWilliams R, et al. Genomic profiling of small-bowel adenocarcinoma. *JAMA Oncol* 2017;3(11):1546–53.
59. Aparicio T, Svrcek M, Zaanan A, et al. Small bowel adenocarcinoma phenotyping, a clinicobiological prognostic study. *Br J Cancer* 2013;109(12):3057–66.
60. Gulhati P, Raghav K, Shroff RT, et al. Bevacizumab combined with capecitabine and oxaliplatin in patients with advanced adenocarcinoma of the small bowel or ampulla of Vater: A single center, open-label, phase 2 study. *Cancer* 2017;123(6):1011–7.
61. Hirao M, Komori M, Nishida T, et al. Clinical use of molecular targeted agents for primary small bowel adenocarcinoma: A multicenter retrospective cohort study by the Osaka Gut Forum. *Oncol Lett* 2017;14(2):1628–36.
62. Overman MJ, Adam L, Raghav K, et al. Phase II study of nab-paclitaxel in refractory small bowel adenocarcinoma and CpG island methylator phenotype (CIMP)-high colorectal cancer. *Ann Oncol* 2018;29:139–44.
63. Marabelle A, Le DT, Ascierto PA, et al. Efficacy of pembrolizumab in patients with noncolorectal high microsatellite instability/mismatch repair-deficient cancer: Results from the phase II KEYNOTE-158 study. *J Clin Oncol* 2020;38:1–10.
64. Pedersen KS, Foster NR, Overman MJ, et al. ZEBRA: A multicenter phase II study of pembrolizumab in patients with advanced small-bowel adenocarcinoma. *Clin Cancer Res* 2021;27:3641–8.
65. Aldrich JD, Raghav KPS, Varadhachary GR, et al. Retrospective analysis of taxane-based therapy in small bowel adenocarcinoma. *Oncologist* 2019;24:e384–6.
66. McWilliams RR, Foster NR, Mahoney MR, et al. North Central Cancer Treatment Group N0543 (Alliance): A phase 2 trial of pharmacogenetic-based dosing of irinotecan, oxaliplatin, and capecitabine as first-line therapy for patients with advanced small bowel adenocarcinoma. *Cancer* 2017;123:3494–501.
67. Overman MJ, Varadhachary GR, Kopetz S, et al. Phase II of capecitabine and oxaliplatin for advanced adenocarcinoma of the small bowel and ampulla of Vater. *J Clin Oncol* 2009;27:2598–603.
68. Cardin DB, Gilbert J, Whisenant JG, et al. Safety and efficacy of avelumab in small bowel adenocarcinoma. *Clin Colorectal Cancer* 2022;21(3):236–43.

4 Pancreatic adenocarcinoma

4.1 INTRODUCTION

4.1.1 EPIDEMIOLOGY

Worldwide, in 2018 the incidence age-adjusted standardized rate (ASR) of pancreatic adenocarcinoma (PDAC) was 4.8/100,000, with the highest rates in Western Europe and North America and similar distribution for mortality [1]. In China in 2022, the estimated new cases were 134,374, accounting for 2.8% of malignancies, with 131,203 deaths (4.1%), while in the US they constituted 3.2% of new cancers and 7.9% of deaths [2]. In Europe in 2022 the ASR was 20.5/100,000, with 100,152 new cases, and a mortality ASR of 19.4/100,000, with 94,952 cancer deaths [3].

A 2017 GLOBOCAN database analysis of 48 countries documented that the highest incidence was in countries with high and very high human development index. Although progressive growth in incidence is expected by 2040 in North America and Europe, where an increase in incidence of 28.7% is estimated [4] and will continue until 2060 [5], some predictions suggest the trend will be much more pronounced for Africa and Latin America [6]. Europe remains an area with a relatively high incidence and prevalence, and PDAC poses the largest healthcare and societal burden in the 55–74 years old population, although the incidence rises again after 80 years [5], and since 2017 the annual number of deaths from PDAC has exceeded that from breast cancer [6].

PDAC can be considered a disease of the elderly with a median age of incidence of 65–69 years among males and 75–79 in women [7]. It is expected that in 2030 70% of PDACs will be in the elderly [8], so population aging is assumed to be the cause of 20% of the PDAC increasing incidence [9]. The slight increase in incidence and mortality over the past 20 years for both sexes is common, with a men-to-women ratio for incidence of 1.4/1 [2].

4.1.2 STAGING OF METASTATIC DISEASE

For diagnosis and staging, chest-abdomen CT is the investigation of choice. It must be carried out according to pancreatic protocol, involving a biphasic examination. Abdominal MRI is employed for evaluating small liver lesions, with higher sensitivity and similar specificity [10]. ^{18}FDG-PET/TC is appropriate for staging, being more efficient in detecting distant metastases [11]. Among imaging methods, EUS is sometimes necessary for pancreatic biopsy of patients eligible for upfront systemic therapy. Other more invasive procedures are not indicated in unresectable or metastatic pancreatic adenocarcinoma (mPDAC).

Baseline complete blood counts, chemistry, and markers, such as albumin, liver enzymes, and carbohydrate antigen 19-9 (CA 19-9) are recommended.

Among patients with mPDAC, the molecular characterization includes BRCA, mismatch repair (MMR), and NTRK status.

The reference staging system is TNM Classification (AJCC 8th edition 2017).

Given the not infrequent possibility of insufficient specimens for histologic diagnosis in patients without metastatic sites readily accessible for biopsy, it could be considered to start treatments without a histologic confirmation whenever imaging and serum CA 19-9 are strongly suggestive of PDAC, and after discussion within the multidisciplinary tumor board.

DOI: 10.1201/9781032703350-4

TABLE S1
Prognostic factors analyzed in selected clinical trials of patients with unresectable or metastatic pancreatic adenocarcinoma receiving upfront treatment

Variable	No. trials	Prognostic relationship	No prognostic relationship
Patient-related			
Performance status	23	18	5
Demographic			
Age	16	4	12
Sex	12	2	10
Geographic area	1	0	1
Ethnicity	3	0	3
Anthropometric			
Body mass index	1	0	1
Clinic			
Pain	5	5	0
Weight loss	4	2	2
Jaundice	1	0	1
Thromboembolism	1	1	0
Laboratory			
Hemoglobin	1	1	0
Neutrophil-lymphocyte ratio	1	1	0
Albumin	7	6	1
Glicemia-related	2	1	1
Alkaline phosphatase	3	2	1
Liver enzymes	2	1	1
Carcinoembryonic antigen	1	1	0
Carbohydrate antigen 19-9	3	2	1
Tumor-related			
Tumor burden			
Tumor size (T4, diameters sum)	2	1	1
No. target lesions	1	1	0
Measurable disease	3	0	3
Disease status	14	13	1
No. sites metastases	3	2	1
Primary tumor location	3	3	0
Timing of metastasis	1	1	0
Site of metastasis			
Liver metastases	8	7	1
Nodal metastases	1	1	0
Extra-abdominal metastases	2	1	1
Pathology			
Histotype	1	1	0
Grading (histologic)	3	2	1
Previous treatments			
Primary tumor resection	4	1	3
Palliative surgery	3	2	1
Other (stent, chemo, radio)	4	0	4

4.1.3 Prognosis of metastatic disease

Survival rates are very poor. Overall, 80–85% of patients at the time of diagnosis have a mPDAC [12], while 70–75% of those with a localized PDAC experience a relapse [13]. Even in patients with resectable disease, mortality from PDAC exceeds that from other causes up to 9 years after diagnosis [14]. Given the poor prognosis of the unresectable disease, even when localized, clinical trials of metastatic PDAC have often enrolled patients with locally advanced unresectable disease.

From 1990 to 2011 the upfront standard of care was mono-chemotherapy. However, compared to the first monotherapy studies, which reported a median overall survival (OS) of 6 months, the most recent studies report a median OS of 9–11 months, somewhat longer for locally advanced tumors. The development of new prognostic factors (PFs) has been slow, and many variables that have been evaluated over time in randomized clinical trials (RCTs), to date have not been standardized.

4.2 ANALYSIS OF PROGNOSTIC VARIABLES IN EARLY METASTATIC DISEASE

A systematic review of phase III RCTs that studied upfront therapies in patients with mPDAC resulted in the selection of 54 studies, published from 1974 to 2022. In 25 an evaluation of PFs was done [15–39], and in 20 a multivariate analysis was performed. The current review is focused on the results of the 25 selected studies. Table S1 lists all PFs that have been reported in at least one study and the number of studies that investigated the relationships between the PFs and OS.

4.3 PATIENT-RELATED PROGNOSTIC FACTORS

4.3.1 Performance status

A meta-analysis of 12 RCTs evaluating mPDAC patients receiving first-line chemotherapy reported a poor prognosis of patients with deteriorated PS and high heterogeneity, that was considerably reduced when only studies that compared PS 1 vs. PS 0 were considered, which were the more recent studies and documented an even stronger relationship of PS to OS [40]. This study suggests that among the mPDAC patients receiving chemotherapy, PS 0 could be more important than PS 2 as a predictor of OS [41], while the hypothesis of reduced activity of chemotherapy in patients with poor PS remains controversial [42, 43].

Evidence from other studies also points toward supporting the negative prognostic role of poor PS. Two population-based studies concluded that PS 2–3 was associated with reduced OS [44] and increased 90-day mortality [45]. Four prospective studies confirmed the relationship between poor PS and reduced OS [46–49], while in another study the relationship was not significant [50]. Of 16 retrospective studies that included PS among the possible PFs in the first-line setting [51–66], 13 confirmed the prognostic role [51–63].

The variables affecting PS and its possible changes following chemotherapy are poorly understood. Likewise, the relationship between PS and increased toxicity from polychemotherapy remains unproven, although the age-related therapeutic index may vary according to the regimen [67, 68].

4.3.1.1 Selected trials

Of 23 RCTs that analyzed PS, 18 documented an effect on OS, as resumed in Table 4.1. For 12 studies, comparing the outcomes of 5,153 patients, it was possible to retrieve the effect size (ES) and perform a meta-analysis, whose forest plot is reported in Figure 4.1. The result was that a poor PS is associated with a reduced OS (HR 1.43, CI 1.25–1.63; Q = 125.00, p-value <0.0001; I^2 = 91.2%).

TABLE 4.1

Prognostic relationships of performance status in selected studies of patients with unresectable or metastatic pancreatic adenocarcinoma receiving upfront treatment

Study [ref]	Phase	No. pts	Scale	Comparison	Prognostic relationship	Effect size
NCCTG 1985 [16]	III	184	ECOG	PS 2–3 vs. PS 0–1	Yes	NR
CALGB-7982 1986 [17]	III	184	NR	PS 2–3 vs. PS 0–1	No	NR
British 1989 [18]	III	108	KPS	KPS ≤ vs. >50	Yes	NR
LiGLA 2001 [19]	III	278	KPS	KPS ≤ vs. >60	Yes	RR by score
ECOG-2297 2002 [21]	III	322	ECOG	PS 2 vs. PS 0–1	Yes	NR
RMH 2002 [22]	III	209	ECOG	continuous	Yes	HR 1.40 (1.07–1.82)
NCIC 2003 [23]	III	277	ECOG	continuous	No	NR
Johnson TIP 2004 [24]	III	688	ECOG	PS 1–2 vs. PS 0	Yes	NR
Eli-Lilly PEM 2005 [25]	III	565	ECOG	PS 2 vs. PS 0–1	Yes	NR
GERCOR 2005 [26]	III	313	WHO	PS 2 vs. PS 0–1	Yes	NR
Italian 2005 [27]	III	99	KPS	KPS ≤ vs. >70	No	HR 1.01 (1.00–1.03)
German 2006 [28]	III	195	KPS	KPS < vs. ≥90	Yes	HR 1.69 (1.18–2.44)
PA.3 2007 [29]	III	569	ECOG	PS 2 vs. PS 0–1	Yes	HR 1.85 (1.47–2.32)
SGCCR 2007 [30]	III	319	KPS	KPS < vs. ≥90	Yes	HR 1.30 (1.02–1.64)
ECOG-6201 2009 [31]	III	824	ECOG	continuous	Yes	NR
Romanian 2009 [32]	III	303	KPS	KPS < vs. ≥80	Yes	NR
GIP-1 2010 [33]	III	400	KPS	KPS < vs. ≥80	Yes	HR 1.41 (1.07–1.85)
Pfizer AXI 2011 [34]	III	632	ECOG	PS 1 vs. PS 0	Yes	HR 2.01 (1.54–2.63)
PRODIGE-4 2011 [35]	III	342	ECOG	PS 1 vs. PS 0	No	HR 1.43 (0.99–2.08)
MPACT 2013 [36, 67]	III	861	KPS	KPS < vs. ≥90	Yes	HR 1.60 (1.35–1.89)
TeloVac 2014 [37]	III	712	ECOG	PS ≥1 vs. PS 0	No	HR 1.05 (0.80–1.30)
GAMMA 2015 [38]	III	640	ECOG	PS ≥1 vs. PS 0	Yes	HR 1.39 (1.10–1.76)
MASI 2015 [39]	III	175	ECOG	PS 1 vs. PS 0	Yes	HR 1.56 (1.24–1.96)

Legend: ECOG, Eastern Cooperative Oncology Group. HR, hazard ratio. KPS, Karnofsky Performance Scale. NR, not reported. PS, performance status. RR, risk ratio. WHO, World Health Organization.

4.3.2 Demographic

4.3.2.1 Age

While analyses of the NCDB [45] and SEER databases [69] support a negative prognostic role for advanced age, prospective studies do not confirm the relationship [46–48, 50, 70], except two [71, 72]. Other two retrospective analyses documented poor outcomes for elderly patients [62, 73], while 17 did not find differences by age [52–61, 63–66, 74–76].

Elderly patients could have a poor prognosis for various reasons, such as the more compromised general conditions and comorbidities [77, 78], but not for age itself, as early stage PDAC studies suggest [79, 80], with a possible role of poor nutritional status and reduced access to adjuvant chemotherapy. According to some authors, advanced age predicts reduced benefit from chemotherapy [81], but despite the reduced tolerance in the elderly, more intensive regimens confer similar OS improvements than in the young [82]. Additionally, the Japanese observational NAPOLEON study confirmed that age >65 does not interfere with the activity or toxicity profiles of upfront regimens, with a need for dose reduction also for gemcitabine+nab-paclitaxel (GnP) in >75 years old patients [83].

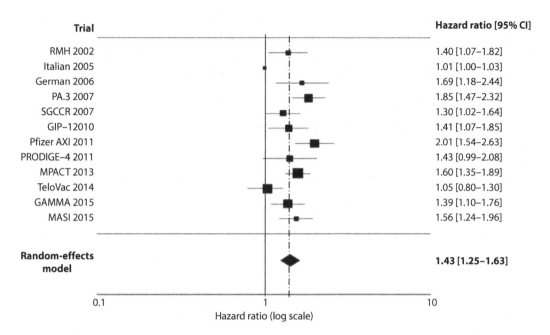

FIGURE 4.1 Forest plot of meta-analysis of performance status in prospective trials of patients with unresectable or metastatic pancreatic adenocarcinoma

4.3.2.2 Sex

In mPDAC patients, the outcome does not seem to be affected by sex. A population-based study [45] and a retrospective analysis [63] showed poor OS in females. However, seven prospective studies [46–50, 70, 71] and 19 retrospective did not find differences [52–62, 64–66, 73–76, 84].

Nevertheless, after the introduction of more intense regimens such as FOLFIRINOX, some authors suggested that female sex may be a prognostic and predictive variable. This hypothesis was supported by a small study of 49 patients, in which females presented superior overall response rates (ORRs) (75% vs. 36%), with numerically longer progression-free survival (PFS) and OS [85]. Similarly, a secondary analysis of the trial PRODIGE-4 detected a favorable trend for females [86]. Such a trend was documented after the GnP regimen too, and if were confirmed in larger studies, sex could become a predictive variable in mPDAC.

4.3.2.3 Other demographic variables

Despite the variable geographic distribution, no prognostic difference associated with geographic origin was reported. Some areas in the US are an exception, such as Arkansas, where mortality rates seem to differ by sex, age, and race [87], and a similar poor prognosis in the UK vs. other European countries has been described [62].

Ethnicity did not affect the survival of patients enrolled in the MPACT study [48], but it has been rarely evaluated as a PF, even though a possible increased risk for Caucasians was shown by a South African cancer registry [88].

4.3.2.4 Selected trials

Sixteen studies evaluated age, as resumed in Table 4.2. Four RCTs documented a significant relationship between age and OS, but with conflicting conclusions, as it was favorable PF for patients >70 years in one study [21] and negative PF among those with >65 years in other two [35, 36], with another trial not specifying [18]. For eight studies, comparing 3,526 patients, ES data were included in a meta-analysis, and the overall ES was not significant (HR 1.01, CI 0.95–1.15; Q = 19.99, p-value = 0.0056; I^2 = 65.0%).

TABLE 4.2
Prognostic relationships of age in selected studies of patients with unresectable or metastatic pancreatic adenocarcinoma receiving upfront treatment

Study [ref]	Phase	No. pts	Comparison	Prognostic relationship	Effect size
CALGB-7982 1986 [17]	III	184	<55 vs. 55–65 vs. >65	No	NR
British 1989 [18]	III	108	NR	Yes	NR
LiGLA 2001 [19]	III	278	> vs. ≤60	No	RR 1.28 (0.95–1.72)
ECOG-2297 2002 [21]	III	322	> vs. ≤70	Yes	NR
RMH 2002 [22]	III	209	NR	No	NR
Johnson TIP 2004 [24]	III	688	≥ vs. <65	No	NR
Eli-Lilly PEM 2005 [25]	III	565	NR	No	NR
Italian 2005 [27]	III	99	continuous	No	HR 0.98 (0.95–1.00)
German 2006 [28]	III	195	continuous	No	HR 1.02 (1.00–1.04)
PA.3 2007 [29]	III	569	≥ vs. <65	No	HR 1.12 (0.93–1.35)
ECOG-6201 2009 [31]	III	824	<55 vs. 55–70 vs. >70	No	NR
GIP-1 2010 [33]	III	400	≥ vs. <65	No	HR 0.89 (0.72–1.12)
PRODIGE-4 2011 [35]	III	342	≥ vs. <65	Yes	HR 1.47 (1.07–2.02)
MPACT 2013 [36, 67]	III	861	≥ vs. <65	Yes	HR 1.23 (1.03–1.45)
TeloVac 2014 [37]	III	712	≥ vs. <60	No	HR 1.10 (0.90–1.30)
MASI 2015 [39]	III	348	≥ vs. <65	No	HR 0.99 (0.79–1.24)

Legend: HR, hazard ratio. NR, not reported. RR, risk ratio.

Of the twelve studies that evaluated the effect of sex on OS, only two documented a significant relationship, as reported in Table 4.3. In both trials, female sex was associated with longer OS [29, 39]. A meta-analysis was performed from the results of three studies, supporting the favorable prognostic role of female sex (HR 1.20, 1.04–1.38; Q = 0.63, p-value = 0.7297; I^2 = 0%).

One study evaluated the geographic area of origin, North America vs. other, and did not find survival differences, while patients from Eastern Europe had shorter OS [46]. Three studies evaluated the ethnicity, and two of them did not document any difference between Caucasians and other races [17, 25], while another negative study compared Hispanics, non-Hispanic Whites, and Blacks [31].

4.3.3 ANTHROPOMETRIC

The body mass index (BMI) of mPDAC patients was associated with the outcome. A meta-analysis of 10 studies documented OS reduction with increasing BMI [89], and other studies support a higher incidence and mortality from PDAC in patients with high BMI [90–93]. On the other hand, three prospective and two retrospective studies did not report any prognostic relationship [47, 48, 59, 70, 84], whereas other two retrospective suggested poor outcomes for a BMI <18.5 kg/m^2 [58, 62]. Cut-off differences among studies could explain some divergent results, but insulin resistance, which is common among PDAC patients [94], is suspected to be involved in the relationship.

Other authors did not find a prognostic role for weight [48] or body surface area [54].

4.3.3.1 Selected trials

One study evaluated patients' baseline weight and BMI and did not report any effect on OS [39].

4.3.4 CLINIC

Various baseline symptoms were evaluated in clinical trials.

TABLE 4.3
Prognostic relationships of sex in selected studies of patients with unresectable or metastatic pancreatic adenocarcinoma receiving upfront treatment

Study [ref]	Phase	No. pts	Comparison	Prognostic relationship	Effect size
CALGB-7982 1986 [17]	III	184	M vs. F	No	NR
LiGLA 2001 [19]	III	278	M vs. F	No	RR 1.05 (0.79–1.39)
RMH 2002 [22]	III	209	M vs. F	No	NR
NCIC 2003 [23]	III	277	M vs. F	No	NR
Johnson TIP 2004 [24]	III	688	M vs. F	No	HR 0.95
German 2006 [28]	III	195	M vs. F	No	NR
PA.3 2007 [29]	III	569	M vs. F	Yes	NR
ECOG-6201 2009 [31]	III	824	M vs. F	No	NR
GIP-1 2010 [33]	III	400	M vs. F	No	HR 1.12 (0.89–1.39)
PRODIGE-4 2011 [35]	III	342	M vs. F	No	NR
TeloVac 2014 [37]	III	712	M vs. F	No	HR 1.20 (1.00–1.41)
MASI 2015 [39]	III	350	M vs. F	Yes	HR 1.27 (1.01–1.56)

Legend: F, females. HR, hazard ratio. M males. NR, not reported. RR, risk ratio.

4.3.4.1   Pain

Abdominal or back pain is present in 50–75% of mPDAC patients [95, 96] so pain control has been an outcome measure for evaluating the activity of antineoplastic agents [97]. Data about the prognostic role of pain are discordant, with retrospective studies suggesting a negative prognosis [74, 98], while others not report OS differences [46, 52, 53].

PDAC-related pain is complex, with visceral, somatic, and neuropathic components, and is frequently related to celiac plexus invasion, increased density of sensory and sympathetic fibers in the territory of tumor-induced neo-angiogenesis, increased number of macrophages in the tumor, and secretion of neuronal growth factors by the tumor micro-environment (TME), which maintains an activation of the inflammatory pathways and a state of immune escape [99].

4.3.4.2   Weight loss

Weight loss (WL) after diagnosis or during first-line chemotherapy has been related to poor OS [53, 74, 100, 101], but not always [60, 70]. The malnutrition risk is present in 85% of mPDAC patients, while cancer-associated cachexia syndrome (CACS) occurs in 70–80% and is associated with reduced OS [102, 103], with one-third of PDAC deaths due to CACS rather than tumor burden (TB).

Tumor relapse is the event that has the greatest impact on the change in body composition, with a rapid decline in skeletal muscle and subcutaneous adipose tissue [104]. In particular, the loss and rate of loss of visceral adipose tissue (VAT) correlates with prognosis. An evaluation of the total psoas area index in mPDAC patients documented a close relationship between sarcopenic psoas and poor OS [105]. Such VAT loss is often associated with diabetes and anemia, but also with the systemic inflammatory response (SIR) [106].

4.3.4.3   Thromboembolism

Among malignant tumors, PDAC presents the highest incidence of thromboembolism (TE) [107, 108], which is asymptomatic in >80% and is thought to be responsible for many early deaths [109]. Therefore, the reported incidence varies [107, 108, 110], with a progressive increase over time up to 19% after one year [111].

The prognostic effect of TE remains unclear, but even in patients with TE, TE-related mortality was always lower than PDAC-related mortality [109, 112–116]. Symptomatic patients and those with an early TE report poor outcomes [111, 117, 118]. Compared to non-cancer patients, TE occurrence in PDAC patients increases hospital mortality 13-fold [119, 120], with a consequent reduction of quality of life that delays cancer treatment and increases costs.

Platelet counts, hyponatremia, and hypoalbuminemia have been suggested among possible predictors of TE. Many authors have reported a PDAC-related increase in the secretion of tissue factor, which was especially expressed in patients receiving chemotherapy [121], platelet factor 4 [122], or a hypercoagulable state [111]. Considering the possible contribution of chemotherapy to TE occurrence [123, 124], the current lack of effective TE risk prediction tools for mPDAC patients remains a major issue [125, 126].

4.3.4.4   Other clinical conditions

Few data relating to jaundice in patients with mPDAC are available, and no relationship between jaundice occurrence and prognosis has been reported [51, 53, 74].

Although the presence of ascites is associated with a trend toward poor OS even without peritoneal metastases, it did not significantly affect OS in retrospective studies [64, 84].

None of the four studies that evaluated diabetes and prognosis of mPDAC documented a relationship [52, 58, 63, 64].

4.3.4.5   Selected trials

All five studies that evaluated pain reported a negative prognostic effect (Table 4.4). Three of these studies evaluated the presentation of pain by a Visual Analogue Scale (VAS) or Numerical Rating Scale (NRS) [23, 32, 39]. Only three RCTs, evaluating 771 patients, expressed an ES, and the pooled HR was comparable to that of the individual studies (HR 1.54, CI 1.30–1.83; Q = 0.54, p-value = 0.7623; I^2 = 0%).

TABLE 4.4
Prognostic relationships of baseline symptoms in selected studies of patients with unresectable or metastatic pancreatic adenocarcinoma receiving upfront treatment

Study [ref]	Phase	No. pts	Comparison	Prognostic relationship	Effect size
Pain					
NCIC 2003 [23]	III	277	NRS ≥ vs. <20	Yes	HR 1.45 (1.11–1.90)
Johnson TIP 2004 [24]	III	688	Yes vs. no	Yes	HR 1.32
SGCCR 2007 [30]	III	319	Yes vs. no	Yes	HR 1.52 (1.17–1.92)
Romanian 2009 [32]	III	303	VAS ≥ vs. <20	Yes	NR
MASI 2015 [39]	III	175	NRS ≥ vs. <20	Yes	HR 1.67 (1.27–2.19)
Weight loss					
VASACC 1981 [15]	III	152	3 groups	No	NR
Johnson TIP 2004 [24]	III	688	≥ vs. <10% 6m	Yes	HR 1.28
ECOG-6201 2009 [31]	III	824	≥ vs. <any 6m	No	NR
Romanian 2009 [32]	III	303	≥ vs. <10% 6m	Yes	NR
Jaundice					
Johnson TIP 2004 [24]	III	688	Yes vs. no	No	HR 1.09
Thromboembolism					
ECOG-6201 2009 [31]	III	824	Yes vs. no	Yes	OS 2.5 vs. 3.1 m

Legend: HR, hazard ratio. m, months. NR, not reported. NRS, Numerical Rating Scale. OS, overall survival. VAS, Visual Analogue Scale.

Of the four RCTs that investigated WL before chemotherapy, two documented poor outcomes for a >10% decrease in the last 6 months [24, 32]. A study evaluated the occurrence of jaundice before chemotherapy and was negative [24]. On the contrary, a previous history of TE was related to OS reduction [31].

4.3.5 LABORATORY

4.3.5.1 Hematology

Among hematologic parameters, an increased count of neutrophils and platelets, and a reduction in red blood cells and lymphocytes were often reported, but changes were unspecific. Hemoglobin reduction has been related to the prognosis of mPDAC, with poor OS for a concentration <12 g/dL [58], but without effects on the outcome in other eight studies evaluating cut-offs in the range of 10–12 g/dL [46, 47, 52–54, 56, 64, 98]. Eight studies examined the increased leukocyte count [47, 51–54, 58, 64, 98], which was confirmed as a PF in two [54, 58]. Of the two studies that examined the increased neutrophil count, it was a negative PF [47, 75]. Conflicting results were reported by the studies investigating the platelet count, with two studies supporting a negative prognostic effect for increased platelet count [47, 76], and two retrospective analyses not [54, 98].

SIR could influence hematologic changes and have a direct effect on prognosis, because of its effects on tumor progression and chemoresistance [127–129], but a standardized measure is not available. Many authors investigated ratios and scores, including neutrophil-to-lymphocyte ratio (NLR) and platelet-to-lymphocyte ratio (PLR). A meta-analysis identified 28 studies, mostly retrospective, and concluded reporting a doubled risk of death for mPDAC patients with high baseline NLR, and a weaker but significant relationship of PLR with OS, despite the presence of considerable heterogeneity [130]. The prognostic effect of NLR is likely to be attributed to neutrophil count [59]. Albeit the contribution of lymphocyte counts on prognosis cannot be excluded, the evolution of the relationships of lymphocyte sub-populations during mPDAC progression deserves further investigation.

4.3.5.2 Chemistry

Serum albumin (SA) level is the most studied laboratory parameter in mPDAC patients. Two population-based articles [44, 45] and various prospective and retrospective analyses support the prognostic negative effect of low albumin on mPDAC outcome. A meta-analysis evaluated the relationship of SA with OS of 42 study cohorts in the first-line setting, including 10,506 mPDAC patients, and reported a significant effect of SA <3.5 g/dL on the risk of death (HR 1.45, CI 1.33–1.59), but the analysis found significant heterogeneity and $I^2 = 83.7\%$. Meta-regression suggested a possible effect of the primary tumor resection (PTR) and poor PS on the relationship of SA with OS [131]. The pathogenesis of hypoalbuminemia may be multifactorial in mPDAC since hepatic synthesis is reduced by SIR [132, 133], which also affects capillary permeability contributing to reduced SA levels. Many albumin-based variables have been developed, among which the modified Glasgow prognostic score (mGPS) has been reported as negative PF by some retrospective studies [65, 73, 134], in addition to being associated with increased 90-day mortality in a population-based study [44]. Other inflammation-related proteins have been studied, and a poor prognosis of mPDAC patients with increased C-reactive protein (CRP) has been reported [44, 45, 50, 52, 64, 73, 98] but not from all studies [57, 58].

Fewer data are available on the relationship between liver enzymes and mPDAC prognosis. Two studies documented poor OS for patients with high alanine aminotransferase (ALT) levels [54, 71] while six found no difference [47, 51, 53, 58, 64, 75]. Similarly, an aspartate aminotransferase (AST) elevation was associated with reduced OS in two studies [53, 54] but no difference in the other six [47, 58, 64, 71, 75, 98]. In contrast, none of the nine studies that assessed baseline bilirubin documented a prognostic effect [46, 47, 52, 53, 58, 64, 73, 75, 98], as for gamma-glutamyl-transpeptidase [53, 75].

One [54] of six studies found a negative prognostic role for increased alkaline phosphatase (ALP) [47, 58, 64, 75, 135], and three [44, 45, 57] of seven studies for increased lactic dehydrogenase (LDH) [47, 52, 75, 98], while other authors detected poor outcomes only beyond a 360 U/L cut-off [84]. Finally, the relationship of baseline glycemia and OS is controversial [136, 137].

4.3.5.3 Tumor markers

Among tumor markers, the CA 19-9, a mucin that 5–10% of subjects are unable to synthesize (sialyl Lewis negative group), has been extensively studied. Some clinical conditions are responsible for false positive results, such as jaundice, cirrhosis, malformations, acute cholangitis, gallstones, etc. However, a relationship of CA 19-9 with prognosis was confirmed in mPDAC [138]. In mPDAC two population-based studies reported a poor prognosis of patients with increased CA 19-9 [44, 45], as three [46, 47, 71] of seven prospective evaluations [48, 50, 70, 72]. Of 19 retrospective studies, eight documented the negative prognostic role of increased CA 19-9 [52, 56, 57, 60, 62, 65, 66, 76] and eleven did not [50, 53, 58, 59, 63, 64, 70, 72, 75, 98], while another study registered a negative effect on OS only for values 10 times higher than normal [84].

The carcinoembryonic antigen (CEA), an oncofetal protein, has been less studied because it is increased in only 30–60% of mPDAC patients [139]. However, increased CEA appeared to be a negative PF in five [46, 57, 58, 75, 140] of nine studies [52, 56, 64, 98]. Contrary to CA 19-9, the reported CEA cut-offs are limited to ranging from 5 to 10 ng/mL.

4.3.5.4 Selected trials

One study documented longer OS for patients with baseline hemoglobin >10 g/dL [24]. Although extensively studied in retrospective studies, the role of NLR was reported in only one RCT, which confirmed the favorable prognostic effect of NLR ≤5 [36, 67].

Seven trials evaluated baseline SA, commonly around a cut-off of 3.2–3.5 g/L, reporting a significant relationship between reduced albumin levels and poor OS in six, as resumed in Table 4.5. A meta-analysis confirmed the unfavorable prognosis of patients with low SA levels (HR 1.69, CI 1.02–2.86; Q = 62.11, p-value <0.0001; I^2 = 93.6%), as shown in Figure 4.2. High serum levels of liver enzymes did not always present a correlation with prognosis. Increased ALP levels were associated with short survival in two studies [22, 38], but not in another [23], and AST did not demonstrate an effect on OS [23]. Conversely, a high serum concentration of the gamma-glutamyltranspeptidase predicted poor OS [39]. Results of the GAMMA trial reported that high blood glucose levels were not prognostic, but high concentrations of glycated hemoglobin correlated with poor OS [38].

TABLE 4.5
Prognostic relationships of serum albumin in selected studies of patients with unresectable or metastatic pancreatic adenocarcinoma receiving upfront treatment

Trial [ref]	Phase	No. pts	Cut-off (ng/mL)	Comparison	Prognostic relationship	Effect size
NCIC 2003 [23]	III	277	NR	low vs. high	No	HR 1.54 (0.97–2.44)
Johnson TIP 2004 [24]	III	688	3.5	< vs. ≥	Yes	HR 1.56
Romanian 2009 [32]	III	297	3.3	< vs. ≥	Yes	NR
PRODIGE-4 2011 [35]	III	342	3.5	< vs. ≥	Yes	HR 1.85 (1.39–2.50)
MPACT 2013 [36, 67]	III	861	3.5	< vs. ≥	Yes	HR 1.06 (1.04–1.08)
GAMMA 2015 (cohort 1) [38]	III	640	ULN	< vs. ≥	Yes	HR 1.61 (1.28–2.04)
GAMMA 2015 (cohort-2) [38]	III	478	ULN	< vs. ≥	Yes	HR 1.75 (1.35–2.33)
MASI 2015 [39]	III	348	3.2	< vs. ≥	Yes	HR 3.33 (2.33–5.00)

Legend: HR, hazard ratio. m, months. NR, not reported. ULN, upper limit normal.

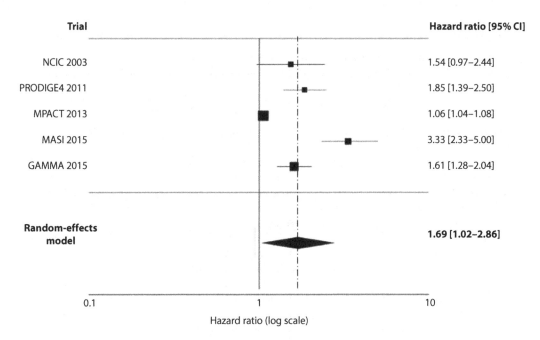

FIGURE 4.2   Forest plot of meta-analysis of baseline serum albumin in prospective trials of patients with unresectable or metastatic pancreatic adenocarcinoma

Data is unclear about the relationship of CA 19-9 with OS. Three studies analyzed CA 19-9, and two reported a negative effect on OS [26, 35, 39], but the cut-offs varied largely. Only one study has documented a negative prognostic role for high CEA [35].

4.4   TUMOR-RELATED PROGNOSTIC FACTORS

4.4.1   TUMOR BURDEN

Although TB is considered a benchmark PF, its determination is difficult. Similarly to other malignancies, the prognosis of oligometastatic disease is better [141], and this is an additional reason why various authors have investigated TB-related measurements.

Primary tumor size was evaluated by fifteen studies [48, 51, 52, 55, 58, 69, 71–77, 84, 90], with four reporting a poor prognosis for longer diameters [48, 55, 69, 71]. The sum of the largest diameters of the target lesions was validated, but has left many doubts because of higher values in patients with multiple sites of metastasis or with more target lesions [48].

At least nineteen studies considered disease status, as locally advanced vs. metastatic, and the occurrence of metastases reduced OS in nine [46, 51, 55, 57, 61, 71, 73, 75, 76] and in seven only after univariate analysis [50, 53, 56, 61, 64, 66, 84], but in four studies it was uninfluent [49, 54, 59, 70].

Even though the number of metastases does not seem an effective PF [84], it was easier to reproduce. Two SEER database analyses were in disagreement about the prognostic role of the number of metastatic sites [142, 143]. Similarly, two population-based studies suggested a better outcome for patients with a single-organ involvement [45, 69], while no differences of OS appeared in other six studies [48, 49, 52, 59, 60, 64].

4.4.1.1   Selected trials

Fourteen studies compared locally advanced versus metastatic PDAC, almost always showing an inverse relationship (Table 4.6). Nine RCTs, including 2,656 patients, reported HR, therefore they

TABLE 4.6

Prognostic relationships of disease status in selected studies of patients with unresectable or metastatic pancreatic adenocarcinoma receiving upfront treatment

Study (ref)	Phase	No. pts	Comparison	Prognostic relationship	Effect size
LiGLA 2001 [19]	III	278	Metastatic vs. LA	Yes	RR 1.97 (1.49–2.60)
ECOG-2297 2002 [21]	III	322	Metastatic vs. LA	No	OS 5.8 vs. 7.5 m
GDFNCLCC 2002 [20]	III	207	Metastatic vs. LA	Yes	HR 1.74 (1.03–2.94)
RMH 2002 [22]	III	209	Metastatic vs. LA	Yes	HR 1.88 (1.31–2.71)
NCIC 2003 [23]	III	277	Metastatic vs. LA	Yes	HR 1.74 (1.32–2.30)
Johnson TIP 2004 [24]	III	688	Metastatic vs. LA	Yes	HR 1.96
GERCOR 2005 [26]	III	313	Metastatic vs. LA	Yes	RR 1.39
Italian 2005 [27]	III	99	Metastatic vs. LA	Yes	HR 2.10 (1.29–3.42)
German 2006 [28]	III	195	Metastatic vs. LA	Yes	HR 1.65 (1.08–2.52)
SGCCR 2007 [30]	III	319	Metastatic vs. LA	Yes	HR 1.49 (1.11–2.00)
ECOG-6201 2009 [31]	III	824	Metastatic vs. LA	Yes	OS 9.2 vs. 5.4 m
GIP-1 2010 [33]	III	399	Metastatic vs. LA	Yes	HR 1.82 (1.34–2.47)
Pfizer AXI 2011 [34]	III	603	Metastatic vs. LA	Yes	HR 2.31 (1.60–3.32)
MASI 2015 [39]	III	348	Metastatic vs. LA	Yes	HR 1.53 (1.10–2.13)

Legend: HR, hazard ratio. LA, locally advanced. m, months. OS, overall survival. RR, risk ratio.

were included in a meta-analysis and an overall ES was calculated (HR 1.76, CI 1.56–1.98; Q = 4.82, p-value = 0.7762; I^2 = 0%) (Figure 4.3).

Other PFs are related to the extent of the disease, such as the number of metastatic sites [24, 35, 37], the extent of T-stage as T4 [26], the size of the metastases [38], the number of target lesions [20]. However, the lack of a standardization has limited their analysis to few studies, which are often not comparable each other.

4.4.2 PRIMARY TUMOR LOCATION

The data are controversial [144]: although a body–tail localization appeared to be associated with poor OS [58, 145, 146], most studies are negative [45–49, 52, 53, 56, 59, 62–64, 71, 73, 84].

The supposed poor prognosis of body–tail mPDAC could be related to a diagnosis at a more advanced stage, but it cannot be excluded that it derives from a different biology, since body–tail tumors more often include tumors of the squamous molecular subtype, with activation of epithelial-mesenchymal transformation genes and other invasive pathways, and less effective immune response [147]. In addition, locoregional growth of body–tail tumors could be faster and associated with high SIR involvement, which would favor chemoresistance [148, 149].

4.4.2.1 Selected trials

Only three RCTs studied the primary tumor location as a PF and found longer median OS for patients with tumors located in the pancreatic head [21, 24, 35].

4.4.3 TIMING OF METASTASIS

The definition of synchronous metastases (SMs) is far from having been standardized, but considering the rapid tumor growth it has been proposed that any metastasis after diagnosis is considered metachronous [150]. Of four retrospective analyses, three reported a poor survival of patients with

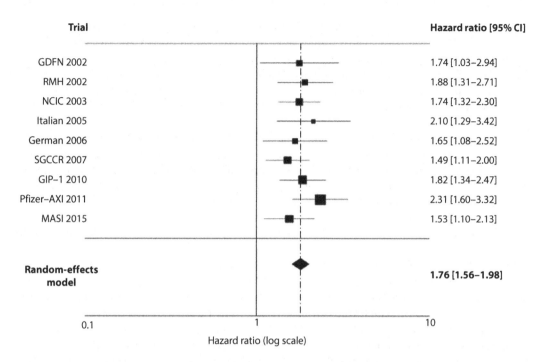

FIGURE 4.3 Forest plot of meta-analysis of disease status in prospective trials of patients with unresectable or metastatic pancreatic adenocarcinoma

SMs only after univariate analysis [56, 59, 65], and another study detected a significantly poor prognosis of patients with unresectable vs. recurrent disease [57].

Some possible effect of surgery on liver metastases (LMs) was suggested for metachronous disease [151, 152] and was poorly studied in SMs [153, 154]. Some effect of metastasectomy for patients with early stage at diagnosis, long disease-free intervals, and single metastasis were documented in SEER data [155].

4.4.3.1 Selected trials
One study investigated the timing of metastasis, and a poor prognosis of SMs was evident [35]. On the other side, other studies that have evaluated the role of previous radical PTR, therefore comparing patients with metachronous vs. SMs, did not find any outcome difference [24, 31, 33].

4.4.4 SITE OF METASTASIS
The most frequent sites of distant metastases of PDAC are the liver and lung, followed by the peritoneum and lymph nodes [143].

LMs occurrence is considered a negative PF [36, 84]. Nine studies documented a significant OS reduction in patients with LMs [45, 47, 48, 59, 62, 64, 65, 84, 98], while the other five did not [52, 53, 58, 61, 70]. A cohort study has suggested that LMs are more frequent at diagnosis in the presence of large PDACs of the pancreatic head with increased liver enzymes and CA 19-9 levels [156].

The lung-limited disease is rare, but published series report good prognosis [157–159], especially for isolated lesions [143]. Other studies confirmed a better OS for patients with lung-limited disease [59, 61, 69], while some authors did not detect any prognostic role [47, 53, 64, 84]. Generally, lung metastases appear later than LMs, and express a different molecular phenotype [160], with higher HER2 amplification rates. The results of the series of patients undergoing resection of lung metastases are promising, but selection biases cannot be excluded [159, 161, 162].

Peritoneal metastases were associated with poor OS [163], albeit they are responsive to modern chemotherapy regimens [164]. Three studies reported a poor prognosis [45, 64, 98], while at least seven experiences were negative [48, 52, 53, 58, 59, 61, 84]. However, given the difficult diagnosis, patients with peritoneal metastases are often excluded from clinical trials. The negative prognostic effect of the peritoneal dissemination could depend on a higher TB or the activation of specific pro-inflammatory pathways, but the measurement of the peritoneal carcinomatosis index (PCI) is limited to a few studies.

The interpretation of the results of studies that have evaluated lymph node metastases is complicated by the need to report the regional or distant site of lymph node involvement separately. While some studies found better outcomes for patients with lymph node limited dissemination [45, 59], other authors suggest poor prognosis for patients with regional [55] or distant lymph node metastases [65], or no prognostic effect [53, 61].

Finally, other sites of metastases, such as bone or brain, are rare and their prognostic role has not been elucidated [69].

4.4.4.1 Selected trials

Seven of eight RCTs reported a negative effect of LMs on OS, and are listed in Table 4.7. An ES of the relationship was available from four articles, comparing 2,018 patients, and a meta-analysis confirmed the reduced OS with LMs occurrence (HR 1.61, CI 1.26–2.07; Q = 3.47, p-value = 0.3241; I^2 = 13.6%) (Figure 4.4).

One study documented a negative prognostic effect of lymph node metastases [39], while two RCTs evaluated extra-abdominal metastases [16, 35], which were related to reduced OS in one [16].

Tumor measurability did not result in any relationship with OS [17, 20, 31].

4.4.5 PATHOLOGY

4.4.5.1 Histology

Rare non-adenocarcinoma histologies did not display different outcomes [84], but some characteristics of adenocarcinoma should be taken into account. In particular, the finding of perineural invasion (PNI) in the PDAC surgical specimen correlated with poor OS [165–167] and was more frequent with advanced stages [168], peritoneal metastases [169] and the prevalence of parasympathetic nerves, that are physiologically absent in the pancreas [170].

TABLE 4.7

Prognostic relationships of liver metastases in selected studies of patients with unresectable or metastatic pancreatic adenocarcinoma receiving upfront treatment

Study [ref]	Phase	No. pts	Comparison	Prognostic relationship	Effect size
NCCTG 1985 [16]	III	184	Yes vs. not	Yes	NR
ECOG-2297 2002 [21]	III	322	Yes vs. not	Yes	NR
Eli-Lilly PEM 2005 [25]	III	565	Yes vs. not	Yes	NR
Romanian 2009 [32]	III	303	Yes vs. not	Yes	NR
PRODIGE-4 2011 [35]	III	342	Yes vs. not	No	HR 1.58 (0.99–2.49)
MPACT 2013 [36, 67]	III	861	Yes vs. not	Yes	HR 1.81 (1.40–2.33)
GAMMA 2015 [38]	III	640	Yes vs. not	Yes	HR 1.82 (1.32–2.53)
MASI 2015 [39]	III	175	Yes vs. not	Yes	HR 1.35 (1.07–1.72)

Legend: HR, hazard ratio. NR, not reported.

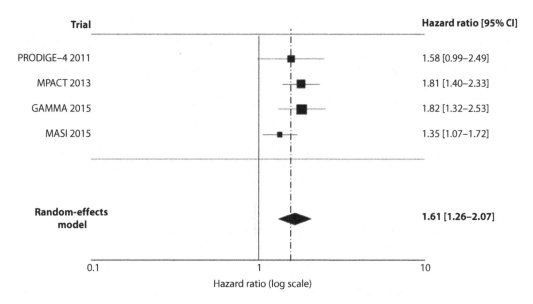

FIGURE 4.4   Forest plot of meta-analysis of liver metastases in prospective trials of patients with unresectable or metastatic pancreatic adenocarcinoma

4.4.5.2   Tumor grade

Considering the frequent difficulty in obtaining large tumor samples at diagnosis in mPDAC, most studies have described short survival for poorly differentiated tumors relying on the previously resected PDAC [171]. Although Ki-67 is associated with aggressive pathologic features and poorly differentiated tumors, its relationship to OS remains debated [172].

In the mPDAC studies, some authors found an association between the tumor grade and the outcome [62, 69], but others did not [53, 64], while a trend towards higher ORRs after FOLFIRINOX has been shown for patients with elevated Ki-67 [85].

4.4.5.3   Molecular biology

Global genomic analyses defined the exome of PDAC [173], and several molecular classifications have been proposed [174–179]. Although two major molecular profiles of PDAC, the classical and the squamous subtype, have been identified with potential therapeutic implications [174], the presence of high heterogeneity at both the inter- and intra-tumoral level limits the relevance of tumor genetics and genomic data [180].

Four frequently mutated genes were identified, such as KRAS, TP53, CDKN2A (p16), and SMAD4 [174], and their coexisting mutations reduced OS [181, 182].

Actionable alterations have been found in up to 25% of PDACs, and in particular, DNA repair dysfunction suggests increased sensitivity to platinum agents and poly-ADP ribose polymerase (PARP) inhibitors [183], but not different outcomes [184]. Other genes have been evaluated in terms of predicting drug response (DPYD, hENT, KRAS, ACOX1), but data on their prognostic role are lacking.

4.4.5.4   Selected trials

One study compared ampulloma with PDAC reporting 56% vs. 31% 6-month survival rates [20]. Three RCTs analyzed the prognostic effect of tumor grade, which correlated with OS in two [21, 24, 28].

4.4.6   PREVIOUS TREATMENTS

The previous radical PTR of patients with metachronous metastases was not prognostic [52, 58, 59, 64, 74, 98], but various authors proposed to reassess the role of the palliative prophylactic

PTR in mPDAC, when feasible, due to the longer median survival of patients after the introduction of new drugs [185, 186]. To date, palliative PTR, vs. bypass procedures, is not clinically justified [187]. A systematic review concluded that in some patients PTR may prolong OS compared to chemotherapy alone, characterizing these patients as having well-differentiated tumors, age <66, tumor size <42 millimeters, and female sex [188]. In addition, a SEER database evaluation of mPDAC patients reported that a partial or complete PTR was associated with improved OS [69].

Although the advantages of managing jaundice and duodenal stenosis by endoscopic procedures compared to surgery are evident [189], placement of a biliary stent for palliation of jaundice, in comparison to patients that did not require a stent, does not appear to affect OS [53, 60].

4.4.6.1   Selected trials

An analysis of the MPACT trial included the previous Whipple procedure among the independent PFs [48], but no prognostic role emerged for a previous PTR in three recent RCTs [24, 31, 33]. Among very old studies evaluating the effect on OS of a palliative surgical approach, two reported a positive relationship [17, 18], and another did not [15].

Similarly, prior treatments such as radiotherapy, adjuvant chemotherapy, or neo-adjuvant chemotherapy [31, 48], as with the placement of a biliary stent, appeared unable to affect mPDAC prognosis [15, 37, 48]. Only in a trial published in 1989 has the prevention or surgical palliation of jaundice and intestinal obstruction shown some favorable effects on OS [18].

4.5   PROGNOSTIC FACTORS IN DECISION-MAKING

The analysis of actionable genomic alterations (MMR, BRCA, NTRK) is recommended for mPDAC patients who are eligible for second-line treatments [190]. Although this indication is based on expert opinions, a small subgroup could benefit from targeted therapies. On the contrary, upfront therapy of mPDAC consists of cytotoxic chemotherapy.

Some PFs should be taken into account in decision-making, as summarized in Table 4.8.

4.5.1   UPFRONT TREATMENT

Two studies documented the superiority of polychemotherapy over gemcitabine [35, 36] and another the superiority of a triplet (NALIRIFOX) over the GnP doublet [191]. However, for patients with ECOG PS >2 best supportive care alone is recommended, while single-agent gemcitabine could be appropriate for some patients with ECOG PS 2.

Generally, the benefit of triplets is more pronounced in patients with good PS and age >65 years. NALIRIFOX does not seem better than GnP in patients with ECOG PS 1, early onset, low number of metastatic sites. If triplet is superior to GnP in the subgroup with at least 3 sites of metastasis, polychemotherapy is always preferred over gemcitabine in patients with 1–2 sites. The toxicity profile of triplets affected the selection criteria of the RCTs, which excluded patients with ECOG PS >1, severe comorbidities, and hyperbilirubinemia (>1.5 ULN) [35, 191]. Similar to the recommendation to reduce doses by 20% for patients >75 years or propose modified triplet regimens, also the alternative GnP doublet requires dose reductions for the elderly [36].

Other variables were under-represented in clinical trials, such as patients with only extra-hepatic or metachronous metastases, with previous biliary stents. Though some authors have suggested a lower efficacy of gemcitabine in tumors of the pancreatic tail [192], generally tail was not analyzed separately from the body. Anyway, body–tail mPDACs reported favorable OS trends after NALIRIFOX vs. GnP, as well as better results of doublet/triplet vs. Gemcitabine.

In addition to the reports from prospective trials, some retrospective analyses support a possible predictive effect of polychemotherapy efficacy for other variables, such as sex, BMI, PTR, NLR, albumin, ALP, and CA 19-9.

TABLE 4.8
Prognostic and predictive variables in clinical decision-making in metastatic pancreatic adenocarcinoma

A. Upfront systemic treatment

1	Performance status

    1. ECOG PS 0: triplet favored (FFX is better than GEM; NFX is better than GnP)

    2. ECOG PS 1: doublet similar to triplet (GnP is similar to NFX)

2	Number of sites of metastasis

    • ≥ 3: triplet favored (NFX is better than GnP)

3	Age

    • <65 years: doublet favored (GnP is better than GEM; GnP is similar to NFX)

B. Treatment of refractory disease (after first-line gemcitabine-based regimens)

1	Performance status

    • ECOG PS 1: doublet favored (nIRI+FU is better than FU)

2	Location

    • Body-tail: doublet favored (nIRI+FU is better than FU)

3	Serum albumin

    • Low (<3.5 g/L): doublet favored (nIRI+FU is better than FU)

4	Age

    • < 65 years: doublet favored (nIRI+FU is better than FU)

5	PFS after first-line chemotherapy

    • short: doublet favored (nIRI+FU is better than FU)

    • long: doublet favored (OXA+FU is better than FU)

6	Timing metastases (at mPDAC diagnosis)

    • Metachronous: doublet favored (nIRI+FU is better than FU)

    • Synchronous: doublet favored (OXA+FU is better than FU)

Legend: ECOG PS, Eastern Cooperative Oncology Group performance status. FFX, FOLFIRINOX. FU, fluorouracil. GEM, gemcitabine. GnP, gemcitabine+nab-paclitaxel. mPDAC, metastatic pancreatic adenocarcinoma. NFX, NALIRIFOX. nIRI, liposomal irinotecan. OXA, oxaliplatin. PFS, progression-free survival.

TABLE 4.9
Prognostic factors evaluated in prospective trials of upfront treatment in patients with unresectable or metastatic pancreatic adenocarcinoma

Suggested	Not suggested	Needing study
Performance status	Age	Sex
Pain	Ethnicity	Body mass index
Weight loss	Geographic area	Hemoglobin
Thromboembolism	Jaundice	NLR
Albumin	Liver enzymes	CEA
	Glycemia	CA 19-9
Disease status	Histotype	Number of metastatic sites
Liver metastases	Tumor grading	Primary tumor location
	Primary tumor resection	Timing of metastases
		Lung metastases
		Nodal metastases

Legend: CA 19-9, Carbohydrate antigen 19-9. CEA, carcino-embryonic antigen. NLR, neutrophil-to-lymphocyte ratio.

In patients with a family history of PDAC and 5–9% of patients with gBRCA1/2 or PALB2 mutations, it is advisable to propose a platinum-based regimen as an upfront regimen. The usefulness of olaparib maintenance for patients with gBRCA mutation after a disease control by platinum-based chemotherapy is still debated, due to the lack of OS improvement [193]. To date, the option to depotentiate the first-line regimen after maximum response should always be evaluated and discussed individually.

4.5.2 TREATMENT OF REFRACTORY DISEASE

Forty percent of patients usually receive second-line, but among them patients with ECOG PS 2, ascites, hypoalbuminemia, and increased ALP report small improvement, if any [135].

In the rare cases of mPDAC with NTRK fusions (>1%), treatment with larotrectinib or entrectinib is recommended, whereas for patients who have MMR-deficient tumors (0.8%), pembrolizumab can be considered. In other cases, the second-line regimen must take into account what drugs were received upfront.

One of the studies that demonstrated a significant OS improvement after progression to upfront gemcitabine-based regimens compared the combination of nanoliposomal irinotecan and fluorouracil with fluorouracil alone [194]. The benefit was more pronounced in patients with poor PS, age <65, male sex, albumin <4 g/L, nonmetastatic disease, body–tail location, and short PFS. In contrast, the results of studies regarding the usefulness of combining oxaliplatin with fluorouracil after gemcitabine-based regimens are conflicting. The only study reporting a benefit suggested a favorable activity in the subgroups of patients with reduced PS, SMs and longer PFS [195].

4.6 CONCLUSION

A large population-based study developed an electronic decision support tool that included most of the above-discussed variables but did not identify individual stratification PFs [48]. On the other hand, a consensus conference defined variables to be measured in mPDAC studies, starting from a list of the most commonly reported PFs in 39 RCTs. After evaluation by 23 experts using a modified Delphi panel, the authors concluded that 12 PFs were mandatory, while 8 were recommended [196].

Considering the evidence that emerged from the 25 selected RCTs and in other studies of mPDAC patients receiving upfront treatments, only seven PFs could be considered evidence-based, while a substantial number deserves further evaluation, as resumed in Table 4.9. We believe that standardization for CA 19-9 cut-off in metastatic disease is urgent. Among the future candidate PFs, BMI, NLR, CEA, primary tumor location and timing of metastases could be the most relevant. At the same time, the relationships between TE and NLR, CEA and LMs in mPDAC patients should be clarified, as well as the role of sex in the patient's immune context and the type of systemic treatment.

Finally, some patient-related variables, such as PS and pain, should be frequently re-evaluated given the remarkable potential as outcome measures.

REFERENCES

1. Huang J, Lok V, Ngai CH, et al. Worldwide burden of, risk factors for, and trends in pancreatic cancer. *Gastroenterology* 2021;160(3):744–54.
2. Xia C, Dong X, Li H, et al. Cancer statistics in China and United States, 2022: Profiles, trends, and determinants. *Chin Med J (Engl)* 2022;135(5):584–90.
3. ECIS – European Cancer Information System, available at: http://ecis.jrc.ec.europa.eu, accessed October 31, 2023.
4. Rawla P, Sunkara T, Gaduputi V. Epidemiology of pancreatic cancer: Global trends, etiology and risk factors. *World J Oncol* 2019;10(1):10–27.

5. Lippi G, Mattiuzzi C. The global burden of pancreatic cancer. *Arch Med Sci* 2020;16(4):820–4.
6. Ferlay J, Partensky C, Bray F. More deaths from pancreatic cancer than breast cancer in the EU by 2017. *Acta Oncol* 2016;55(9–10):1158–60.
7. GBD 2017 Pancreatic Cancer Collaborators. The global, regional, and national burden of pancreatic cancer and its attributable risk factors in 195 countries and territories, 1990–2017: A systematic analysis for the Global Burden of Disease Study 2017. *Lancet Gastroenterol Hepatol* 2019;4:934–47.
8. Smith BD, Smith GL, Hurria A, et al. Future of cancer incidence in the United States: Burdens upon an aging, changing nation. *J Clin Oncol* 2009;27(17):2758–65.
9. Chen X, Yi B, Liu Z, et al. Global regional and national burden of pancreatic cancer 1990 to 2017: Results from the global burden of disease study 2017. *Pancreatol* 2020;20(3):462–9.
10. Hong SB, Choi SH, Kim KW, et al. Meta-analysis of MRI for the diagnosis of liver metastasis in patients with pancreatic adenocarcinoma. *J Magn Reson Imaging* 2020;51(6):1737–44.
11. Wang L, Dong P, Wang WG, Tian BL. Positron emission tomography modalities prevent futile radical resection of pancreatic cancer: A meta-analysis. *Int J Surg* 2017;46:119–25.
12. Li D, Xie K, Wolff R, Abbruzzese JL. Pancreatic cancer. *Lancet* 2004;363(9414):1049–57.
13. Katz MH, Wang H, Fleming JB, et al. Long-term survival after multidisciplinary management of resected pancreatic adenocarcinoma. *Ann Surg Oncol* 2009;16(4):836–47.
14. Swords D, Mulvihill SJ, Firpo MA, et al. Causes of death and conditional survival estimates of medium- and long-term survivors of pancreatic adenocarcinoma. *JAMA Oncol* 2018;4(8):1129–30.
15. Frey C, Twomey P, Keehn R, et al. Randomized study of 5-FU and CCNU in pancreatic cancer: Report of the Veterans Administration Surgical Adjuvant Cancer Chemotherapy Study Group. *Cancer* 1981;47:27–31.
16. Cullinan S, Moertel CG, Wieand HS, et al. A phase III trial on therapy of advanced pancreatic cancer. *Cancer* 1990;65:2207–12.
17. Oster MW, Gray R, Panasci L, et al. Chemotherapy for advanced pancreatic cancer. A comparison of 5-fluorouracil, adriamycin, and mitomycin (FAM) with 5-fluorouracil, streptozotocin, and mitomycin (FSM). *Cancer* 1986;57:29–33.
18. Keating JJ, Johnson PJ, Cochrane AMG, et al. A prospective randomised controlled trial of tamoxifen and cyproterone acetate in pancreatic carcinoma. *Br J Cancer* 1989;60:789–92.
19. Johnson CD, Puntis M, Davidson N, et al. Randomized, dose-finding phase III study of lithium gamolenate in patients with advanced pancreatic adenocarcinoma. *Br J Surg* 2001;88:662–8.
20. Ducreux M, Rougier P, Pignon J-P, et al. A randomised trial comparing 5-FU with 5-FU plus cisplatin in advanced pancreatic carcinoma. *Ann Oncol* 2002;13:1185–91.
21. Berlin JD, Catalano P, Thomas JP, et al. Phase III study of gemcitabine in combination with fluorouracil versus gemcitabine alone in patients with advanced pancreatic carcinoma: Eastern Cooperative Oncology Group Trial E2279. *J Clin Oncol* 2002;20:3270–5.
22. Maisey N, Chau I, Cunningham D, et al. Multicenter randomized phase III trial comparing protracted venous infusion (PVI) fluorouracil (5-FU) with PVI 5-FU plus mitomycin in inoperable pancreatic cancer. *J Clin Oncol* 2002;20:3130–6.
23. Moore MJ, Hamm J, Dancey J, et al. Comparison of gemcitabine versus the matrix metalloproteinase inhibitor BAY 12-9566 in patients with advanced or metastatic adenocarcinoma of the pancreas: A phase III trial of the National Cancer Institute of Canada Clinical Trial Group. *J Clin Oncol* 2003;21:3296–302.
24. Van Cutsem E, van de Velde H, Karasek P, et al. Phase III trial of gemcitabine plus tipifarnib compared with gemcitabine plus placebo in advanced pancreatic cancer. *J Clin Oncol* 2004;22(8):1430–8.
25. Oettle H, Richards D, Ramanathan RK, et al. A phase III trial of pemetrexed plus gemcitabine versus gemcitabina in patients with unresectable or metastatic pancreatic cancer. *Ann Oncol* 2005;16:1639–45.
26. Louvet C, Labianca R, Hammel P, et al. Gemcitabine in combination with oxaliplatin compared with gemcitabine alone in locally advanced or metastatic pancreatic cancer: Results of a GERCOR and GISCAD phase III trial. *J Clin Oncol* 2005;23(15):3509–16.
27. Reni M, Cordio S, Milandri C, et al. Gemcitabine versus cisplatin, epirubicin, fluorouracil, and gemcitabine in advanced pancreatic cancer: A randomised controlled multicentre phase III trial. *Lancet Oncol* 2005;6:369–76.
28. Heinemann V, Quietzsch D, Gieseler F, et al. Randomized phase III trial of gemcitabine plus cisplatin compared with gemcitabine alone in advanced pancreatic cancer. *J Clin Oncol* 2006;24:3946–52.
29. Moore MJ, Goldstein D, Hamm J, et al. Erlotinib plus gemcitabine compared with gemcitabine alone in patients with advanced pancreatic cancer: A phase III trial of the National Cancer Institute of Canada Clinical Trials Group. *J Clin Oncol* 2007;25:1960–6.

30. Herrmann R, Bodoky G, Ruhstaller T, et al. Gemcitabine plus capecitabine compared with gemcitabine alone in advanced pancreatic cancer: A randomized, multicenter, phase III trial of the Swiss Group for Clinical Cancer Research and the Central European Cooperative Oncology Group. *J Clin Oncol* 2007;25:2212–7.

31. Poplin E, Feng Y, Berlin J, et al. Phase III, randomized study of gemcitabine and oxaliplatin versus gemcitabine (fixed-dose rate infusion) compared with gemcitabine (30-minute infusion) in patients with pancreatic carcinoma E6201: A trial of the Eastern Cooperative Oncology Group. *J Clin Oncol* 2009;27:3778–85.

32. Ciuleanu TE, Pavlovsky AV, Bodoky G, et al. A randomised phase III trial of glufosfamide compared with best supportive care in metastatic pancreatic adenocarcinoma previously treated with gemcitabine. *Eur J Cancer* 2009;45:1589–96.

33. Colucci G, Labianca R, Di Costanzo F, et al. Randomized phase III trial of gemcitabine plus cisplatin compared with single-agent gemcitabine as first-line treatment of patients with advanced pancreatic cancer: The GIP-1 study. *J Clin Oncol* 2010;28:1645–51.

34. Kindler HL, Ioka T, Richel D, et al. Axitinib plus gemcitabine versus placebo plus gemcitabine in patients with advanced pancreatic adenocarcinoma: A double-blind randomised phase 3 study. *Lancet Oncol* 2011;12:256–62.

35. Gourgou-Bourgade S, Bascoul-Mollevi C, Desseigne F, et al. Impact of FOLFIRINOX compared with gemcitabine on quality of life in patients with metastatic pancreatic cancer: Results from the PRODIGE 4/ACCORD 11 randomized trial. *J Clin Oncol* 2013;31(1):23–9.

36. Von Hoff DD, Ervin T, Arena FP, et al. Increased survival in pancreatic cancer with nab-paclitaxel plus gemcitabine. *N Engl J Med* 2013;369:1691–703.

37. Middleton G, Silcocks P, Cox T, et al. Gemcitabine and capecitabine with or without telomerase paptide vaccine GV1001 in patients with locally advanced or metastatic pancreatic cancer (TeloVac): An open-label, randomised, phase 3 trial. *Lancet Oncol* 2014;15:829–40.

38. Fuchs CS, Azevedo S, Okusaka T, et al. A phase 3 randomized, double-blind, placebo-controlled trial of ganitumab or placebo in combination with gemcitabine as first-line therapy for metastatic adenocarcinoma of the pancreas: The GAMMA trial. *Ann Oncol* 2015;26:921–7.

39. Deplanque G, Demarchi M, Hebbar M, et al. A randomized, placebo-controlled phase III trial of masitinib plus gemcitabine in the treatment of advanced pancreatic cancer. *Ann Oncol* 2015;26:1194–200.

40. Colloca G. Performance status as prognostic factor in phase III trials of first-line chemotherapy of unresectable or metastatic pancreatic cancer: A trial-level meta-analysis. *Asia Pac J Clin Oncol* 2021;18(3):232–9.

41. Cheng S, Qureshi M, Pullenayegum E, et al. Do patients with reduced or excellent performance status derive the same clinical benefit from novel systemic cancer therapies? A systematic review and meta-analysis. *ESMO Open* 2017;2:e000225.

42. Storniolo AM, Enas NH, Brown CA, et al. An investigational new drug treatment program for patients with gemcitabine. *Cancer* 1999;85:1261–8.

43. Tabernero J, Chiorean G, Infante JR, et al. Prognostic factors of survival in a randomized phase III trial (MPACT) of weekly nab-paclitaxel plus gemcitabine versus gemcitabine alone in patients with metastatic pancreatic cancer. *Oncologist* 2015;20:143–50.

44. Strijker M, van Veldhuisen E, van der Geest LG, et al. Readily available biomarkers predict poor survival in metastatic pancreatic cancer. *Biomarkers* 2021;26(4):325–34.

45. van den Boorn HG, Dijksterhuis WPM, van der Geest LGM, et al. SOURC-PANC: A prediction model for patients with metastatic pancreatic ductal adenocarcinoma based on nationwide population-based data. *J Natl Compr Canc Netw* 2021;19(9):1045–53.

46. Ishii H, Okada S, Nose H, et al. Prognostic factors in patients with advanced pancreatic cancer treated with systemic chemotherapy. *Pancreas* 1996;12(3):267–71.

47. Hang J, Wu L, Zhu L, et al. Prediction of overall survival for metastatic pancreatic cancer: Development and validation of a prognostic nomogram with data from open clinical trial and real-world study. *Cancer Med* 2018;7(7):2974–84.

48. Goldstein D, Von Hoff DD, Chiorean EG, et al. Nomogram for estimating overall survival in patients with metastatic pancreatic cancer. *Pancreas* 2020;49:744–50.

49. Nordgård O, Lapin M, Tjensvoll K, et al. Prognostic value of disseminated tumor cells in unresectable pancreatic ductal adenocarcinoma: A prospective observational study. *BMC Cancer* 2022;22(1):609.

50. Lim SH, Yun J, Lee MY, et al. Gemcitabine and erlotinib with or without oxaliplatin in previously untreated advanced pancreatic cancer: A randomized phase II trial. *Yonsei Med J* 2021;62(8):671–8.

51. Cubiella J, Castells A, Fondevila C, et al. Prognostic factors in nonresectable pancreatic adenocarcinoma: A rationale to design therapeutic trials. *Am J Gastroenterol* 1999;94(5):1271–8.

52. Ueno H, Okada S, Okusaka T, Ikeda M. Prognostic factors in patients with metastatic pancreatic adenocarcinoma receiving systemic chemotherapy. *Oncology* 2000;59:296–301.

53. Maréchal R, Demols A, Gay F, et al. Prognostic factors and prognostic index for chemonaïve and gemcitabine-refractory patients with advanced pancreatic cancer. *Oncology* 2007;73(1–2):41–51.

54. Matsubara J, Ono M, Honda K, et al. Survival prediction for pancreatic cancer patients receiving gemcitabine treatment. *Mol Cell Proteomics* 2010;9(4):695–704.

55. Hamada T, Nakai Y, Yasunaga H, et al. Prognostic nomogram for nonresectable pancreatic cancer treated with gemcitabine-based chemotherapy. *Br J Cancer* 2014;110(8):1943–9.

56. Xue P, Zhu L, Wan Z, et al. A prognostic index model to predict the clinical outcomes for advanced pancreatic cancer patients following palliative chemotherapy. *J Cancer Res Clin Oncol* 2015;141(9):1653–60.

57. Kou T, Kanai M, Yamamoto M, et al. Prognostic model for survival based on readily available pretreatment factors in patients with advanced pancreatic cancer receiving palliative chemotherapy. *Int J Clin Oncol* 2016;21(1):118–25.

58. Park HS, Lee HS, Park JS, et al. Prognostic scoring index for patients with metastatic pancreatic adenocarcinoma. *Cancer Res Treat* 2016;48(4):1253–63.

59. Colloca GA, Venturino A, Guarneri D. Second-generation inflammation-related scores are more effective than systemic inflammation ratios in predicting prognosis of patients with unresectable or metastatic pancreatic cancer receiving cytotoxic chemotherapy. *Med Oncol* 2018;35(12):158.

60. Fernández A, Salgado M, García A, et al. Prognostic factors for survival with nab-paclitaxel plus gemcitabine in metastatic pancreatic cancer in real-life practice: The ANICE-PaC study. *BMC Cancer* 2018;18(1):1185.

61. Lecuelle J, Aarnink A, Tharin Z, et al. Using exome sequencing to improve prediction of FOLFIRINOX first efficacy for pancreatic adenocarcinoma. *Cancers* 2021;13:1851.

62. Taieb J, Seufferlein T, Reni M, et al. Treatment sequences and prognostic/predictive factors in metastatic pancreatic ductal adenocarcinoma: Univariate and multivariate analyses of a real-world study in Europe. *BMC Cancer* 2023;23(1):877.

63. Varzaru B, Iacob RA, Croitoru AE, et al. Real-life results of palliative chemotherapy in metastatic pancreatic ductal adenocarcinoma. *Cancers* 2023;15:3500.

64. Yi JH, Lee J, Park SH, et al. A prognostic model to predict clinical outcomes with first-line gemcitabine-based chemotherapy in advanced pancreatic cancer. *Oncology* 2011;80(3–4):175–80.

65. Hwang I, Kang J, Ip HNN, et al. Prognostic factors in patients with metastatic or recurrent pancreatic cancer treated with first-line nab-paclitaxel plus gemcitabine: Implication of inflammation-based scores. *Invest New Drugs* 2019;37(3):584–90.

66. Tingle SJ, Severs GR, Goodfellow M, et al. NARCA: A novel prognostic scoring system using neutrophil-albumin ratio and Ca19-9 to predict overall survival in palliative pancreatic cancer. *J Surg Oncol* 2018;118(4):680–6.

67. Goldstein D, El-Maraghi RH, Hammel P, et al. *nab*-paclitaxel plus gemcitabine for metastatic pancreatic cancer: Long-term survival from a pgase III trial. *J Natl Cancer Inst* 2015;107(2):dju413.

68. Scheithauer W, Tamanathan RK, Moore M, et al. Dose modification and efficacy of nab-paclitaxel plus gemcitabine vs. gemcitabine for patients with metastatic pancreatic cancer: Phase III MPACT trial. *J Gastrointest Oncol* 2016;7:469–78.

69. Ma X, Guo J, Zhang C, Bai J. Development of a prognostic nomogram for metastatic pancreatic ductal adenocarcinoma integrating marital status. *Sci Rep* 2022;12(1):7124.

70. Alpertunga I, Sadiq R, Pandya D, et al. Glycemic control as an early prognostic marker in advanced pancreatic cancer. *Front Oncol* 2021;11:571855.

71. Deng QL, Dong S, Wang L, et al. Development and validation of a nomogram for predicting survival in patients with advanced pancreatic ductal adenocarcinoma. *Sci Rep* 2017;7(1):11524.

72. Comito T, Massaro M, Teriaca MA, et al. Can STEreotactic Body Radiation Therapy (SBRT) improve the prognosis of unresectable locally advanced pancreatic cancer? long-term clinical outcomes, toxicity and prognostic factors on 142 patients (STEP Study). *Curr Oncol* 2023;30:7073–88.

73. Glen P, Jamieson NB, McMillan DC, et al. Evaluation of an inflammation-based prognostic score in patients with inoperable pancreatic cancer. *Pancreatology* 2006;6(5):450–3.

74. Jamal MH, Doi SA, Simoneau E, et al. Unresectable pancreatic adenocarcinoma: Do we know who survives? *HPB* 2010;12(8):561–6.

75. Gao S, Wu M, Chen Y, et al. Lactic dehydrogenase to albumin ratio in prediction of unresectable pancreatic cancer with intervention chemotherapy. *Future Oncol* 2018;14(14):1377–86.

76. Zhang K, Gao HF, Mo M, et al. A novel scoring system based on hemostatic parameters predicts the prognosis of patients with advanced pancreatic cancer. *Pancreatol* 2019;19(2):346–51.

77. Berger AK, Abel U, Komander C, et al. Chemotherapy for advanced pancreatic adenocarcinoma in elderly patients (>70 years of age): A retrospective cohort study at the national center for tumor diseases Heidelberg. *Pancreatol* 2014;14(3):211–5.

78. Macchini M, Chiaravalli M, Zanon S, et al. Chemotherapy in elderly patients with pancreatic cancer; efficacy, feasibility and future perspectives. *Cancer Treat Rev* 2019;72:1–6.

79. Van der Geest LGM, Besselink MGH, van Gestel YRBM, et al. Pancreatic cancer surgery in elderly patients: Balancing between short-term harm and long-term benefit. A population-based study in the Netherlands. *Acta Oncol* 2016;55(3):278–85.

80. van Dongen JC, van der Geest LGM, de Meijer VE, et al. Age and prognosis in patients with pancreatic cancer: A population-based study. *Acta Oncol* 2022;61(3):286–93.

81. Marechal R, Delmos A, Fay F, et al. Tolerance and efficacy of gemcitabine and gemcitabine-based regimens in elderly patients with advanced pancreatic cancer. *Pancreas* 2008;36(3):e16–21.

82. Garcia G, Odaimi M. Systemic combination chemotherapy in elderly pancreatic cancer: A review. *J Gastrointest Cancer* 2017;48:121–8.

83. Nakazawa J, et al. A multicenter retrospective study of gemcitabine plus nab-paclitaxel or FOLFIRINOX in metastatic pancreatic cancer: NAPOLEON study. *Ann Oncol* 2019;30:iv17–18.

84. Shibuki T, Mizuta T, Shimokawa M, et al. Prognostic nomogram for patients with unresectable pancreatic cancer treated with gemcitabine plus nab-paclitaxel or FOLFIRINOX: A post-hoc analysis of a multicenter retrospective study in Japan (NAPOLEON study). *BMC Cancer* 2022;22:19.

85. Hohla F, Hopfinger G, Romeder F, et al. Female gender may predict response to FOLFIRINOX in patients with unresectable pancreatic cancer: A single institution retrospective review. *Int J Oncol* 2014;44(1):319–26.

86. Lambert A, Jarlier M, Gourgou Bourgade S, et al. Response to FOLFIRINOX by gender in patients with metastatic pancreatic cancer: Results from the PRODIGE 4/ACCORD 11 randomized trial. *PLoS ONE* 2017;12(9):e0183288.

87. Zhang J, Dhakal I, Ning B, et al. Patterns and trends of pancreatic cancer mortality rates in Arkansas, 1969–2002: A comparison with the US population. *Eur J Cancer Prev* 2008;17:18–27.

88. CAoSA. Factsheet on Pancreatic Cancer [Fact Sheet]. 2014 [cited 2020 2 April], available at: https://www.cansa.org.za/files/2020/02/Fact-Sheet-on-Pancreatic-Cancer-NCR-2014-web-February-2020.pdf

89. Shi Y-Q, Yang J, Du P, et al. Effect of body mass index on overall survival of pancreatic cancer: A meta-analysis. *Medicine* 2016;95(14):e3305.

90. Larsson SC, Orsini N, Wolk A. Body mass index and pancreatic cancer risk: A meta-analysis of prospective studies. *Int J Cancer* 2007;120:1993–8.

91. Stolsenberg-Solomon RZ, Graubard BI, Chiari S, et al. Insulin, glucose, insulin resistance, and pancreatic cancer in male smokers. *J Am Med Assoc* 2005;294:2872–8.

92. Yuan C, Bao Y, Wu C, et al. Prediagnostic body mass index and pancreatic cancer survival. *J Clin Oncol* 2013;31:4229–34.

93. Carreras-Torres R, Johansson M, Gaborieau V, et al. The role of obesity, Type 2 diabetes, and metabolic factors in pancreatic cancer: A Mendelian randomization study. *J Natl Cancer Inst* 2017;109(9):djx012.

94. Dalal S, Hui D, Bidaut L, et al. Relationship among body mass index, longitudinal body composition alterations, and survival in patients with locally advanced pancreatic cancer receiving chemoradiation: A pilot study. *J Pain Symptom Manage* 2012;44(2):181–91.

95. D'Haese JG, Hartel M, Demir IE, et al. Pain sensation in pancreatic diseases is not uniform: The different facets of pancreatic pain. *World J Gastroenterol* 2014;20(27):9154–61.

96. Mercadante S, Tirelli W, David F, et al. Morphine versus oxycodone in pancreatic cancer pain: A randomized controlled study. *Clin J Pain* 2010;26:794–7.

97. Burris HA, Moore MJ, Andersen J, et al. Improvement in survival and clinical benefit with gemcitabine as first-line therapy for patients with advanced pancreas cancer: A randomized trial. *J Clin Oncol* 1997;15:2403–13.

98. Morizane C, Okusaka T, Morita S, et al. Construction and validation of a prognostic index for patients with metastatic pancreatic adenocarcinoma. *Pancreas* 2011;40:415–21.

99. Chatterjee D, Katz MH, Rashid A, et al. Perineural and intraneural invasion in post-therapy pancreaticoduodenectomy specimens predicts poor prognosis in patients with pancreatic ductal adenocarcinoma. *Am J Surg Pathol* 2012;36(3):409–17.

100. Choi Y, Kim T-Y, Lee K-H, et al. The impact of body mass index dynamics on survival of patients with advanced pancreatic cancer receiving chemotherapy. *J Pain Symptom Manage* 2014;48(1):13–25.
101. Vasconcelos de Matos L, Coelho A, Cunha R, et al. Association of weight change, inflammation markers and disease staging with survival of patients undergoing chemotherapy for pancreatic adenocarcinoma. *Nutr Cancer* 2022;74(2):546–54.
102. Bachmann J, Buchler MW, Friess H, et al. Cachexia in patients with chronic pancreatitis and pancreatic cancer: Impact on survival and outcome. *Nutr Cancer* 2013;65:827–33.
103. Bachmann J, Heiligensetzer M, Krakowski-Roosen H, et al. Cachexia worsens prognosis in patients with resectable pancreatic cancer. *J Gastrointest Surg* 2008;12:1193–201.
104. Kong H-H, Kim K-W, Ko Y-S, et al. Longitudinal changes in body composition of long-term survivors of pancreatic head cancer and factors affecting the changes. *J Clin Med* 2021;10:3436.
105. Williet N, Fovet M, Maoui K, et al. A low total psoas muscle area index is a strong prognostic factor in metastatic pancreatic cancer. *Pancreas* 2021;50(4):579–86.
106. Martignoni ME, Kunze P, Hildebrandt W, et al. Role of mononuclear cells and inflammatory cytokines in pancreatic cancer-related cachexia. *Clin Cancer Res* 2005;11:5802–8.
107. Epstein AS, Soff GA, Capanu M, et al. Analysis of incidence and clinical outcomes in patients with thromboembolic events and invasive exocrine pancreatic cancer. *Cancer* 2012;118(12):3053–61.
108. Ishigaki K, Nakai Y, Isayama H, et al. Thromboembolisms in advanced pancreatic cancer: A retrospective analysis of 475 patients. *Pancreas* 2017;46(8):1069–75.
109. Suzuki T, Hori R, Takeuchi K, et al. Venous thromboembolism in Japanese patients with pancreatic cancer. *Clin Appl Thromb Hemost* 2021;27:1–6.
110. Blom JW, Osanto S, Rosendaal FR, et al. High risk of venous thrombosis in patients with pancreatic cancer: A cohort study of 202 patients. *Eur J Cancer* 2006;42(3):410–4.
111. Frere C, Bournet B, Gourgou S, et al. Incidence of venous thromboembolism in patients with newly diagnosed pancreatic cancer and factors associated with outcomes. *Gastroenterol* 2020;158(5):1346–58.
112. Khorana AA, Francis CW, Culakova E, et al. Thromboembolism is a leading cause of death in cancer patients receiving outpatient chemotherapy. *J Thromb Hemost* 2007;5:632–4.
113. Menapace LA, Peterson DR, Berry A, et al. Symptomatic and incidental thromboembolism are both associated with mortality in pancreatic cancer. *Thromb Hemost* 2011;106:371–8.
114. Sorensen HT, Mellemkjaer L, Olsen JH, et al. Prognosis of cancer associated with venous thromboembolism. *N Engl J Med* 2000;343:1846–50.
115. Kim JS, Kang EJ, Kim DS, et al. Early venous thromboembolism at the beginning of palliative chemotherapy is a poor prognostic factor in patients with metastatic pancreatic cancer: A retrospective study. *BMC Cancer* 2018;18:1260.
116. Yamashita Y, Morimoto T, Amano H, et al. Anticoagulation therapy for venous thromboembolism in the real world – from the COMMAND VTE registry. *Circ J* 2018;82(5):1262–70.
117. Ueno H, Ikeda M, Ueno M, et al. Phase I/II study of nab-paclitaxel plus gemcitabine for chemotherapy-naive Japanese patients with metastatic pancreatic cancer. *Cancer Chemother Pharmacol* 2016;77(3):595–603.
118. Barrau M, Maoui K, Le Roy B, et al. Early venous thromboembolism is a strong prognostic factor in patients with advanced pancreatic ductal adenocarcinoma. *J Cancer Res Clin Oncol* 2021;147(1):3447–54.
119. Okushi Y, Kusunose K, Okayama Y, et al. Acute hospital mortality of venous thromboembolism in patients with cancer from registry data. *J Am Heart Assoc* 2021;10:e019373.
120. Ohashi Y, Ikeda M, Kunitoh H, et al. Venous thromboembolism in cancer patients: Report of baseline data from the multicentre, prospective Cancer-VTE Registry. *Jpn J Clin Oncol* 2020;50(11):1246–53.
121. Khorana AA, Francis CW, Menzies KE, et al. Plasma tissue factor may be predictive of venous thromboembolism in pancreatic cancer. *J Thromb Hemost* 2008;6:1983–5.
122. Poruk KE, Firpo MA, Huerter LM, et al. Serum platelet factor 4 is an independent predictor of survival and venous thromboembolism in patients with pancreatic adenocarcinoma. *Cancer Epidemiol Biomarkers* 2010;19(10):2605–10.
123. Kasthuri RS, Hisada Y, Ilich A, et al. Effect of chemotherapy and longitudinal analysis of circulating extracellular vesicle tissue factor activity in patients with pancreatic and colorectal cancer. *Res Pract Thromb Haemost* 2020;4:636–43.
124. Giustozzi M, Curcio A, Weijs B, et al. Variation in the association between antineoplastic therapies and venous thromboembolism in patients with active cancer. *Thromb Haemost* 2020;120(5):847–56.
125. Munoz Martin AJ, Font Puig C, Navarro Martin LM, et al. Clinical guide SEOM on venous thromboembolism in cancer patients. *Clin Transl Oncol* 2014;16(10):927–30.

126. van Es N, Franke VF, Middeldorp S, et al. The Khorana score for the prediction of venous thromboembolism in patients with pancreatic cancer. *Thromb Res* 2017;150:30–2.

127. Kadokura M, Ishida Y, Tatsumi A, et al. Performance status and neutrophil-lymphocyte ratio are important prognostic factors in elderly patients with unresectable pancreatic cancer. *J Gastrointest Oncol* 2016;7(6):982–8.

128. Dolan RD, Laird BJA, Klepstad P, et al. An exploratory study examining the relationship between performance status and systemic inflammation frameworks and cytokine profiles in patients with advanced cancer. *Medicine* 2019;98(37):e17019.

129. Kobayashi S, Ueno M, Kameda R, et al. Duodenal stenting followed by systemic chemotherapy for patients with pancreatic cancer and gastric outlet obstruction. *Pancreatol* 2016;16:1085–91.

130. Colloca G, Venturino A. Peripheral blood cell variables related to systemic inflammation in patients with unresectable or metastatic pancreatic cancer: A systematic review and meta-analysis. *Pancreas* 2021;50(8):1131–6.

131. Colloca GA, Venturino A. Baseline serum albumin as a prognostic factor of patients receiving systemic chemotherapy for metastatic pancreatic adenocarcinoma: A systematic review and meta-analysis. *Acta Oncol* 2024; in press.

132. Kowalski-Saunders PW, Winwood PJ, Arthur MJ, et al. Reversible inhibition of albumin production by rat hepatocytes maintained on a laminin-rich gel (Engelbreth-Holm-Swarm) in response to secretory products of Kuppfer cells and cytokines. *Hepatol* 1992;16:733–41.

133. Barber MD, Ross JA, Fearon KC. Changes in nutritional, functional, and inflammatory markers in advanced pancreatic cancer. *Nutr Cancer* 1999;35:106–10.

134. Wu D, Wang X, Shi G, et al. Prognostic and clinical significance of modified Glasgow prognostic score in pancreatic cancer: A meta-analysis of 4,629 patients. *Aging* 2021;13(1):1410–21.

135. Yu K, Ozer M, Cockrum P, et al. Real-world prognostic factors for survival among treated patients with metastatic pancreatic ductal adenocarcinoma *Cancer Med* 2021;10:8934–43.

136. Ma J, Wang J, Ge L, et al. The impact of diabetes mellitus on clinical outcomes following chemotherapy for the patients with pancreatic cancer: A meta-analysis. *Acta Diabetol* 2019;56(10):1103–11.

137. Pretta A, Ziranu P, Puzzoni M, et al. Retrospective survival analysis in patients with metastatic pancreatic ductal adenocarcinoma with insulin-treated type 2 diabetes mellitus. *Tumori* 2021;107(6):550–5.

138. Ballehaninna UK, Chamberlain RS. The clinical utility of serum CA 19–9 in the diagnosis, prognosis and management of pancreatic adenocarcinoma: An evidence based appraisal. *J Gastrointest Oncol* 2012;3:105–19.

139. Satake K, Chung YS, Yokomatsu H, et al. A clinical evaluation of various tumor markers for the diagnosis of pancreatic cancer. *Int J Pancreatol* 1990;7:25–36.

140. Imaoka H, Mizuno N, Hara K, et al. Prognostic impact of carcinoembryonic antigen (CEA) on patients with metastatic pancreatic cancer. A retrospective cohort study. *Pancreatol* 2016;16(5):859–64.

141. Takeda T, Sasaki T, Okamoto T, et al. Outcomes of pancreatic cancer with oligometastasis. *J Hepatobiliary Pancreat Sci* 2023;30(2):229–39.

142. Feng F, Cai W, Wang G, et al. Metastatic pancreatic adenocarcinomas could be classified into M1a and M1b category by the number of metastatic organs. *BMC Gastroenterol* 2020;20:89.

143. Oweira H, Petrausch U, Helbling D, et al. Prognostic value of site-specific metastases in pancreatic adenocarcinoma: A Surveillance Epidemiology and End Results database analysis. *World J Gastroenterol* 2017;23(10):1872–80.

144. Sohn TA, Yeo CJ, Camerol JL, et al. Resected adenocarcinoma of the pancreas – 616 patients: Results, outcomes, and prognostic indicators. *J Gastrointest Surg* 2000;4(6):567–79.

145. Artinyan A, Soriano PA, Prendergast C, et al. The anatomic location of pancreatic cancer is a prognostic factor for survival. *HPB* 2008;10(5):371–6.

146. Dreyer SB, Jamieson NB, Upstill-Goddard R, et al. Defining the molecular pathology of pancreatic body and tail adenocarcinoma. *Br J Surg* 2018;105(2):e183–91.

147. Ling Q, Xu X, Zheng SS, et al. The diversity between pancreatic head and body/tail cancers: Clinical parameters and in vitro models. *Hepatobiliary Pancreat Dis Int* 2013;12(5):480–7.

148. Colloca GA, Venturino A, Guarneri D. Retrospective analysis by site of primary tumor of patients with unresectable locally advanced or metastatic pancreatic adenocarcinoma receiving chemotherapy. *Clin Exp Metastasis* 2019;36(6):519–25.

149. Mukhija D, Sohal DPS, Khorana AA. Adjuvant treatment in potentially curable pancreatic cancer need to include tumor location in the equation? *Pancreas* 2018;47(8):e50–2.

150. Dong S, Wang L, Guo YB, et al. Risk factors of liver metastasis from advanced pancreatic adenocarcinoma: A large multicenter cohort study. *World J Surg Oncol* 2017;15:120.

151. Dunschede F, Will L, von Langsdorf C, et al. Treatment of metachronous and simultaneous liver metastases of pancreatic cancer. *Eur Surg Res* 2010;44:209–13.

152. Gleisner AL, Assumpcao L, Cameron JL, et al. Is resection of periampullary or pancreatic adenocarcinoma with synchronous hepatic metastasis justified? *Cancer* 2007;110(11):2484–92.

153. Hackert T, Niesen W, Hinz U, et al. Radical surgery of oligometastatic pancreatic cancer. *Eur J Surg Oncol* 2017;43(2):358–63.

154. Tachezy M, Gebauer F, Janot M, et al. Synchronous resections of hepatic oligometastatic pancreatic cancer: Disputing a principle in a time of safe pancreatic operations in a retrospective multicenter analysis. *Surgery* 2016;160(1):136–44.

155. Liu Q, Zhang R, Michalski CW, et al. Surgery for synchronous and metachronous single-organ metastasis of pancreatic cancer: A SEER database analysis and systematic literature review. *Sci Rep* 2020;10:4444.

156. Zang Y, Fan Y, Gao Z. Pretreatment C-reactive protein/albumin ratio for predicting overall survival in pancreatic cancer. A meta-analysis. *Medicine* 2020;99:23.

157. Arnaoutakis GJ, Rangachari D, Laheru DA, et al. Pulmonary resection for isolated pancreatic adenocarcinoma metastasis: An analysis of outcomes and survival. *J Gastrointest Surg* 2011;15:1611–7.

158. Thomas RM, Truty MJ, Nogueras-Gonzalez GM, et al. Selective reoperation for locally recurrent or metastatic pancreatic ductal adenocarcinoma following primary pancreatic resection. *J Gastrointest Surg* 2012;16:1696–704.

159. Ilmer M, Schiergens TS, Renz BW, et al. Oligometastatic pulmonary metastasis in pancreatic cancer patients: Safety and outcome of resection. *Surg Oncol* 2019;31:16–21.

160. Yachida S, Jones S, Bozic I, et al. Distant metastasis occurs late during the genetic evolution of pancreatic cancer. *Nature* 2010;467:1114–7.

161. Groot VP, Blair AB, Gemenetzis G, et al. Isolated pulmonary recurrence after resection of pancreatic cancer: The effect of patient factors and treatment modalities on survival. *HPB* 2019;21(8):998–1008.

162. Okui M, Yamamichi T, Asakawa A, et al. Resection for pancreatic cancer lung metastases. *Korean J Thorac Cardiovasc Surg* 2017;50:326–8.

163. Thomassen I, Lemmens VEPP, Nienhuijs SW, et al. Incidence, prognosis, and possible treatment strategies of peritoneal carcinomatosis of pancreatic origin: A population-based study. *Pancreas* 2013;42:72–5.

164. Takeda T, Sasaki T, Mie T, et al. Improved prognosis of pancreatic cancer patients with peritoneal metastasis. *Pancreatol* 2021;21(5):903–11.

165. Mitsunaga S, Hasebe T, Kinoshita T, et al. Detail histologic analysis of nerve plexus invasion in invasive ductal carcinoma of the pancreas and its prognostic impact. *Am J Surg Pathol* 2007;31(11):1636–44.

166. Chen JW, Bhandari M, Astill DS, et al. Predicting patient survival after pancreatico-duodenectomy for malignancy: Histopathological criteria based on perineural infiltration and lymphovascular invasion. *HPB* 2010;12(2):101–8.

167. Garcea G, Dennison AR, Ong SL, et al. Tumour characteristics predictive of survival following resection for ductal adenocarcinoma of the head of pancreas. *Eur J Surg Oncol* 2007;33(7):892–7.

168. Crippa S, Pergolini I, Javed AA, et al. Implications of perineural invasion on disease recurrence and survival after pancreatectomy for pancreatic head ductal adenocarcinoma. *Ann Surg* 2022;276(2):378–85.

169. Tanaka M, Mihaljevic AL, Probst P, et al. Meta-analysis of recurrence pattern after resection for pancreatic cancer. *Br J Surg* 2019;106(12):1590–601.

170. Zhang L, Guo L, Tao M, et al. Parasympathetic neurogenesis is strongly associated with tumor budding and correlates with an adverse prognosis in pancreatic ductal adenocarcinoma. *Chin J Cancer Res* 2016;28(2):180–6.

171. Hartwig W, Hackert T, Hinz U, et al. Pancreatic cancer surgery in the new millennium: Better prediction of outcome. *Ann Surg* 2011;254:311–9.

172. Ansari D, Rosendahl A, Elebro J, et al. Systematic review of immunohistochemical biomarkers to identify prognostic subgroups of patients with pancreatic cancer. *Br J Surg* 2011;98:1041–55.

173. Jones S, Zhang X, Parsons DW, et al. Core signaling pathways in human pancreatic cancers revealed by global genomic analyses. *Science* 2008;321(5897):1801–6.

174. Aung KL, Fischer SE, Denroche RE, et al. Genomics-driven precision medicine for advanced pancreatic cancer: Early results from the COMPASS Trial. *Clin Cancer Res* 2018;24(6):1344–54.

175. Bailey P, Chang DK, Nones K, et al. Genomic analyses identify molecular subtypes of pancreatic cancer. *Nature* 2016;531(7592):47–52.

176. Collisson EA, Sadanandam A, Olson P, et al. Subtypes of pancreatic ductal adenocarcinoma and their differing responses to therapy. *Nat Med* 2011;17(4):500–3.

177. Moffitt RA, Marayati R, Flate EL, et al. Virtual microdissection identifies distinct tumor- and stroma-specific subtypes of pancreatic ductal adenocarcinoma. *Nat Genet* 2015;47(10):1168–78.
178. Puleo F, Nicolle R, Blum Y, et al. Stratification of pancreatic ductal adenocarcinomas based on tumor and microenvironment features. *Gastroenterology* 2018;155(6):1999–2013.e3.
179. Birnbaum DJ, Finetti P, Birnbaum D, et al. Validation and comparison of the molecular classifications of pancreatic carcinomas. *Mol Cancer* 2017;16(1):168.
180. Gutiérrez ML, Muñoz-Bellvís L, Orfao A. Genomic heterogeneity of pancreatic ductal adenocarcinoma and its clinical impact. *Cancers* 2021;13:4451.
181. Rachakonda PS, Bauer AS, Xie H, et al. Somatic mutations in exocrine pancreatic tumors: Association with patient survival. *PLoS ONE* 2013;8(4):e60870.
182. Yachida S, White CM, Naito Y, et al. Clinical significance of the genetic landscape of pancreatic cancer and implications for identification of potential long-term survivors. *Clin Cancer Res* 2012;18(22):6339–47.
183. Hayashi H, Higashi T, Miyata T, et al. Recent advances in precision medicine for pancreatic ductal adenocarcinoma. *Ann Gastroenterol Surg* 2021;5(4):457–66.
184. Lowery MA, Wong W, Jordan EJ, et al. Prospective evaluation of germline alterations in patients with exocrine pancreatic neoplasms. *J Natl Cancer Inst* 2018;110(10):1067–74.
185. Perinel J, Adham M. Palliative therapy in pancreatic cancer – Palliative surgery. *Transl Gastroenterol Hepatol* 2019;4:28.
186. Sakaguchi T, Valente R, Tanaka K, et al. Surgical treatment of metastatic pancreatic ductal adenocarcinoma: A review of current literature. *Pancreatol* 2019;19(5):672–80.
187. Gillen S, Schuster T, Friess H, et al. Palliative resections versus bypass procedures in pancreatic cancer – A systematic review. *Am J Surg* 2012;203(4):496–502.
188. Nie D, Lai G, An G, et al. Individualized prediction of survival benefits of pancreatectomy plus chemotherapy in patients with simultaneous metastatic pancreatic cancer. *Front Oncol* 2021;11:719253.
189. Azemoto N, Ueno M, Yanagimoto H, et al. Endoscopic duodenal stent placement versus gastrojejunostomy for unresectable pancreatic cancer patients with duodenal stenosis before introduction of initial chemotherapy (GASPACHO study): A multicenter retrospective study. *Jpn J Clin Oncol* 2022;52(2):134–42.
190. Sohal DPS, Kennedy EB, Cinar P, et al. Metastatic pancreatic cancer: ASCO guideline update. *J Clin Oncol* 2020;38(27):3217–30.
191. Wainberg ZA, Melisi D, Macarulla T, et al. NALIRIFOX versus nab-paclitaxel and gemcitabine in treatment-naive patients with metastatic pancreatic ductal adenocarcinoma (NAPOLI 3): A randomised, open-label, phase 3 trial. *Lancet* 2023;402(10409):1272–81.
192. Mukhija D, Sohal DPS, Khorana AA. Adjuvant treatment in potentially curable pancreatic cancer need to include tumor location in the equation? *Pancreas* 2018;47(8):e50–e52.
193. Golan T, Hammel P, Reni M, et al. Maintenance Olaparib for germline *BRCA*-mutated metastatic pancreatic cancer. *N Engl J Med* 2019;381(4):317–27.
194. Wang-Gillam A, Li CP, Bodoky G, et al. Nanoliposomal irinotecan with fluorouracil and folinic acid in metastatic pancreatic cancer after previous gemcitabine-based therapy (NAPOLI-1): A global, randomised, open-label, phase 3 trial. *Lancet* 2016;387(10018):545–57.
195. Pelzer U, Schwaner I, Stieler J, et al. Best supportive care (BSC) versus oxaliplatin, folinic acid and 5-fluorouracil (OFF) plus BSC in patients for second-line advanced pancreatic cancer: A phase III-study from the German CONKO-study group. *Eur J Cancer* 2011;47(11):1676–81.
196. ter Veer E, van Rijssen LB, Besselink MG, et al. Consensus statement on mandatory measurements in pancreatic cancer trials (COMM-PACT) for systemic treatment of unresectable disease. *Lancet Oncol* 2018;19(3):e151–60.

5 Hepatocellular carcinoma

5.1 INTRODUCTION

5.1.1 EPIDEMIOLOGY

A report from the GLOBOCAN 2020 database showed an estimated 905,700 new cases and 830,200 deaths from hepatocellular carcinoma (HCC) worldwide, with age-adjusted standardized rates (ASRs) of 9.5 and 8.7/100,000 new cases and deaths. Incidence and mortality were higher in males [1]. The incidence ASR for liver cancer in Europe in 2022 was 13.9/100,000, with 62,124 new cases, and mortality ASR of 12.1/100,000 and 54,165 cancer deaths, with higher prevalence in males [2].

HCC was among the top five causes of death in 90/185 countries, with the highest incidences in Eastern Asia, Northern Africa, and South-Eastern Asia.

A meta-analysis of 31 studies documented an annual percentage change of +2.6%, particularly pronounced in North America, Europe, and Australia, and a downward trend in Asia [3]. The annual number of cases is predicted to increase by 55% between 2020 and 2040, with mortality increasing by 56% [1].

The risk of developing HCC is age-dependent [4] with a peak of >70 years in the US [5], and it remains doubtful that the incidence declines after age 75 [6, 7], although age is strongly affected by the prevalence of the etiologic factors.

5.1.2 STAGING OF METASTATIC DISEASE

Although in the absence of liver cirrhosis, biopsy is necessary for diagnosis, for HCC arising on cirrhosis LI-RADS radiologic criteria are sufficient [8, 9]. Various LI-RADS algorithms have been defined according to the context. However, CT/MRI with extracellular agents or with hepatobiliary agents is required for staging [8].

Moreover, many studies have found higher sensitivity and predictive positive values for MRI compared with CT [10–12]. On the other hand, it should be remembered that an HCC bioptic sampling is increasingly recommended for the molecular characterization of the tumor [9].

Many factors contribute to the staging, prognosis, and treatment strategies of HCC. Initial staging involves a chest-abdomen CT, omitting liver MRI if there is no indication of curative resection or locoregional treatments (LR-TR) [9], and an assessment of liver function. In contrast to other malignancies, some variables independent of tumor spread, such as liver function, have been included in staging systems.

The TNM Classification (AJCC 8th edition 2017) [13] does not define distinct features within M1 disease, which is considered to include all patients with extra-hepatic disease (EHD). BCLC is the most widely used staging system, and is functional for directing treatment choices: in addition to the extent of HCC, BCLC staging includes performance status (PS) and liver function [14]. Over time, not only it is increasingly affirming its prognostic value, but also its role in therapeutic choices, as confirmed in the latest version which reclassified into 3 groups the BCLC B stage [15].

Liver function often synthetized by the Child–Pugh score, supplemented by albumin-bilirubin (ALBI) grade in Child A [16], has predictive value concerning systemic treatment efficacy, and almost all systemic antineoplastic treatments have been studied in patients with Child score A. Other variables related to portal hypertension are rarely altered in patients with good liver function. However, in suspected portal hypertension an EGDS with the treatment of esophageal varices should precede treatment with anti-angiogenic drugs, although the extended Baveno VI criteria seem to be able to predict the status of varices in 40% of cases [17].

DOI: 10.1201/9781032703350-5

TABLE S1
Prognostic factors analyzed in selected clinical trials of patients with unresectable or metastatic hepatocellular carcinoma receiving upfront treatment

Variable	No. trials	Prognostic relationship	No prognostic relationship
Patient-related			
Performance status	8	2	6
Demographic			
Age	7	1	6
Sex	6	2	4
Geo & ethnic			
Geographic area	1	0	1
Race	1	0	1
Anthropometric			
Child–Pugh score	8	7	1
Body weight	1	0	1
Clinic			
Cirrhosis	5	1	4
Ascites	1	1	0
Alcohol abuse	3	0	3
Smoking status	1	1	0
HBV	5	2	3
HCV	3	0	3
Lab			
Hemoglobin	1	0	1
Prothrombin time	1	0	1
Neutrophil-lymphocyte ratio	1	1	0
Albumin	3	2	1
Bilirubin	3	3	0
Alkalyne phosphatase	1	1	0
Alanine transaminase	1	1	0
Reactive C-protein	1	1	0
Creatinine	1	0	1
Alfa-feto protein	8	6	2
CA 125	1	1	0
CYFRA 21.1	1	1	0
Tumor-related			
Tumor burden			
Tumor stage	4	1	3
Tumor size	3	1	2
Disease status	1	0	1
No. sites metastases	1	1	0
No. tumor foci	2	1	1
SHARP composite variable	1	1	0
Portal invasion/thrombosis	6	5	1
Site of metastasis			
Extra-epatic metastases	4	1	3
Pathology			
Macroscopic appearance	2	1	1
Intratumor viability	1	0	1
Previous treatment			
Previous treatments	3	1	2
Concomitant antiviral therapy	1	0	1

In 2017 LI-RADS released a treatment response algorithm after LR-TR with the intent to standardize clinical practice [8], reporting better performance than mRECIST [18], but currently, the most widely used remain RECIST1.1 criteria [19, 20], with mRECIST criteria that appear to be superimposable in the assessment of progression [21].

Serum alpha-fetoprotein (AFP) levels should always be measured before treatment. In cases with increased levels, serologic responses have demonstrated prognostic value [22–26], but standardization is not available [27, 28].

5.1.3 PROGNOSIS OF METASTATIC DISEASE

Over the past 15 years, the prognosis of unresectable loco-regional or metastatic hepatocellular carcinoma (mHCC) has improved with a median overall survival (OS) from 6.8 months in 2005 [29] to 13.2 in 2020 [30]. After the introduction of immunotherapy and its integration with existing treatments, median OS is expected to increase further, compared with the 19.2 months reported in the IMbrave150 trial [30]. In addition, it is necessary to consider the continuous improvements in oligometastatic disease (OMD) control. Therefore, improved treatment performance is expected in mHCC.

5.2 ANALYSIS OF PROGNOSTIC VARIABLES IN EARLY METASTATIC DISEASE

A systematic review of prospective trials that studied upfront treatments in mHCC resulted in the selection of 43 studies, published from 1995 to 2022. In 11 trials an analysis of prognostic factors (PFs) was done (6 phase III, 5 phase II), with all studies reporting the results of the analysis [29, 31–40]. Beyond all the limitations related to the biases of analysis and reporting of the PFs, the present systematic review evaluated the results of these studies as summarized in Table S1. It lists all the evaluated PFs that have been reported in at least one study and the number of studies that found or did not find a relationship between PFs and OS. Due to the limited number of studies available, two studies with partial eligibility concerning inclusion criteria were evaluated in the analysis [36, 39].

5.3 PATIENT-RELATED PROGNOSTIC FACTORS

5.3.1 PERFORMANCE STATUS

Few reports have focused on PS in mHCC. A 2010 meta-analysis evaluated OS in the control arms of 30 trials, which had evaluated untreated patients or those receiving a placebo, and documented a 2-year survival of 17.5%, noting that some variables correlated independently with OS, including PS [41]. In a recent trial-level analysis evaluating mHCC patients undergoing systemic treatments, among the baseline variables, only PS showed a prognostic role ($\beta = -0.636$; p-value = 0.048) [26]. Similarly, an analysis of 40 cohorts of patients who had received immune checkpoint inhibitors (ICIs) concluded that ECOG PS correlated with OS [42]. However, PS appears to be under-reported also in immunotherapy trials.

5.3.1.1 Selected trials

Eight trials evaluated PS. Only two trials documented a significant prognostic relationship [31, 35], while other two reported the effect size (ES), and in those studies, no OS change emerged by PS [37, 40] (Table 5.1).

5.3.2 DEMOGRAPHIC

5.3.2.1 Age

A SEER database evaluation reported a poor prognosis in the elderly [43]. In addition to expectations about aging societies, with an increase of cirrhosis unrelated to viral infections [44], and the

TABLE 5.1

Prognostic relationships of performance status in selected studies of patients with unresectable or metastatic hepatocellular carcinoma receiving upfront treatment

Study [ref]	Phase	No. pts	Scale	Comparison	Prognostic relationship	Effect size
MDACC 2004 [36]	II	37	Zubrod	PS 2–3 vs. PS 0–1	No	NR
PIAF 2005 [29]	III	188	ECOG	PS 1 vs. PS 0	No	NR
FFCD 0303 2007 [37]	II	50	WHO	PS 1–2 vs. PS 0	No	HR 1.76 (0.95–3.26)
SHARP 2008 [31]	III	602	ECOG	PS 1–2 vs. PS 0	Yes	NR
Korean 2009 [38]	II	32	ECOG	PS 2 vs. PS 0–1	No	NR
AGEO 2013 [40]	II	204	WHO	PS 1 vs. PS 0	No	HR 0.99 (0.62–1.58)
				PS 2–3 vs. PS 0	No	HR 1.75 (0.93–3.26)
REFLECT 2018 [34]	III	954	ECOG	PS 1 vs. PS 0	No	NR
SoraHAIC 2019 [35]	III	247	ECOG	High vs. low	Yes	NR

Legend: ECOG, Eastern Cooperative Oncology Group. HR, hazard ratio. NR, not reported. PS, performance status. WHO, World Health Organization.

current burden of HCV, typical of older age [45], an age-dependent risk of developing HCC itself must be taken into account [4]. NAFLD, which can evolve into NASH in the presence of oxidative stress and inflammation, is a risk factor for cirrhosis and HCC [46]. Even though the incidence of HCC could decrease after 70, because the liver becomes resistant to the development of damage [46], other cancerogenesis pathways, such as the p16 promoter methylation, are associated with aggressive HCC among patients >50 years old [47].

Fortunately, recent clinical trials have recruited older patients [48, 49], although frailty assessment is unfrequent [50].

The efficacy of some mHCC treatments by age is also controversial. Among LR-TRs, radiofrequency ablation is less effective in the elderly [51], yet some doubt of efficacy also exists for targeted therapies [52–54].

5.3.2.2 Sex

Several studies have confirmed the previously reported differences in HCC incidence and mortality by sex, which could be a consequence of the differences observed in the predisposing liver diseases [55–57].

The liver is a sexually dimorphic organ, exhibiting different gene expressions, mitochondrial functions, microsomal enzyme activities, and immune responses according to sex [58]. Some data support the hypothesis that the sex disparity could be mediated by the stimulatory effects of androgens and the protective effects of estrogen in the development and progression of HCC, and a possible protective action of estrogen signaling pathways, both on HCC and hepatitis infection, was reported [59]. The interactions are complex and partly mediated by the activation of systemic immune response (SIR) [59–61] or to drug detoxification pathways and HCC-related DNA methylation changes that show gender-related disparities, as well as sex chromosomes involvement in HCC development [62–66]. Sex significantly contributes to shaping the immune responses, explaining some differences [67]. Sexual dimorphism has been particularly studied in HBV-related diseases [55]. Also, NAFLD is considered a sexual dimorphic disease [57], and androgen receptor activation could be involved in the pathogenesis of NASH-related HCC [68–70].

It follows that sexual dimorphism might interfere with the different activity of immunotherapy in the two sexes [71, 72], because of the control of PD1 and PD-L1 transcription operated by sex hormones [73] and other possible reasons, such as epigenetic factors and immune environment [74].

5.3.2.3   Other demographic variables

The risk of mortality among patients with recurrent HCC is significantly more consistent among Asians [75]. In the US, HCC incidence and mortality are not equally distributed, and the more advanced stage at diagnosis can explain the poor OS for Blacks and the longer OS for Asians and Hispanics [76]. In contrast, in the context of autoimmune hepatitis and related cirrhosis, higher rates of HCC incidence were registered in Asia [56].

Although the prevalence of some risk factors may account for some of these different geographic and ethnic distributions, such as HBV in Asia, further studies are needed to understand the causes of the different mortality risks in various regions of the world [77], but also the role of population genetics of HCC-related DNA methylation changes and various predisposing gene polymorphisms [78–83].

A SEER analysis did not identify any difference in OS by race, yet a poor prognosis of unmarried patients [84].

5.3.2.4   Selected trials

Seven trials assessed age. A cut-off was used in three studies and varied considerably between the Asian studies (50–53 years) [35, 38] and the European study (70 years) [40] (Table 5.2). Only in one trial after univariate analysis, a prognostic relationship between age and OS was found [35].

Six studies evaluated sex (Table 5.3). Two trials documented a significant prognostic relationship, with longer median OS among females [34, 40].

Two trials evaluated variables related to geographic origin and ethnicity, without reporting relationships with OS, but the study that assessed ethnicity had enrolled predominantly White patients [36].

5.3.3   Anthropometric

Various measures related to body mass and liver function have shown a relationship with OS.

5.3.3.1   Body mass index and body composition

Obesity is associated with an increased risk of HCC and HCC-related mortality [85]. A Korean database of HBV-related HCC patients reported a negative prognostic role for BMI in females [86]. The hypothesis that could explain this difference lies in the different relationship of BMI with total body fat in the two sexes [87], but there could also be racial differences [88]. Obesity and the

---

TABLE 5.2
Prognostic relationships of age in selected studies of patients with unresectable or metastatic hepatocellular carcinoma receiving upfront treatment

Study [ref]	Phase	No. pts	Comparison	Prognostic relationship	Effect size
MDACC 2004 [36]	II	37	NR	No	NR
PIAF 2005 [29]	III	188	NR	No	NR
FFCD 0303 2007 [37]	II	50	NR	No	NR
Korean 2009 [38]	II	32	> vs. <53	No	NR
AGEO 2013 [40]	II	204	> vs. <70	No	HR 1.27 (0.75–2.13)
BRISK-FL 2013 [32]	III	1155	NR	No	NR
SoraHAIC 2019 [35]	III	247	> vs. <50	Yes	NR

Legend: HR, hazard ratio. NR, not reported.

TABLE 5.3

Prognostic relationships of sex in selected studies of patients with unresectable or metastatic hepatocellular carcinoma receiving upfront treatment

Study [ref]	Phase	No. pts	Comparison	Prognostic relationship	Effect size
MDACC 2004 [36]	II	37	M vs. F	No	NR
PIAF 2005 [29]	III	188	M vs. F	No	NR
Korean 2009 [38]	II	32	M vs. F	No	NR
AGEO 2013 [40]	II	204	M vs. F	Yes	HR 2.22 (1.18–4.35)
REFLECT 2018 [34]	III	954	M vs. F	Yes	HR 1.24 (1.01–1.52)
SoraHAIC 2019 [35]	III	247	M vs. F	No	NR

Legend: F, females. HR, hazard ratio. M, males. NR, not reported.

associated hepatopathy (NAFLD) favor immune dysfunction and tumor progression, but also a more pronounced anti-tumor activity and longer survival after immunotherapy [89].

Sarcopenia has been reported as a negative PF in patients with mHCC receiving sorafenib (L3 SMI ≤39.2 cm²/m²) [90, 91], and confirmed in other studies [92–94].

5.3.3.2   Liver function

Most of the anthropometric indicators used in patients with HCC concern liver function since OS is independently affected by underlying liver disease and cirrhosis [95]. Although a standardized measurement of liver function is not available, liver function parameters have been included in the definition of the tumor stage, such as in the BCLC system, and often were not evaluated separately.

Child–Pugh score, a variable associated with liver failure, has been used in defining the subgroup of mHCC patients who benefit from sorafenib [31, 96]. Despite the overlap in objective response rates and side effects from sorafenib between Child-A and Child-B patients, a significantly poor OS of the Child-B subgroup has been reported [97].

Recently, the ALBI grade, an index of liver function that has been developed to evaluate the prognosis of HCC patients, has been investigated. It has been reported as being of prognostic value outside of liver disease [98–100]. Subsequent modifications have been proposed [101, 102], and it sometimes reported better discriminative ability than the Child–Pugh score for predicting the prognosis of HCC patients [103, 104].

5.3.3.3   Selected trials

Only one study evaluated body weight as a possible PF at a 60 kg cut-off, without finding any relationship with OS [34].

Eight trials evaluated Child scores. Seven studies documented a significant prognostic role, as reported in Table 5.4. The pooled analysis of the six studies that reported an ES of Child A vs. Child B confirmed the favorable outcomes of Child A (HR 0.46, CI 0.30–0.72; Q = 9.66, p-value = 0.0855; I^2 = 48.2%) (Figure 5.1).

5.3.4   Clinic

5.3.4.1   Liver diseases and cirrhosis

Liver cirrhosis is the condition that is most frequently associated with HCC [105]. Usually, the underlying pathology on which HCC occurs affects biology and prognosis of HCC. Though HBV and

TABLE 5.4

Prognostic relationships of Child–Pugh score in selected studies of patients with unrecectable or metastatic hepatocellular carcinoma receiving upfront treatment

Study [ref]	Phase	No. pts	Comparison	Prognostic relationship	Effect size
PIAF 2005 [29]	III	188	A vs. B-C	Yes	HR 0.52 (0.34–0.80)
FFCD 0303 2007 [37]	II	50	A vs. B	Yes	HR 0.33 (0.14–0.80)
SHARP 2008 [31]	III	602	NR	Yes	NR
Korean 2009 [38]	II	32	A vs. B	No	HR 0.24 (0.04–1.35)
Singapore 2012 [39]	II	44	A vs. B	Yes	HR 0.11 (0.03–0.41)
AGEO 2013 [40]	II	204	A vs. B	Yes	HR 0.46 (0.30–0.71)
			A vs. C	Yes	HR 0.39 (0.18–0.85)
BRISK-FL 2013 [32]	III	1155	NR	Yes	NR
REFLECT 2018 [34]	III	954	A vs. B	Yes	HR 0.60 (0.50–0.71)

Legend: HR, hazard ratio. NR, not reported.

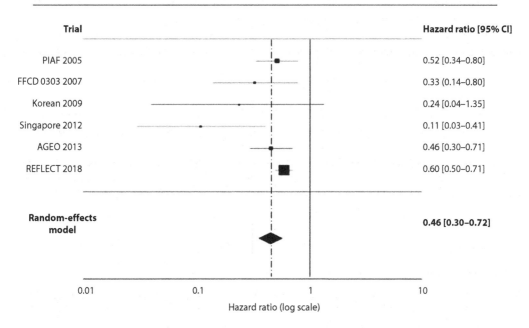

FIGURE 5.1 Forest plot of meta-analysis of Child–Pugh score in prospective trials of patients with unresectable or metastatic hepatocellular carcinoma

HCV are the main risk factors of HCC, their treatment and the HBV vaccine suggest a reduction of virus-related HCC. On the other hand, despite the stable frequency of other risk factors, metabolic risk factors (metabolic syndrome, obesity, type 2 diabetes mellitus, NAFLD) are on the rise [106, 107].

5.3.4.2 Hepatitis

HCC arising on HBV is more aggressive than HCC arising on HCV or NASH [75, 108]. Disease with active viral replication for a long time, with associated inflammation, appears to be the major risk factor, and HBV treatment by reducing viral load reduces inflammation and HCC risk [109]. Patients with HBV-related hepatitis in the immune-tolerant stage have an increased risk of HCC and HCC-related death [110, 111]. Although antiviral therapy does not affect the course of HCC

[112], the sensitivity of HCC to antineoplastic treatments may change. In the subgroup of patients with HBV-related HCC, a meta-analysis of 16 trials reported longer OS after lenvatinib and with regorafenib [113], in contrast to atezolizumab [114]. There is also consistent evidence that the effect of sorafenib on OS is dependent on patients' hepatitis status, without any improvement in HBV-positive patients [115, 116]. After resection of HCC, HBV, or HCV-positive serology is associated with poor prognosis [117], and the prevalence of recurrent HCC was higher among HBV patients [75]. As suggested by the epidemiologic finding of increased HCC from aflatoxin in HBV-carrier males, a study of 110 Chinese patients confirmed the presence of genomic and transcriptional differences between males and females [118].

HCC arising from HCV liver infection is generally caused through indirect pathways, and is almost exclusively diagnosed in cirrhotic patients [119]. After HCV is cured, HCC incidence is reduced, and when follow-up increases, there is a reduction in the risk of HCC [120]. It was estimated that treatment of 90% of HCV infections could reduce the incidence of HCC by 15%.

Patients with HCC on chronic non-B non-C hepatitis reported outcomes similar to HBV-related HCC [121].

In the US, alcohol was associated with an annual incidence of HCC of 1.44% in patients with cirrhosis, and HCC-related deaths are expected to nearly double [122, 123]. Degree of alcohol intake, sex, older age, obesity, type 2 diabetes mellitus, gut microbial dysbiosis, and genetic variants are key factors in the development of alcohol-associated cirrhosis and HCC.

NAFLD is currently the most common form of chronic liver disease worldwide and is a growing risk factor for HCC, involving 25% of the global population. The annual incidence rate of HCC in NAFLD-cirrhosis is greater than 1% [124].

5.3.4.3   Selected trials

Five trials evaluated the presence of cirrhosis (Table 5.5). In the PIAF study, the definition of cirrhosis was histologic or radiologic [29], while in the others it was not specified. In one of the five studies, a significant prognostic relationship was documented [40].

Five studies evaluated HBsAg, but only two reported a negative prognostic role, as described in Table 5.6. Three studies evaluated serum positivity for HCV antibodies, without a significant relationship to OS [29, 32, 40]. One study documented a prognostic effect of alcoholic liver disease, while in the same study viral etiology did not affect the outcome [40].

5.3.5   Laboratory

5.3.5.1   Hematology

Various laboratory abnormalities have been associated with the prognosis of mHCC, and many of them can be attributed to SIR activation in the localized HCC [125–127]. Although the relationships

---

TABLE 5.5

Prognostic relationships of liver cirrhosis in selected studies of patients with unresectable or metastatic hepatocellular carcinoma receiving upfront treatment

Study [ref]	Phase	No. pts	Comparison	Prognostic relationship	Effect size
MDACC 2004 [36]	II	37	Yes vs. no	No	NR
PIAF 2005 [29]	III	188	Yes vs. no	No	NR
FFCD 0303 2007 [37]	II	50	Yes vs. no	No	NR
AGEO 2013 [40]	II	204	Yes vs. no	Yes	HR 2.83 (1.74–4.60)
REFLECT 2018 [34]	III	954	Yes vs. no	No	NR

Legend: HR, hazard ratio. NR, not reported.

TABLE 5.6

Prognostic relationships of hepatitis B infection in selected studies of patients with unresectable or metastatic hepatocellular carcinoma receiving upfront treatment

Study [ref]	Phase	No. pts	Comparison	Prognostic relationship	Effect size
PIAF 2005 [29]	III	188	Yes vs. no	No	NR
Korean 2009 [38]	II	32	Yes vs. no	No	NR
BRISK-FL 2013 [32]	III	1155	Yes vs. no	No	NR
REFLECT 2018 [34]	III	954	Yes vs. no	Yes	HR 1.25 (1.07–1.46)
SoraHAIC 2019 [35]	III	247	Yes vs. no	Yes	NR

Legend: HR, hazard ratio. NR, not reported.

between inflammation and immunity are complex, the balance of the primary tumor microenvironment (TME) is changed from immuno-surveillance toward stimulation of HCC growth [128, 129].

5.3.5.2 Chemistry

A systematic review analyzed 28 prognostic models for outcome prediction in mHCC and documented that albumin and bilirubin were commonly reported [130]. Many laboratory variables, such as albumin or C-reactive protein (CRP), have been frequently evaluated as part of ratios [131] or within prognostic scores [132, 133]. Similar composite variables have included bilirubin [134], and alkaline phosphatase (ALP) [135, 136].

Despite multiple studies in localized disease, poor data are available in mHCC patients for serum albumin [95], bilirubin [95, 125] and aspartate aminotransferase (AST) [125, 137].

5.3.5.3 Tumor markers

The most studied marker is AFP, a tumor-associated fetal glycoprotein, whose concentration drops at birth and remains low throughout life, below 5 ng/mL [138]. Unfortunately, about one-third of HCC patients do not express it [139], and generally a normal AFP predicts better outcomes [43].

AFP expression is correlated with potentially more angiogenic tumors and could define aggressive subgroups of HCC [140]. Although the presence of the receptor for AFP in tumor cells and cells of the immune system may be involved in promoting immune escape and a paracrine stimulus for HCC growth, pro-angiogenic activity seems more relevant in metastatic disease, as high concentrations of AFP (>400 mg/L) activate VEGF signaling [141]. About 30–50% of the patients on systemic therapy have serum levels >400 ng/mL [142, 143], which are often associated with EHD [144]. A posthoc analysis of the REACH and REACH-2 trials documented the prognostic role of high AFP levels in the first-line setting and after sorafenib therapy [145], while a pooled analysis of two studies of sorafenib documented an independent relationship with OS [54].

5.3.5.4 Selected trials

One study documented a prognostic role for NLR at cut-off 3 [35], while another did not for anemia and prothrombin time [29]. CRP was found to be inversely related to OS [39].

Three studies evaluated serum albumin, whose increase in two cases was associated with longer OS [29, 31], while in a third study with a 4 g/L cut-off did not [35].

Three studies evaluated bilirubin, reporting a negative prognostic effect for increased bilirubin [29, 31, 35]. Similarly, ALP [31] and ALT [29] elevations were associated with poor prognosis.

Seven trials investigated AFP, with a cut-off ranging from 15 to 1,000 ng/mL. Of these, five found a significant prognostic relationship (Table 5.7). From four studies the HR was available, then

TABLE 5.7

Prognostic relationships of alpha-fetoprotein in selected studies of patients with unresectable or metastatic hepatocellular carcinoma receiving upfront treatment

Trial	Phase	No. pts	Comparison	Prognostic relationship	Effect size
PIAF 2005 [29]	III	188	NR	No	NR
SHARP 2008 [31]	III	602	< vs. >200	Yes	NR
Korean 2009 [38]	II	32	< vs. >705	Yes	HR 4.70 (1.73–12.8)
AGEO 2013 [40]	II	204	< vs. >15	No	HR 1.49 (0.90–2.48)
BRISK-FL 2013 [32]	III	1155	< vs. >200	Yes	NR
REFLECT 2018 [34]	III	954	< vs. >200	Yes	HR 1.72 (1.47–2.00)
SoraHAIC 2019 [35]	III	247	< vs. >1000	Yes	HR 1.52 (1.12–2.07)

Legend: HR, hazard ratio. NR, not reported.

a meta-analysis was performed, which confirmed the unfavorable prognostic role of high AFP (HR 1.70, CI 1.11–2.60; Q = 4.76, p-value = 0.1904; I^2 = 37.0%).

5.4   TUMOR-RELATED PROGNOSTIC FACTORS

5.4.1   TUMOR BURDEN

5.4.1.1   Tumor stage

No single criterion has been established to define tumor burden (TB), and studies have often used stage and primary tumor size.

Although the stage is important in defining prognosis (CLIP, Okuda, BCLC classification) and in selecting treatments (BCLC), staging systems often include other variables. Due to the mixing of the TB parameters with other patient-related variables (liver function, PS, etc.), various staging systems have been proposed [146–149]. Even BCLC classification, which is the most widely used, has critical issues, such as the differentiation of stage C according to PS or level of portal vein thrombosis involvement in Child A patients [150] and the heterogeneity of stage B [151, 152].

5.4.1.2   Tumor size

Primary tumor size is widely used to evaluate TB. Tumor diameter correlates with microvascular invasion, tumor grade, regional spread, and distant metastasis [153]. A SEER analysis documented that the frequency of metastases increased 5-fold for tumors sized >58 vs. <30 mm [154], and the independent prognostic role of the primary tumor size was confirmed by other studies of mHCC [95, 125, 155].

Composite prognostic indicators have associated tumor size with other variables such as the number and size of the other liver lesions, defined by the Milan criteria or up-to-seven criteria [156, 157], the TB score [158], or the total tumor volume [159]. Others have associated tumor size with AFP, as the up-to-seven criteria integrated with AFP [160], yet have not been validated in patients with EHD.

5.4.1.3   Oligometastatic disease

The distinction between locally advanced and metastatic disease is rarely used in studies of HCC, whereas an improved OS for the OMD is presumable. Numerous experiences of complete resection of EHD are reported in the literature, and the OMD prognosis is likely more favorable. In particular, the benefit of aggressive treatments was evident for isolated metastases with good liver function and primary tumor control [161].

Similarly to the number of metastases, a good prognosis has been suggested for a low number of involved metastatic sites [43].

5.4.1.4   Portal vein tumor thrombosis

Portal vein tumor thrombosis (PVTT) is a frequent complication of cirrhosis (14%) [162] and HCC (10–40%) [163, 164], for which various classifications are reported [165–168].

In addition to altering the hepatic circulation, PVTT reduces nutrient supply to the liver and consequently hepatic functional reserve, with increased hepatogenic liver metastasis and portal hypertension. This is associated with very low median OS and aggressive tumors, high TB, elevated AFP, deterioration of liver function tests, and PS.

PVTT might indicate a biologically advanced stage, in which multiple molecular events may contribute to its development [169]. PVTT is more frequent among patients with proliferative HCC, extracellular matrix receptor expression [170], active HBV, tumor size >3 cm, absent/incomplete capsule, and high des-gamma-carboxy pro-thrombin levels [171].

PVTT-associated HCCs have a poor prognosis after local and systemic therapy, including immunotherapy [42, 95, 172], with some guidelines and small studies supporting surgery for limited PVTT, in particular when distal to the right and left portal branches [173]. On the other hand, the results of sorafenib have been disappointing, suggesting to explore the feasibility of LR-TR in combination with sorafenib [174], with a meta-analysis reporting that the most effective approach might be TACE+sorafenib compared with hepatectomy or other options [175].

5.4.1.5   Selected trials

Three trials evaluated tumor size [29, 32, 35], but only in one study, this variable was prognostic [32]. Four trials evaluated stage, by CLIP score [37, 40], BCLC [34], or Okuda stage system [29], and only in the last case a significant relationship of advanced stage (III vs. I-II) with reduced OS was found. Disease status, locally advanced vs. metastatic, did not influence outcomes [36]. While a significant relationship between the increasing number of metastatic sites and poor prognosis was reported [34], the prognosis of multifocal HCC appears controversial [34, 35]. Finally, in the SHARP study, a TB variable was identified, defined according to the presence of macrovascular invasion (MVI), EHD, or both, and was significantly associated with OS [31].

Six studies evaluated the PVTT effect on OS (Table 5.8). A pooled analysis of the three studies that reported an ES suggests a trend to unfavorable prognosis for PVTT (HR 1.36, CI 0.93–2.00; Q = 2.61, p-value = 0.2705; I^2 = 23.5%).

5.4.2   PRIMARY TUMOR LOCATION

Right-sided HCCs are 2–3 times more frequent than left-sided, and present a better prognosis, supporting the hypothesis that the more liver was left over, the more recurrences there are.

A Chinese study investigated the right vs. left liver origin (74.7% vs. 25.3%) after hepatectomy, and in 650 matched pairs, OS was significantly longer for patients with right-sided tumors (72 vs. 66 months) [155]. Similar findings were reported by other authors [176, 177].

5.4.3   TIMING OF METASTASIS

SEER database reported that 14.8% of HCC patients have metastases at diagnosis [84]. In the context of cirrhotic disease, it is a frequent diagnostic dilemma to distinguish between multifocal disease or synchronous liver metastases (LMs). Various studies have documented better outcomes for patients with multicentric disease than with synchronous metastases [178–180]. One study evaluated 42 patients separating multicentric HCC from intrahepatic metastases and reported a median

TABLE 5.8

Prognostic relationships of portal vein tumor thrombosis in selected studies of patients with unresectable or metastatic hepatocellular carcinoma receiving upfront treatment

Study [ref]	Phase	No. pts	Comparison	Prognostic relationship	Effect size
PIAF 2005 [29]	III	188	Yes vs. no	Yes	HR 1.53 (1.12–2.08)
SHARP 2008 [31]	III	602	Yes vs. no	Yes	NR
Korean 2009 [38]	II	32	Yes vs. no	No	NR
BRISK-FL 2013 [32]	III	1155	Yes vs. no	Yes	NR
REFLECT 2018 [34]	III	954	Yes vs. no	Yes	HR 1.22 (1.02–1.46)
SoraHAIC 2019 [35]	III	247	Vp4 vs. Vp1–2	Yes	HR 2.27 (1.51–3.44)
			Vp3 vs. Vp1–2	Yes	HR 1.63 (1.08–2.46)

Legend: HR, hazard ratio. NR, not reported. Vp1, third branch portal vein invasion. Vp2, second branch portal vein invasion. Vp3, first branch portal vein invasion. Vp4, main portal vein invasion.

OS of 25.7 vs. 8.9 months. The characteristics of the two subpopulations differed, with cirrhosis and PVTT differentiating the two groups after multivariate analysis [181].

Some authors suggest that after HCC resection a relapse-free survival longer than 18–24 months is more probably associated with multicentric disease than with metachronous LMs [179, 182]. An analysis of 661 resected HCC patients documented a recurrence in 356 (54%) after 22 months. Median survival from the time of recurrence to death was 21 months, and time from primary resection to recurrence was an independent PF [183].

5.4.4 SITE OF METASTASIS

The site of metastasis was poorly studied, and data are conflicting [42, 84]. A survey of the SEER database documented that the liver, lung, and bone were the most frequent sites, while brain metastases were rare [154]. The liver is the most common site of recurrence, especially in the first two years [184]. Other studies have confirmed the prevalence of pulmonary localization for EHD, affecting 39–55% of mHCCs [185, 186], while they are synchronous in only 3.6% of cases [187]. According to other studies, nodal metastases would also be considered a frequent site of distant tumor spread [188]. Although peritoneal metastases have been found in 18% of autopsy series [189], their occurrence at the time of surgery is 6.3% [190], and are rarely evident at imaging. Adrenal metastases have a very low frequency of 0.4–0.8% [191, 192], although they may affect 10% of patients during an mHCC course.

Some evidence suggests a negative prognostic effect for LMs. Even among patients with EHD, 66% die from hepatic causes and only 22% from EHD progression [193, 194]. Even though the presence of EHD is the variable often used in the definition of prognostic models [130], some studies suggest that EHD patients could have a better prognosis [42].

SEER database reported that lung metastases were an independent PF, reducing OS [84]. In contrast, in patients with resectable metastatic disease, lung metastases might be associated with a favorable prognosis after surgery [195]. Among patients with synchronous pulmonary metastasis, the outcome is worse for males, those with larger primary tumor size, and bone metastasis, while it is better if AFP levels are normal, and patients received hepatectomy, radiotherapy, or chemotherapy [187].

Controversial findings are available about the prognosis of patients with bone metastases. A single-center retrospective analysis identified 20/1,017 cases with bone metastases, whose prognosis ranged around three months [196]. On the other hand, an evaluation of 1,778 patients with bone metastases from the SEER database, including 987 bone-only diseases, documented a median OS superior to that of patients with brain or lung metastases [84].

A SEER analysis reported longer OS for patients with exclusive nodal disease compared with all other extra-hepatic sites [43, 197].

Some Asian series of mHCC patients with peritoneal metastases suggested a possible improved OS after surgery, but the prognosis was largely dependent on the Child–Pugh score [198] and on extra-peritoneal tumor control [199].

Though the prognosis of brain metastases is poor [84], LR-TR can affect the outcome [200], which improves also according to the number of brain metastases, the presence of hemorrhage, and ALBI [201].

Even for patients with adrenal metastases, the expected OS is around 6 months. However, some studies suggest a positive effect of adrenalectomy, with a median OS of 15.8 months [192]. A study of 16 patients who underwent adrenalectomy documented a median OS of 35 months, which was even longer in patients who had previously undergone OLT [188, 192, 202]. A recent single-institution retrospective analysis of 16 patients confirmed better outcomes after adrenalectomy, supporting prospective trials [203].

5.4.4.1 Selected trials

Four trials investigated the outcome of patients with EHD [34, 36, 40], and only one study found a negative prognostic relationship [35].

5.4.5 PATHOLOGY

5.4.5.1 Histology

Atypical histotypes are rare, although they would account for 20–30% of cases, with more than 12 subtypes [204]. Despite the limited reports on mHCC and the scarce evidence about their prognosis, a review documented that scirrhous HCC accounts for 4% of HCC, and has been associated with poor outcomes [205].

5.4.5.2 Tumor grade

Edmondson-Steiner grading system is a classification that considers the morphology and size of tumor cells [206] and is the most widely used grading system in HCC. It was related to the outcome of localized disease [207, 208] but remains poorly studied in mHCC. Some SEER database analyses including a percentage of mHCC confirmed the negative prognostic effect for poorly differentiated tumors [84, 209].

Similarly, a meta-analysis found an inverse relationship with OS for Ki-67, which was more frequently high in patients with stage III/IV vs. I/II HCC (53% vs. 43%), and its association with grade, size, number of lymph nodes, presence of metastasis, cirrhosis, and venous invasion [210].

5.4.5.3 Other pathologic variables

Patterns of vascular invasion have been associated with HCC outcomes, for both macrovascular and microvascular invasion [155].

MVI is easy to detect at baseline radiologic evaluation and predicted OS in a pooled analysis of two mHCC trials [54]. The type of affected vessel, portal or venous, also influenced the intrahepatic or systemic tumor spread.

Microscopic vascular invasion is diagnosed on histologic examination, reflects dissemination of tumor cells, and is associated with poor disease-free survival after resection. Some authors argue that it is the only PF after OLT, but there are no predictive markers to diagnose microscopic vascular invasion before surgery [211].

The clinical significance of tertiary lymphoid structures (TLSs) in HCC is controversial, but an analysis of two cohorts suggested that intra-tumoral TLSs are associated with low early recurrence rates [212].

5.4.5.4 Molecular biology

HCC accounts for 90% of primary liver cancer. A molecular classification has identified two subgroups, proliferation, and nonproliferation [213, 214], corresponding the former to iCluster-1 and -3, the latter to iCluster-2 of the TCGA classification [121, 215]. These molecular subgroups correlate with clinical and pathological characteristics, etiology, and prognosis. HCCs in the proliferation group are characterized by signal activation of AKT/mTOR, MET, TGF-beta, IGF, and NOTCH, and have a poor prognosis, while the nonproliferation subgroup remains a highly heterogeneous class. In particular, NGS has shown that specific mutation signatures are associated with individual risk factors [216] and has provided a map of HBV integrations in the genome [217]. The nonproliferative subgroup is characterized by an altered WNT pathway, usually a CTNNB1 mutation, and has a better prognosis, preserving the zonation program that distributes metabolic functions along the porto-central axis. Two types of well-differentiated nonproliferative, the periportal type and the perivenous type, have been identified, with the former associated with a reduced risk of recurrence after resection [218].

Unfortunately, to date, the most frequent mutations in HCC, such as those at TERT promoter, TP53, and CTNNB1, are not targetable [219]. In addition, a high degree of molecular heterogeneity, intertumoral but also intratumoral, with a difficult distinction between trunk mutations and branch mutations, is typical of HCC [219, 220]. Various molecular markers have been tested in small studies, but none predicted response to treatments [214].

5.4.5.5 Selected trials

Two trials evaluated MVI [29, 32], and one reported a significant correlation with OS [32].

The SEARCH study evaluated VEGF-A and HGF serum levels and found that they correlated with reduced OS while VEGF-C and KIT were associated with better outcomes [33]. Another study also confirmed the findings about KIT [34].

5.4.6 PREVIOUS TREATMENTS

Due to the multiple available LR-TR options and the concomitant impaired liver function, palliative surgery of the primary tumor generally is not indicated. On the other hand, LR-TR of recurrent OMD is the rule, either with surgical or ablative techniques and is associated with increased OS. Despite recurrences in >50% of patients, long-term survival can be achieved after resection of the relapsing HCC. Therefore, aggressive management with combined resection or LR-TR for intrahepatic recurrence and resection of isolated extra-hepatic metastases may offer long-term survival in selected patients [221]. SEER database confirmed the better prognosis both after LR-TR of the primary tumor and after surgery of the metastatic disease [43].

5.4.6.1 Selected trials

Three studies analyzed the possible effects of previous treatments of mHCC. Some studies did not document a relationship with OS for prior LR-TR or surgery [32], or TACE [40], but no data are available for prior OLT [38].

5.5 PROGNOSTIC FACTORS IN DECISION-MAKING

No systemic antineoplastic treatment is recommended for patients with BCLC D stage, poor general conditions (PS ECOG ≥2) and/or impaired liver function (Child B or C).

It remains difficult to draw reliable conclusions about the relevance of individual PFs within the studies and treatments, in terms of expected efficacy. This is because of heterogeneous inclusion criteria of trials, different staging systems, recurrent under-representation of some subgroups (female sex, BCLC B), and variability of characteristics of study cohorts (HBV prevalent in Asians, advanced age prevalent in Western countries). Therefore, to date in clinical practice, the drug toxicity profiles often support clinical decisions, especially in the setting of refractory disease.

However, some RCT results suggest a predictive role concerning the activity of various treatment modalities for several PFs, as summarized in Table 5.9.

TABLE 5.9

Prognostic and predictive variables in clinical decision-making in metastatic hepatocellular carcinoma

A. Upfront systemic treatment

1	HBV-related liver disease
	• HBV-related HCC: ICI-based favored (ATEZ+BEV/STRIDE are better than SOR)
	• HBV-related HCC: LENV [ICI not feasible] favored (LENV is better than SOR)
2	Tumor burden
	• Low: consider TARE/TACE when feasible, before systemic treatment
	• Low: consider HAIC (unresectable HCC >7 cm with PVI and without EHD/MVI)
3	AFP
	• <200 ng/mL: LENV favored (LENV is better than SOR)
4	PVTT
	• HAIC could be considered (HAIC+SOR is better than SOR)

B. Treatment of refractory disease

1	AFP
	• >400 ng/mL: RAMU or CABO favored (RAMU/CABO are better than placebo)
	• >200 ng/mL: LENV favored (LENV is better than SOR)
2	Tumor burden
	• EHD: CABO, RAMU, or REG favored (CABO/RAMU/REG are more active)
	• MVI: CABO favored (CABO is better than placebo)
	• No MVI: RAMU favored (RAMU is better than placebo)
3	HBV-related liver disease
	• HBV-related HCC: REG favored (REG is better than placebo)
	• Non-HCV-related: CABO favored (CABO is better than placebo)
4	Age
	• ≥65 years old: CABO or RAMU favored (CABO/RAMU are better than placebo)
	• <65 years old: REG favored (REG is better than placebo)
5	ECOG PS
	• ECOG PS 0: CABO or REG favored (CABO/REG are better than placebo)
6	Child–Pugh score
	• Child–Pugh A5: REG favored (REG is better than placebo)

Legend: AFP, alpha-fetoprotein. ATEZ, atezolizumab. BEV, bevacizumab. CABO, cabozantinib. ECOG PS, Eastern Cooperative Oncology Group performance status. EHD, extra-hepatic disease. HAIC, FOLFOX-based hepatic artery infusion chemotherapy. HBV, hepatitis B virus. HCC, hepatocellular carcinoma. HCV, hepatitis C virus. ICI, immune checkpoint inhibitor. LENV, lenvatinib. MVI, macrovascular invasion. PVI, portal vein invasion. PVTT, portal vein tumor thrombosis. RAMU, ramucirumab. REG, regorafenib. SOR, sorafenib. STRIDE, single tremelimumab regular interval durvalumab regimen. TACE, trans-arterial chemo-embolization. TARE, trans-arterial radio-embolization.

5.5.1 UPFRONT TREATMENT

The current recommended upfront treatment of mHCC patients with ECOG PS 0–1 and Child–Pugh A, who are no longer amenable to surgery and LR-TR, consists of the combination of atezolizumab+bevacizumab, which reported a median OS of 19.2 vs. 13.4 months achieved with sorafenib [30, 222], or durvalumab+tremelimumab [223]. Of the three trials that evaluated the combination of ICIs+antiangiogenic drugs [30, 48, 224], two demonstrated a significant improvement of OS over sorafenib [30, 224].

However, the enrollment criteria of the trials were very selective and excluded many groups, often for safety reasons, which over time have not been confirmed (e.g., immunotherapy in immunosuppressed patients with previous OLT). Taking into account the statistical limitations, the IMbrave150 trial did not detect a better OS of the association in the subgroups of patients with ECOG PS 0, females, low TB, AFP >400 ng/mL, and non-viral etiology. In contrast, the ORIENT-32 study found no differences based on ECOG PS or AFP >400 ng/mL, but improved outcomes in patients with HBV-related hepatopathy and EHD. Differently than the IMbrave150 trial, HBV etiology was more represented (94% vs. 48%). Despite the negative result of the COSMIC-312 study, which was reflected in all subgroups, among patients with HBV-related HCC the combination atezolizumab+cabozantinib was shown to be superior to sorafenib, and is interesting that in this trial the HBV subgroup was limited to the 29% of enrolled patients [48].

The single tremelimumab regular interval durvalumab (STRIDE) combination may be considered a viable alternative in patients not candidates for bevacizumab, given its superiority over sorafenib [239]. While the outcome improvement is confirmed in the various subgroups, this is more pronounced for those aged <65, Asians, EHD, non-HCV-related liver disease and serum AFP >400 ng/mL. Upfront mono-therapy with anti-PD-L1 antibody vs. sorafenib appeared more active among patients with high TB [49, 223].

Possible alternatives for patients not eligible for immunotherapy regimens are lenvatinib [34] or sorafenib [31]. Although statistically equivalent, again the subgroup analysis of the REFLECT study opens reflections for future studies more than giving answers for the choice of the drug. It reports the better performance of lenvatinib in patients with high TB (MVI+/-EHD), HBV-related liver disease, and serum AFP ≥200 ng/mL. The two original studies that led to approval of sorafenib vs. placebo in the first-line setting reported differences too. The SHARP study found a better OS in the subgroup with MVI and without EHD, and among patients with HCV-related liver disease [31]. In the Asia-Pacific study better outcomes of patients with low TB after sorafenib vs. placebo were confirmed, but longer OS was reported in other subgroups, such as ECOG PS 1–2, age <65, increased serum AFP, no previous hepatectomy or TACE [53].

Recently, upfront systemic therapy has been supported by some guidelines and experts even at an early stage, especially in relapsed disease after therapy with curative intent or after progression to LR-TR [9, 15]. However, patients with BCLC B stage in immunotherapy trials are underrepresented, and the BCLC B subgroup in the IMbrave150 and HYMALAIA trials did not perform better in the experimental arm than sorafenib, contrary to what was observed in the ORIENT-32 trial, which, however, included a low number of patients with BCLC B. Therefore, it appears necessary to understand whether in the subgroups of poor prognosis BCLC B, identified by the BCLC guidelines [15], an early systemic approach could improve the outcome. This is because a more extensive integration of LR-TR with systemic therapy might be more effective in terms of OS [225], by replacing TACE with TARE [226] or supplementing TACE with SBRT [227] rather than with sorafenib or other systemic therapies. In this context, some studies have documented a favorable outcome after FOLFOX-HAIC [35, 228], and an Asian FOLFOX-HAIC trial defined some characteristics of patients with low TB concluding that LR-TR with FOLFOX-HAIC performed better than TACE [228], which is usually ineffective for tumors >5 cm. Therefore, a preliminary evaluation of patients with tumor diameter >7 cm without MVI/

EHD could suggest a discussion about the feasibility of upfront LR-TR with FOLFOX-HAIC (or TACE/TARE for smaller lesions) [228], considering the absence of direct comparison with systemic therapy. The HAIC-FOLFOX study in patients with unresectable HCC >7 cm, without MVI/EHD, reported a better OS in all subgroups, but the improvement was more pronounced in patients <50 years, with <3 lesions, and serum AFP >400 ng/mL. On the other hand, the study findings should be confirmed in some underrepresented subgroups (females, HBV-unrelated liver disease, Child A6). The SoraHAIC study recruited only patients with portal vein invasion, including patients with EHD, and confirmed better outcomes after the HAIC+sorafenib association vs. sorafenib alone in all the analyzed subgroups, though some patients were underrepresented (females, HBV-unrelated) [35].

5.5.2 TREATMENT OF REFRACTORY DISEASE

It is even more difficult to define the role of PFs in refractory mHCC. Aside from the clear difference detected after ramucirumab in the subgroup of patients with serum AFP >400 ng/mL in the REACH trials [33, 229], the subgroup results usually follow those of the studies. Consequently, often the choice of drug in the second-line setting is based on the drug toxicity profile and previous treatments. In addition to lenvatinib and sorafenib, regorafenib [142], cabozantinib [230], and ramucirumab can be proposed, but the latter only in the presence of AFP values >400 ng/mL [229]. As much as from a regulatory point of view the three drugs are appropriate, the trial eligibility criteria and toxicity profiles are different, but even the most susceptible sub-populations showed differences suggesting that some PFs should also be taken into account in decision-making. For example, in the REACH study, ramucirumab was not shown to be superior to placebo, except in the subgroup with pretreatment serum AFP ≥400 ng/mL and in EHD. The REACH 2 trial was designed to enroll only patients with AFP ≥400 ng/mL and led to drug approval, but it also reported a better OS in some subgroups, such as >65 years, EHD, no MVI, or who had not received previous LR-TR [229]. In contrast, the CELESTIAL study documented an advantage of cabozantinib vs. placebo, which appeared more pronounced in ECOG PS 0, elderly, non-Asian area (and non-Asian race), with more extensive TB, HCV-unrelated liver disease, AFP ≥400 ng/mL [230]. The RESORCE study also reported better outcomes after regorafenib vs. placebo in refractory disease, but the longer OS appeared more pronounced in the ECOG PS 0, <65 years, EHD, HBV-related liver disease, and Child A5 subgroups [142].

5.6 CONCLUSION

A synthesis of the findings about the examined PFs is reported in Table 5.10.

As repeatedly pointed out, RCTs have frequently excluded clinically relevant subgroups of patients, such as PVTT, Child B, and OLT. Frequently, studies reflect the epidemiologic imbalances of mHCC characteristics in different geographic areas, such as age and cause of hepatopathy, as well as a general underrepresentation of the female sex.

In addition, some variables such as PS and inflammatory parameters have been poorly analyzed, especially in immunotherapy trials.

Molecular heterogeneity and the wide OS fluctuations suggest further investigation of the molecular and TME composition of HCC both at the time of upfront and refractory treatments. In this context, studies on the composition of the immune subpopulations of TME, the role of androgen receptor, methylation status and the two molecular subgroups, as well as the molecular characteristics of cases with PVTT and liver- or lung-limited disease deserve special attention.

However, already simple parameters such as the timing of metastasis, or tumor growth kinetics during treatments as well as NLR, AFP, albumin, and their changes, could help detect important signals to guide treatment plans.

TABLE 5.10

Prognostic factors evaluated in prospective trials of upfront treatment in patients with unresectable or metastatic hepatocellular carcinoma

Suggested	Not suggested	Needing study
Child–Pugh score	Performance status	Sex
HBV infection	Age	NLR
Albumin	Geo & ethnic	L3 SMI
Bilirubin	Cirrhosis	
Liver enzymes		
Alpha-fetoprotein		
Stage (BCLC classification)	Number of sites of metastasis	Tumor diameter
PVTT	Number of metastases	Tumor sidedness
	Site of metastasis	Timing of metastasis
	Previous local treatments	Vascular invasion
		Previous OLT

Legend: BCLC, Barcelona Clinic Liver Cancer. HCC, hepatocellular carcinoma. L3 SMI, L3 skeletal muscle index. NLR, neutrophil-to-lymphocyte ratio. OLT, orthotopic liver transplantation. PVTT, portal vein tumor thrombosis.

REFERENCES

1. Rumgay H, Arnold M, Ferlay J, et al. Global burden of primary liver cancer in 2020 and predictions to 2040. *J Hepatol* 2022;77:1598–606.
2. ECIS – European Cancer Information System, available at: https://ecis.jrc.ec.europa.eu, accessed March 14, 2023.
3. Dasgupta P, Henshaw C, Youlden DR, et al. Global trends in incidence rates of primary adult liver cancers: A systematic review and meta-analysis. *Front Oncol* 2020;10:171.
4. Cho S-J, Yoon J-H, Hwang S-S, et al. Do young hepatocellular carcinoma patients with relatively good liver function have poorer outcomes than elderly patients? *J Gastroenterol Hepatol* 2007;22:1226–31.
5. Nordenstedt H, White DL, El-Serag H. The changing pattern of epidemiology in hepatocellular carcinoma. *Dig Liver Dis* 2010;42(S3):S206–14.
6. Cohen MJ, Bloom AI, Barak O, et al. Trans-arterial chemo-embolization is safe and effective for very elderly patients with hepatocellular carcinoma. *World J Gastroenterol* 2013;19(16):2521–8.
7. El-Serag HB. Epidemiology of hepatocellular carcinoma in USA. *Hepatol Res* 2007;37:S88–94.
8. Chernyak V, Fowler KJ, Kamaya A, et al. Liver imaging reporting and data system (LI- RADS) version 2018: imaging of hepatocellular carcinoma in at-risk patients. *Radiology* 2018;289:816–30.
9. Ducreux M, Abou-Alfa GK, Bekaii-Saab T, et al. The management of hepatocellular carcinoma. Current expert opinion and recommendations derived from the 24th ESMO/World Congress on Gastrointestinal Cancer, Barcelona, 2022. *ESMO Open* 2023;8(3):101567.
10. Hanna RF, Vesselin Z, Miloushev VZ, et al. Comparative 13-year meta-analysis of the sensitivity and positive predictive value of ultrasound, CT, and MRI for detecting hepatocellular carcinoma. *Abdom Radiol* 2016;41:71–90.
11. Kim SY, An J, Lim YS, et al. MRI with liver-specific contrast for surveillance of patients with cirrhosis at high risk of hepatocellular carcinoma. *JAMA Oncol* 2017;3(4):456–63.
12. Kim Y-Y, Lee S, Shin J, et al. Diagnostic performance of CT versus MRI liver imaging reporting and data system category 5 for hepatocellular carcinoma: A systematic review and meta-analysis of comparative studies. *Eur Radiol* 2022;32(10):6723–9.
13. Amin MB, Edge S, Greene F, et al. *AJCC Cancer Staging Manual*. 8th Ed. New York: Springer; 2017.
14. Llovet JM, Brú C, Bruix J. Prognosis of hepatocellular carcinoma: The BCLC staging classification. *Semin Liver Dis* 1999;19(3):329–38.

15. Reig M, Forner A, Rimola J, et al. BCLC strategy for prognosis prediction and treatment recommendation: The 2022 update. *J Hepatol* 2022;76:681–93.
16. Johnson PJ, Berhane S, Kagebayashi C, et al. Assessment of liver function in patients with hepatocellular carcinoma: A new evidence-based approach—The ALBI grade. *J Clin Oncol* 2015;33:550–8.
17. Augustin S, Pons M, Maurice JB, et al. Expanding the Baveno VI criteria for the screening of varices in patients with compensated advanced chronic liver disease. *Hepatol* 2017;66:1980–8.
18. Seo N, Myoung Soo Kim MS, Park M-S, et al. Evaluation of treatment response in hepatocellular carcinoma in the explanted liver with liver imaging reporting and data system version 2017. *Eur Radiol* 2020;30(1):261–71.
19. Gillmore R, Stuart S, Kirkwood A, et al. EASL and mRECIST responses are independent prognostic factors for survival in hepatocellular cancer patients treated with transarterial embolisation. *J Hepatol* 2011;55:1309–16.
20. Prajpati HJ, Spivey JR, Hanish SI, et al. mRECIST and EASL responses at early time point by contrast-enhanced dynamic MRI predict survival in patients with unresectable hepatocellular carcinoma (HCC) treated by doxorubicin drug-eluting beads transarterial chemoembolization (DEB TACE). *Ann Oncol* 2013;24:965–73.
21. Yu H, Bai Y, Xie X, et al. RECIST 1.1 versus mRECIST for assessment of tumour response to molecular targeted therapies and disease outcomes in patients with hepatocellular carcinoma: A systematic review and meta-analysis. *BMJ Open* 2022;12(6):e052294.
22. Yau T, Merle P, Rimassa L, et al. Assessment of tumor response, alpha-fetoprotein response, and time to progression in the phase III CELESTIAL trial of cabozantinib versus placebo in advanced hepatocellular carcinoma. *Ann Oncol* 2018;29:ix46.
23. Bruix J, Reig M, Merle P, et al. Alpha-fetoprotein (AFP) response in patients with unresectable hepatocellular carcinoma (HCC) in the phase III RESORCE trial. *Ann Oncol* 2019;30:v291.
24. Shao YY, Liu TH, Hsu C, et al. Early alpha-foetoprotein response associated with treatment efficacy of immune checkpoint inhibitors for advanced hepatocellular carcinoma. *Liver Int* 2019;39(11):2184–9.
25. Zhu AX, Dayyani F, Yen CJ, et al. Alpha-fetoprotein as a potential surrogate biomarker for atezolizumab + bevacizumab treatment of hepatocellular carcinoma. *Clin Cancer Res* 2022;28(16):3537–45.
26. Colloca GA, Venturino A. Radiographic and serologic response in patients with unresectable hepatocellular carcinoma receiving systemic antineoplastic treatments: A trial-level analysis. *Cancer* 2024;130(10):1773–83.
27. Tian BW, Yan LJ, Ding ZN, et al. Early alpha-fetoprotein response predicts prognosis of immune checkpoint inhibitor and targeted therapy for hepatocellular carcinoma: A systematic review with meta-analysis. *Expert Rev Gastroenterol Hepatol* 2023;17(1):73–83.
28. He C, Peng W, Liu X, et al. Post-treatment alpha-fetoprotein response predicts prognosis of patients with hepatocellular carcinoma: A meta-analysis. *Medicine (Baltimore)* 2019;98(31):e16557.
29. Yeo W, Mok TS, Zee B, et al. A randomized phase III study of doxorubicin versus cisplatin/interferon α-2b/doxorubicin/fluorouracil (PIAF) combination chemotherapy for unresectable hepatocellular carcinoma. *J Natl Cancer Inst* 2005;97:1532–8.
30. Finn RS, Qin S, Ikeda M, et al. Atezolizumab plus bevacizumab in unresectable hepatocellular carcinoma. *N Engl J Med* 2020;382(20):1894–905.
31. Llovet JM, Ricci S, Mazzaferro V, et al. Sorafenib in advanced hepatocellular carcinoma. *N Engl J Med* 2008;359:378–90.
32. Johnson PJ, Qin S, Park J-W, et al. Brivanib versus sorafenib as first-line therapy in patients with unresectable, advanced hepatocellular carcinoma: Results from the randomized phase III BRISK-FL study. *J Clin Oncol* 2013;31:3517–24.
33. Zhu AX, Rosmorduc O, Evans TRJ, et al. SEARCH: A phase III, randomized, double-blind, placebo-controlld trial of sorafenib plus erlotinib in patients with advanced hepatocellula carcinoma. *J Clin Oncol* 2015;33:559–66.
34. Kudo M, Finn RS, Qin S, et al. Overall survival and objective response in advanced unresectable hepatocellular carcinoma: A subanalysis of the REFLECT study. *J Hepatol* 2023;78(1):133–41.
35. He MK, Li QJ, Zou RH, et al. Sorafenib plus hepatic arterial infusion of oxaliplatin, fluorouracil, and leucovorin vs sorafenib alone for hepatocellular carcinoma with portal vein invasion. *JAMA Oncol* 2019;5(7):953–60.
36. Patt YZ, Hassan MM, Aguayo A, et al. Oral capecitabine for the treatment of hepatocellular carcinoma, cholangiocarcinoma, and gallbladder carcinoma. *Cancer* 2004;101:578–86.
37. Boige V, Raoul J-L, Pignon J-P, et al. Multicentre phase II trial of capecitabine plus oxaliplatin (XELOX) in patients with advanced hepatocellular carcinoma: FFCD 03-03 trial. *Br J Cancer* 2007;97:862–7.

38. Lee JO, Lee KW, Oh DY, et al. Combination chemotherapy with capecitabine and cisplatin for patients with metastatic hepatocellular carcinoma. *Ann Oncol* 2009;20:1402–7.
39. Toh HC, Chen P-J, Carr BI, et al. Phase 2 trial of linifanib (ABT-869) in patients with unresectable or metastatic hepatocellular carcinoma. *Cancer* 2013;119(2):380–7.
40. Zaanan A, Williet N, Hebbar M, et al. Gemcitabine plus oxaliplatin in advanced hepatocellular carcinoma: A large multicenter AGEO study. *J Hepatol* 2013;58:81–8.
41. Cabibbo G, Enea M, Attanasio M, et al. A meta-analysis of survival rates of untreated patients in randomized clinical trials of hepatocellular carcinoma. *Hepatol* 2010;51(4):1274–83.
42. Wang R, Lin N, Mao B, et al. The efficacy of immune checkpoint inhibitors in advanced hepatocellular carcinoma: A meta-analysis based on 40 cohorts incorporating 3697 individuals. *J Cancer Res Clin Oncol* 2022;148(5):1195–210.
43. Oweira H, Petrausch U, Helbling D, et al. Prognostic value of site-specific extra-hepatic disease in hepatocellular carcinoma: A SEER database analysis. *Expert Rev Gastroenterol Hepatol* 2017;11(7):695–701.
44. Oishi J, Itamoto T, Kobayashi T, et al. Hepatectomy for hepatocellular carcinoma in elderly patients aged 75 years or more. *Gastrointest Surg* 2009;13(4):695–701.
45. Asahina Y, Tsuchiya K, Tamaki N, et al. Effect of aging on risk for hepatocellular carcinoma in chronic hepatitis C virus infection. *Hepatol* 2010;52:518–27.
46. Sheedfar F, Di Biase S, Koonen D, et al. Liver disease and aging: Friends or foes? *Aging Cell* 2013;12:950–4.
47. Lv X, Ye G, Zhang X, et al. P16 methylation was associated with the development, age, hepatic viruses infection of hepatocellular carcinoma, and p16 expression had a poor survival. *Medicine* 2017;96:38(e8106).
48. Kelley RK, Rimassa L, Cheng A-L, et al. Cabozantinib plus atezolizumab versus sorafenib for advanced hepatocellular carcinoma (COSMIC-312): A multicentre, open-label, randomised, phase 3 trial. *Lancet Oncol* 2022;23:995–1008.
49. Yau T, Park J-W, Finn RS, et al. Nivolumab versus sorafenib in advanced hepatocellular carcinoma (CheckMate 459): A randomised, muticentre, open-label, phase 3 trial. *Lancet Oncol* 2022;23:77–90.
50. Kapacee ZA, McNamara MG, de Liguori Carino N, et al. Systemic therapies in advanced hepatocellular carcinoma: How do older patients fare? *Eur J Surg Oncol* 2021;47:583–90.
51. Hung AK, Guy J. Hepatocellular carcinoma in the elderly: Meta-analysis and systematic literature review. *World J Gastroenterol* 2015;21(42):12197–210.
52. Du J, Mao Y, Liu M, et al. Dose age affect the efficacy of molecular targeted agents in the treatment of hepatocellular carcinoma: A systematic review and meta-analysis. *Oncotarget* 2017;8(60):102413–9.
53. Cheng AL, Kang Y-K, Chen Z, et al. Efficacy and safety of sorafenib in patients in the Asia-Pacific region with advanced hepatocellular carcinoma: A phase III randomised, double-blind, placebo-controlled trial. *Lancet Oncol* 2009;10:25–34.
54. Bruix J, Cheng A-L, Meinhardt G, et al. Prognostic factors and predictors of sorafenib benefit in patients with hepatocellular carcinoma: Analysis of two phase III studies. *J Hepatol* 2017;67:999–1008.
55. Zheng B, Zhu Y-J, Wang H-Y, et al. Gender disparity in hepatocellular carcinoma (HCC): Multiple underlying mechanisms. *Sci China Life Sci* 2017;60(6):575–84.
56. Yan L-J, Yao S-Y, Meng G-X, et al. Sex and regional disparities in incidence of hepatocellular carcinoma in autoimmune hepatitis: A systematic review and meta-analysis. *Hepatol Int* 2021;15(6):1413–20.
57. Burra P, Bizzaro D, Gonta A, et al. Clinical impact of sexual dimorphism in non-alcoholic fatty liver disease (NAFLD) and non-alcoholic steatohepatitis (NASH). *Liver Int* 2021;41(8):1713–33.
58. Dhir RN, Dworakowski W, Thangavel C, et al. Sexually dimorphic regulation of hepatic isoforms of human cytochrome p450 by growth hormone. *J Pharmacol Exp Ther* 2006;316(1):87–94.
59. Shi L, Feng Y, Lin H, et al. Role of estrogen in hepatocellular carcinoma: Is inflammation the key? *J Transl Med* 2014;12:93.
60. Liu W-C, Liu Q-Y. Molecular mechanisms of gender disparity in hepatitis B virus-associated hepatocellular carcinoma. *World J Gastroenterol* 2014;20(20):6252–61.
61. Yeh Y-T, Chang C-W, Wei R-J, et al. Progesterone and related compounds in hepatocellular carcinoma: Basic and clinical aspects. *BioMed Res Int* 2013;2013:290575.
62. Shen J, Wang S, Zhang Y-J, et al. Exploring genome-wide DNA methylation profiles altered in hepatocellular carcinoma using Infinium Human Methylation 450 Bead Chips. *Epigenetics* 2013;8(1):34–43.
63. Li X, Hui A-M, Sun L, et al. p16INK4A hypermethylation is associated with hepatitis virus infection, age, and gender in hepatocellular carcinoma. *Clin Cancer Res* 2004;10(22):7484–9.

64. Lee HS, Kim B-H, Cho N-Y, et al. Prognostic implications of and relationship between CpG island hypermethylation and repetitive DNA hypomethylation in hepatocellular carcinoma. *Clin Cancer Res* 2009;15(3):812–20.
65. Park S-J, Jeong S-Y, Kim HJ. Y chromosome loss and other genomic alterations in hepatocellular carcinoma cell lines analyzed by CGH and CGH array. *Cancer Genet Cytogenet* 2006;166(1):56–64.
66. Liu J, Wang Z-M, Zhen S-F, et al. Aberration of X chromosome in liver neoplasm detected by fluorescence in situ hybridization. *Hepatobiliary Pancreat Dis Int* 2004;3(1):110–4.
67. Ruggieri A, Gagliardi MC, Anticoli S. Sex-dependent outcome of hepatitis B and C viruses infections: Synergy of sex hormones and immune responses? *Front Immunol* 2018;9:2302.
68. Ali MA, Lacin S, Abdel-Wahab R, et al. Nonalcoholic steatohepatitis-related hepatocellular carcinoma: Is there a role for the androgen receptor pathway? *Onco Targets Ther* 2017;10:1403–12.
69. Ma W-L, Lai H-C, Yeh S, et al. Androgen receptor roles in hepatocellular carcinoma, cirrhosis and hepatitis. *Endocr Relat Cancer* 2014;21(3):R165–82.
70. Kalra M, Mayes J, Assefa S, et al. Role of sex steroid receptors in pathobiology of hepatocellular carcinoma. *World J Gastroenterol* 2008;14(39):5945–61.
71. Wang S, Cowley LA, Liu X-S. Sex differences in cancer immunotherapy efficacy, biomarkers, and therapeutic strategy. *Molecules* 2019;24(18):3214.
72. Conforti F, Pala L, Bagnardi V, et al. Cancer immunotherapy efficacy and patients' sex: A systematic review and meta-analysis. *Lancet Oncol* 2018;19(6):737–46.
73. Wang C, Dehghani B, Li Y, et al. Membrane estrogen receptor regulates experimental autoimmune necephalomyelitis through up-regulation of programmed death 1. *J Immunol* 2009;182(5):3294–303.
74. Sayaf K, Gabbia D, Russo FP, et al. The role of sex in acute and chronic liver damage. *Int J Mol Sci* 2022;23:10654.
75. Tan DJH, Wong C, Ng CH, et al. A meta-analysis on the rate of hepatocellular carcinoma recurrence after liver transplant and associations to etiology, alpha-fetoprotein, income and ethnicity. *J Clin Med* 2021;10:238.
76. Rich NE, Carr C, Yopp AC, et al. Racial and ethnic disparities in survival among patients with hepatocellular carcinoma in the United States: A systematic review and meta-analysis. *Clin Gastroenterol Hepatol* 2022;20(2):e267–88.
77. Thylur RP, Roy SK, Shrivastava A, et al. Assessment of risk factors, and racial and ethnic differences in hepatocellular carcinoma. *JGH Open* 2020;4:351–9.
78. Zhang S, Jiang J, Tang W, et al. Methylenetetrahydrofolate reductase C677T (Ala>Val, rs1801133 C>T) polymorphism decreases the susceptibility of hepatocellular carcinoma: A meta-analysis involving 12,628 subjects. *Biosci Rep* 2020;40:BSR20194229.
79. Su H. Correlation between MTHFR polymorphisms and hepatocellular carcinoma: A meta-analysis. *Nutr Cancer* 2019;71(7):1055–60.
80. Quan Y, Yang J, Qin T, et al. Associations between twelve common gene polymorphisms and susceptibility to hepatocellular carcinoma: Evidence from a meta-analysis. *World J Surg Oncol* 2019;17:216.
81. Luo Y-Y, Zhang H-P, Huang A-L, et al. Association between KIF1B rs17401966 genetic polymorphism and hepatocellular carcinoma susceptibility: An updated meta-analysis. *BMC Med Genet* 2019;20:59.
82. Zhang C, Ye Z, Zhang Z, et al. A comprehensive evaluation of single nucleotide polymorphisms associated with hepatocellular carcinoma risk in Asian populations: A systematic review and network meta-analysis. *Gene* 2020;735:144365.
83. Wang C, Liu W, Zhao L, et al. Association of cytotoxic T-lymphocyte antigen-4 + 49A/G gene polymorphism with hepatocellular carcinoma risk in Chinese. *J Cancer Res Ther* 2018;14(S):S1117–20.
84. Chen J. The prognostic analysis of different metastatic patterns in advanced liver cancer patients: A population based analysis. *PLoS ONE* 2018;13(8):e0200909.
85. Gupta A, Das A, Majumder K, et al. Obesity is independently associated with increased risk of hepatocellular cancer-related mortality: A systematic review and meta-analysis. *Am J Clin Oncol* 2018;41(9):874–81.
86. Kim K, Choi S, Park SM. Association of high body mass index and hepatocellular carcinoma in patients with chronic hepatitis B virus infection: A Korean population-based cohort study. *JAMA Oncol* 2018;4(5):737–9.
87. Camhi SM, Bray GA, Bouchard C, et al. The relationship of waist circumference and BMI to visceral, subcutaneous, and total body fat: Sex and race differences. *Obesity* 2011;19(2):402–8.
88. Fahira A, Hanifah RS, Wardoyo MP, et al. Is higher BMI associated with worse overall mortality in hepatocellular carcinoma patients? An evidence based case report. *Acta Med Indones* 2019;51(4):356–63.

89. Wang Z, Aguilar EG, Luna JI, et al. Paradoxical effects of obesity on T cell function during tumor progression and PD-1 checkpoint blockade. *Nat Med* 2019;25:141–51.
90. Imai K, Takai K, Hanai T, et al. Skeletal muscle depletion predicts the prognosis of patients with hepatocellular carcinoma treated with sorafenib. *Int J Mol Sci* 2015;16(5):9612–24.
91. Baadran H, Elsabaawy MM, Ragab A, et al. Baseline sarcopenia is associated with lack of response to therapy, liver decompensation and high mortality in hepatocellular carcinoma patients. *Asian Pac J Cancer Prev* 2020;21(11):3285–90.
92. Antonelli G, Gigante E, Iavarone M, et al. Sarcopenia is associated with reduced survival in patients with advanced hepatocellular carcinoma undergoing sorafenib treatment. *United Eur Gastroenterol J* 2018;6(7):1039–48.
93. Nishikawa H, Nishijima N, Enomoto H, et al. Prognostic significance of sarcopenia in patients with hepatocellular carcinoma undergoing sorafenib therapy. *Oncol Lett* 2017;14(2):1637–47.
94. Saeki I, Yamasaki T, Maeda M, et al. No muscle depletion with high visceral fat as a novel beneficial biomarker of sorafenib for hepatocellular carcinoma. *Liver Cancer* 2018;7(4):359–71.
95. Baek KK, Kim JK, Uhm JE, et al. Prognostic factors in patients with advanced hepatocellular carcinoma treated with sorafenib: A retrospective comparison with previously known prognostic models. *Oncology* 2011;80(3–4):167–74.
96. Shen A, Tang C, Wang Y, et al. A systematic review of sorafenib in Child-Pugh A patients with unresectable hepatocellular carcinoma. *J Clin Gastroenterol* 2013;47(10):871–80.
97. McNamara MG, Slagter AE, Nuttall C, et al. Sorafenib as first-line therapy in patients with advanced Child-Pugh B hepatocellular carcinoma – A meta-analysis. *Eur J Cancer* 2018;105:1–9.
98. Toyoda H, Lai PBS, O'Beirne J, et al. Long-term impact of liver function on curative therapy for hepatocellular carcinoma: Application of the ALBI grade. *Br J Cancer* 2016;114:744–50.
99. Toyoda H, Johnson PJ. The ALBI score: from liver function in patients with HCC to a general measure of liver function. *JHEP Rep* 2022;4:100557.
100. Feng D, Wang M, Hu J, et al. Prognostic value of the albumin-bilirubin grade in patients with hepatocellular carcinoma and other liver disease. *Ann Transl Med* 2020;8(8):553.
101. Demirtas CO, D'Alessio A, Rimassa L, et al. ALBI grade: Evidence for an improved model for liver functional estimation in patients with hepatocellular carcinoma. *JHEP Rep* 2021;3:100347.
102. Hsu W-F, Hsu S-C, Chen T-H, et al. Modified albumin-bilirubin model for stratifying survival in patients with hepatocellular carcinoma receiving anticancer therapy. *Cancers* 2022;14:5083.
103. Peng Y, Wei Q, He Y, et al. ALBI versus Child-Pugh in predicting outcome of patients with HCC: A systematic review. *Exp Rev Gastroenterol Hepatol* 2020;14(5):383–400.
104. Bannaga A, Arasaradnam RP. Neutrophil to lymphocyte ratio and albumin bilirubin grade in hepatocellular carcinoma: A systematic review. *World J Gastroenterol* 2020;26(33):5022–49.
105. Singal AG, Pillai A, Tiro J. Early detection, curative treatment, and survival rates for hepatocellular carcinoma surveillance in patients with cirrhosis: A meta-analysis. *PLOS Med* 2014;11(4):e1001624.
106. McGlynn KA, Petrick JL, El-Serag HB. Epidemiology of hepatocellular carcinoma. *Hepatol* 2021;73(Suppl 1):4–13.
107. Llovet JM, Kelley RK, Villanueva A, et al. Hepatocellular carcinoma. *Nat Rev Dis Primers* 2021;7(1):6.
108. Pazgan-Simon M, Simon KA, Jarowicz E, et al. Hepatitis B virus treatment in hepatocellular carcinoma patients prolongs survival and reduces the risk of cancer recurrence. *Clin Exp Hepatol* 2018;4(3):210–6.
109. Kaur SP, Talat A, Karimi-Sari H, et al. Hepatocellular carcinoma in hepatitis B virus-infected patients and the role of hepatitis B surface antigen (HbsAg). *J Clin Med* 2022;11:1126.
110. Kim G-A, Lim Y-S, Han S, et al. High risk of hepatocellular carcinoma and death in patients with immune-tolerant-phase chronic hepatitis B. *Gut* 2017;945–52.
111. Premkumar M, Chawla YK. Should we treat immune tolerant chronic hepatitis B? Lessons from Asia. *J Clin Exp Hepatol* 2022;12(1):144–54.
112. Sapena V, Enea M, Torres F, et al. Hepatocellular carcinoma recurrence after direct-acting antiviral therapy: An individual patient data meta-analysis. *Gut* 2022;71(3):593–604.
113. Park J, Cho J, Lim JH, et al. Relative efficacy of systemic treatments for patients with advanced hepatocellular carcinoma according to viral status: A systematic review and network meta-analysis. *Target Oncol* 2019;14(4):395–403.
114. Hatanaka T, Kakizaki S, Hiraoka A, et al. Comparative efficacy and safety of atezolizumab and bevacizumab between hepatocellular carcinoma patients with viral and non-viral infection: A Japanese multicenter observational study. *Cancer Med* 2023;12(5):5293–303.

115. Jackson R, Psarelli E-E, Berhane S, et al. Impact of viral status on survival in patients receiving sorafenib for advanced hepatocellular cancer: A meta-analysis of randomized phase III trials. *J Clin Oncol* 2017;35(6):622–8.

116. Kolamunnage-Dona R, Berhane S, Potts H, et al. Sorafenib is associated with a reduced rate of tumor growth and liver function deterioration in HCV-induced hepatocellular carcinoma. *J Hepatol* 2021;75(4):879–87.

117. Zhou Y, Si X, Wu L, et al. Influence of viral hepatitis status on prognosis in patients undergoing hepatic resection for hepatocellular carcinoma: A meta-analysis of observational studies. *World J Surg Oncol* 2011;9:108.

118. Xu C, Cheng S, Chen K, et al. Sex differences in genomic features of hepatitis B-associated hepatocellular carcinoma with distinct antitumor immunity. *Cell Molec Gastroenterol Hepatol* 2023;15(2):327–54.

119. Lee M-H, Yang H-I, Lu S-N, et al. Hepatitis C virus seromarkers and subsequent risk of hepatocellular carcinoma: Long-term predictors from a community-based cohort study. *J Clin Oncol* 2010;28(30):4587–93.

120. Lockart I, Yeo MGH, Hajarizadeh B, et al. HCC incidence after hepatitis C cure among patients with advanced fibrosis or cirrhosis: A meta-analysis. *Hepatol* 2022;76:139–54.

121. Wu S-S, Shan Q-Y, Xie W-X, et al. Outcomes after hepatectomy of patients with positive HbcAb Non-B Non-C hepatocellular carcinoma compared to overt hepatitis B virus hepatocellular carcinoma. *Clin Transl Oncol* 2020;22:401–10.

122. Ioannou GN, Green P, Kerr KF, et al. Models estimating risk of hepatocellular carcinoma in patients with alcohol or NAFLD-related cirrhosis for risk stratifications. *J Hepatol* 2019;71(3):523–33.

123. Julien J, Ayer T, Bethea ED, et al. Projected prevalence and mortality associated with alcohol-related liver disease in the USA, 2019–40: A modelling study. *Lancet Publ Health* 2020;5(6):e316–23.

124. Fassio E, Barreyro FJ, Perez MS, et al. Hepatocellular carcinoma in patients with metabolic dysfunction-associated fatty liver disease: Can we stratify at-risk populations? *World J Hepatol* 2022;14(2):354–71.

125. Marasco G, Poggioli F, Colecchia A, et al. A nomogram-based prognostic model for advanced hepatocellular carcinoma patients treated with sorafenib: A multicenter study. *Cancers* 2021;13:2677.

126. Nakano M, Kuromatsu R, Nilzeki T, et al. Immunological inflammatory biomarkers as prognostic predictors for advanced hepatocellular carcinoma. *ESMO Open* 2021;6(1):100020.

127. Wang S, Deng Y, Yu X, et al. Prognostic significance of preoperative systemic inflammatory biomarkers in patients with hepatocellular carcinoma after microwave ablation and establishment of a nomogram. *Sci Rep* 2021;11:13814.

128. Yang YM, Kim SY, Seki E. Inflammation and liver cancer: Molecular mechanisms and therapeutic targets. *Semin Liver Dis* 2019;39(1):26–42.

129. Li X, Wu S, Yu Y. Aspirin use and the incidence of hepatocellular carcinoma in patients with hepatitis B virus or hepatitis C virus infection: A meta-analysis of cohort studies. *Front Med* 2021;7:569759.

130. Li L, Li X, Li W, et al. Prognostic models for outcome prediction in patients with advanced hepatocellular carcinoma treated by systemic therapy: A systematic review and critical appraisal. *BMC Cancer* 2022;22(1):750.

131. Tian G, Li G, Guan L, et al. Pretreatment albumin-to-alkalyne phosphatase ratio as a prognostic indicator in solid cancers: A meta-analysis with trial sequential analysis. *Int J Surg* 2020;81:66–73.

132. Scheiner B, Pomej K, Kirstein MM, et al. Prognosis of patients with hepatocellular carcinoma treated with immunotherapy – Development and validation of the CRAFITY score. *J Hepatol* 2022;76:353–63.

133. Takagi K, Domagala P, Polak WG, et al. Prognostic significance of the controlling nutritional status (CONUT) score in patients undergoing hepatectomy for hepatocellular carcinoma: A systematic review and meta-analysis. *BMC Gastroenterol* 2019;19:211.

134. Kuo Y-H, Wang J-H, Hung C-H, et al. Albumin-bilirubin grade predicts prognosis of HCC patients with sorafenib use. *J Gastroenterol Hepatol* 2017;32(12):1975–81.

135. Li Q, Lyu Z, Wang L, et al. Albumin-to-alkalyne phosphatase ratio associates with good prognosis of hepatitis B virus-positive HCC patients. *Onco Targets Ther* 2020;13:2377–84.

136. Chan AWH, Chan SL, Mo FKF, et al. Albumin-to-alkalyne phosphatase ratio: A novel prognostic index for hepatocellular carcinoma. *Dis Markers* 2015;2015:564057.

137. Pinter M, Sieghart W, Hucke F, et al. Prognostic factors in patients with advanced hepatocellular carcinoma treated with sorafenib. *Aliment Pharmacol Ther* 2011;34:949–59.

138. Nomura F, Ohnishi K, Tanabe Y. Clinical features and prognosis of hepatocellular carcinoma with reference to serum alpha-fetoprotein levels. Analysis of 606 patients. *Cancer* 1989;64(8):1700–7.

139. Zong J, Fan Z, Zhang Y. Serum tumor markers for early diagnosis of primary hepatocellular carcinoma. *J Hepatocell Carcinoma* 2020;7:413–22.

140. Llovet JM, Montal R, Sia D, et al. Molecular therapies and precision medicine for hepatocellular carcinoma. *Nat Rev Clin Oncol* 2008;15(10):599–616.

141. Montal R, Andreu-Oller C, Bassaganyas L, et al. Molecular portrait of high alpha-fetoprotein in hepatocellular carcinoma: Implications for biomarker-driven clinical trials. *Br J Cancer* 2019;121:340–3.

142. Bruix J, Qin S, Merle P, et al. Regorafenib for patients with hepatocellular carcinoma who progressed on sorafenib treatment (RESORCE): A randomised, double-blind, placebo-controlled, phase 3 trial. *Lancet* 2017;389(10064):56–66.

143. Zhu AX, Park JO, Ryoo B-Y, et al. Ramucirumab versus placebo as second-line treatment in patients with advanced hepatocellular carcinoma following first-line therapy with sorafenib (REACH): A randomised, double-blind, multicentre, phase 3 trial. *Lancet Oncol* 2015;16(7):859–70.

144. Yokoo T, Patel AD, Lev-Cohain N, et al. Extrahepatic metastasis risk of hepatocellular carcinoma based on α-fetoprotein and tumor staging parameters at cross-sectional imaging. *Cancer Manage Res* 2017;9:503–11.

145. Zhu AX, Finn RS, Kang Y-K, et al. Serum alpha-fetoprotein and clinical outcomes in patients with advanced hepatocellular carcinoma treated with ramucirumab. *Br J Cancer* 2021;124:1388–97.

146. Kudo M, Chung H, Osaki Y. Prognostic staging system for hepatocellular carcinoma (CLIP score): Its value and limitations, and a proposal for a new staging system, the Japan Integrated Staging Score (JIS score). *J Gastroenterol* 2003;38(3):207–15.

147. Faria SC, Szklaruk J, Kaseb AO, et al. TNM/Okuda/Barcelona/UNOS/CLIP international multidisciplinary classification of hepatocellular carcinoma: Concepts, perspectives, and radiologic implications. *Abdom Imaging* 2014;39(5):1070–87.

148. Ueno S, Tanabe G, Sako K, et al. Discrimination value of the new western prognostic system (CLIP score) for hepatocellular carcinoma in 662 japanese patients. *Hepatol* 2001;34:529–34.

149. Levy I, Sherman M, LCSG. Staging of hepatocellular carcinoma: Assessment of the CLIP, Okuda, and Child-Pugh staging systems in a cohort of 257 patients in Toronto. *Gut* 2002;50:881–5.

150. Golfieri R, Bargellini I, Spreafico C, et al. Patients with Barcelona Clinic Liver Cancer stages B and C hepatocellular carcinoma: Time for a subclassification. *Liver Cancer* 2019;8:78–91.

151. Kudo M, Arizumi T, Ueshima K, et al. Subclassification of BCLC B stage hepatocellular carcinoma and treatment strategies: Proposal of a modified Bolondi's subclassification (Kinki criteria). *Dig Dis* 2015;33(6):751–8.

152. Bolondi L, Burroughs A, Dufour J-F, et al. Heterogeneity of patients with intermediate (BCLC B) hepatocellular carcinoma: Proposal for a subclassification to facilitate treatment decisions. *Semin Liv Dis* 2012;32(4):348–59.

153. Usta S, Kayaalp C. Tumor diameter for hepatocellular carcinoma: Why should size matter? *J Gastrointest Cancer* 2020;51(4):1114–7.

154. Yan B, Bai D-S, Zhang C, et al. Characteristics and risk differences of different tumor sizes on distant metastases of hepatocellular carcinoma: A retrospective cohort study in the SEER database. *Int J Surg* 2020;80:94–100.

155. Tang S-C, Lin K-Y, Huang T-F, et al. Association of primary tumor location with long-term oncological prognosis following hepatectomy for hepatocellular carcinoma: A multicenter propensity score matching analysis. *Eur J Surg Oncol* 2023;49(7):1234–41.

156. Sotiropoulos GC, Molmenti EP, Lang H. Milan criteria, up-to-seven criteria, and the illusion of a rescue package for patients with liver cancer. *Lancet Oncol* 2009;10(3):208–9.

157. Mazzaferro V, Llovet JM, Miceli R, et al. Predicting survival after liver transplantation in patients with hepatocellular carcinoma beyond the Milan criteria: A retrospective, exploratory analysis. *Lancet Oncol* 2009;10(1):35–43.

158. Sasaki K, Morioka D, Conci S, et al. The tumor burden score: A new "metro-ticket" prognostic tool for colorectal liver metastases based on tumor size and number of tumors. *Ann Surg* 2018;267(1):132–41.

159. Huo TI, Hsu CY, Huang YH, et al. Prognostic prediction across a gradient of total tumor volume in patients with hepatocellular carcinoma undergoing locoregional therapy. *BMC Gastroenterol* 2010;10(1):146.

160. Iida H, Kalbori M, Hirokawa F, et al. New hepatic resection criteria for intermediate-stage hepatocellular carcinoma can improve long-term survival: A retrospective, multicenter collaborative study. *Asia-Pac J Cancer Prev* 2020;21(10):2903–11.

161. Chua TC, Morris DL. Exploring the role of resection of extrahepatic metastases from hepatocellular carcinoma. *Surg Oncol* 2012;21(2):95–101.

162. Pan J, Wang L, Gao F, et al. Epidemiology of portal vein thrombosis in liver cirrhosis: A systematic review and meta-analysis. *Eur J Intern Med* 2022;104:21–32.

163. Llovet JM, Bustamante J, Castells A, et al. Natural history of untreated nonsurgical hepatocellular carcinoma: Rationale for the design and evaluation of therapeutic trials. *Hepatol* 1999;29(1):62–7.
164. Minagawa M, Makuuchi M. Treatment of hepatocellular carcinoma accompanied by portal vein tumor thrombus. *World J Gastroenterol* 2006;12(47):7561–7.
165. Shi J, Lai ECH, Li N, et al. A new classification for hepatocellular carcinoma with portal vein tumor thrombus. *J Hepatobiliary Pancreat Sci* 2011;18(1):74–80.
166. Spreafico C, Sposito C, Vaiani M, et al. Development of a prognostic score to predict response to Yttrium-90 radioembolization for hepatocellular carcinoma with portal vein invasion. *J Hepatol* 2018;68(4):724–32.
167. Zhang X-P, Gao Y-Z, Chen Z-H, et al. An eastern hepatobiliary surgery hospital / portal vein tumor thrombus scoring system as an aid to decision making on hepatectomy for hepatocellular carcinoma patients with portal vein tumor thrombus: A multicenter study. *Hepatol* 2019;69(5):2076–90.
168. Hwang S, Moon D-B, Kim K-H, et al. Prognostic accuracy of the ADV score following resection of hepatocellular carcinoma with portal vein tumor thrombosis. *J Gastrointest Surg* 2021;25(7):1745–59.
169. Zhou XH, Li JR, Zheng TH, et al. Portal vein tumor thrombosis in hepatocellular carcinoma: Molecular mechanisms and therapy. *Clin Exp Metastasis* 2023;40(1):5–32.
170. Zhang H, Ye J, Weng X, et al. Comparative transcriptome analysis reveals that the extracellular matrix receptor interaction contributes to the venous metastases of hepatocellular carcinoma. *Cancer Genet* 2015;208(10):482–91.
171. Khan AR, Wei X, Xu X. Portal vein tumor thrombosis and hepatocellular carcinoma – The changing tides. *J Hepatocell Carcinoma* 2021;8:1089–115.
172. Lee HA, Seo YS, Shin I-S, et al. Efficacy and feasibility of surgery and external radiotherapy for hepatocellular carcinoma with portal invasion: A meta-analysis. *Int J Surg* 2022;104:106753.
173. Sena G, Paglione D, Gallo G, et al. Surgical resection of a recurrent hepatocellular carcinoma with portal vein thrombosis: Is it a good treatment option? A case report and systematic review of the literature. *J Clin Med* 2022;11:5287.
174. Tao Z-W, Cheng B-Q, Zhou T, et al. Management of hepatocellular carcinoma patients with portal vein tumor thrombosis: A narrative review. *Hepatobiliary Pancreat Dis Int* 2022;21(2):134–44.
175. Luo J, Xu L, Li L, et al. Comparison of treatments for hepatocellular carcinoma patients with portal vein thrombosis: A systematic review and network meta-analysis. *Ann Transl Med* 2021;9(18):1450.
176. Valenzuela A, Ha NB, Gallo A, et al. Recurrent hepatocellular carcinoma and poorer overall survival in patients undergoing left-sided compared with right-sided partial hepatectomy. *J Clin Gastroenterol* 2015;49(2):158–64.
177. Sakuraoka Y, Kubota K, Tanaka G, et al. Is left-sided involvement of hepatocellular carcinoma an important preoperative predictive factor of poor outcome? *World J Surg Oncol* 2020;18(1):317.
178. Yasui M, Harada A, Nonami T, et al. Potentially multicentric hepatocellular carcinoma: Clinicopathologic characteristics and postoperative prognosis. *World J Surg* 1997;21(8):860–5.
179. Huang Z-Y, Liang B-Y, Xiong M, et al. Long-term outcomes of repeat hepatic resection in patients with recurrent hepatocellular carcinoma and analysis of recurrent types and their prognosis: A single-center experience in China. *Ann Surg Oncol* 2012;19(8):2515–25.
180. Wang J, Li Q, Sun Y, et al. Clinicopathologic features between multicentric occurrence and intrahepatic metastasis of multiple hepatocellular carcinomas related to HBV. *Surg Oncol* 2009;18(1):25–30.
181. Li S-L, Su M, Peng T, et al. Clinicopathologic characteristics and prognoses for multicentric occurrence and intrahepatic metastasis in synchronous multinodular hepatocellular carcinoma patients. *Asian Pacific J Cancer Prev* 2013;14(1):217–23.
182. Portolani N, Coniglio A, Ghidoni S, et al. Early and late recurrence after liver resection for hepatocellular carcinoma: Prognostic and therapeutic implications. *Ann Surg* 2006;243:229–35.
183. Tabrizian P, Jibara G, Shrager B, et al. Recurrence of hepatocellular cancer after resection: Patterns, treatments, and prognosis. *Ann Surg* 2015;261(5):947–55.
184. Zhang H, Liu F, Wen N, et al. Patterns, timing, and predictors of recurrence after laparoscopic liver resection for hepatocellular carcinoma: Results from a high-volume HPB center. *Surg Endosc* 2022;36(2):1215–23.
185. Li Z, Zhang K, Lin S-M, et al. Radiofrequency ablation combined with percutaneous ethanol injection for hepatocellular carcinoma: A systematic review and meta-analysis. *Int J Hyperthermia* 2017;33(3):237–46.
186. Cheung FP-Y, Alam NZ, Wright GM. The past, present and future of pulmonary metastasectomy: A review article. *Ann Thorac Cardiovasc Surg* 2019;25(3):129–41.

187. Zhou Y, Zhou X, Ma J, et al. Nomogram for predicting the prognosis of patients with hepatocellular carcinoma presenting with pulmonary metastasis. *Cancer Manage Res* 2021;13:2083–94.
188. Staubitz JI, Hoppe-Lotichius M, Baumgart J, et al. Survival after adrenalectomy for metastatic hepatocellular carcinoma: A 25-year institutional experience. *World J Surg* 2021;45:1118–25.
189. Ikai I, Arli S, Ichida T, et al. Report of the 16th follow-up survey of primary liver cancer. *Hepatol Res* 2005;32(3):163–72.
190. Nakashima T, Okuda K, Kojiro M, et al. Pathology of hepatocellular carcinoma in Japan. 232 consecutive cases autopsied in ten years. *Cancer* 1983;51(5):863–74.
191. Park JS, Yoon DS, Kim KS, et al. What is the best treatment modality for adrenal metastasis from hepatocellular carcinoma? *J Surg Oncol* 2007;96(1):32–6.
192. Teegen EM, Mogl MT, Pratschke J, et al. Adrenal metastasis of hepatocellular carcinoma in patients following liver resection or liver transplantation: Experience from a tertiary referral center. *Int J Surg Oncol* 2018;2018:4195076.
193. Hiraki T, Yamakado K, Ikeda O, et al. Percutaneous radiofrequency ablation for pumonary metastases from hepatocellular carcinoma: Results of a multicenter study in Japan. *J Vasc Interv Radiol* 2011;22(6):741–8.
194. Okusaka T, Okada S, Ishii H, et al. Prognosis of hepatocellular carcinoma patients with extrahepatic metastases. *Hepatogastroenterol* 1997;44(13):251–7.
195. Kitano K, Murayama T, Sakamoto M, et al. Outcome and survival analysis of pulmonary metastasectomy for hepatocellular carcinoma. *Eur J Cardiothorac Surg* 2012;41:376–82.
196. Bathia R, Ravulapati S, Befeler A, et al. Hepatocellular carcinoma with bone metastases: Incidence, prognostic significance, and management – Single-center experience. *J Gastrointest Cancer* 2017;48(4):321–5.
197. Zhang K, Tao C, Wu F, et al. A practical nomogram from the SEER database to predict the prognosis of hepatocellular carcinoma in patients with lymph node metastasis. *Ann Palliat Med* 2021;10(4):3847–63.
198. Lin C-C, Liang H-P, Lee H-S, et al. Clinical manifestations and survival of hepatocellular carcinoma patients with peritoneal metastasis. *J Gastroenterol Hepatol* 2009;24(5):815–20.
199. Hashimoto M, Sasaki K, Moriyama J, et al. Resection of peritoneal metastases in patients with hepatocellular carcinoma. *Surgery* 2013;153:727–31.
200. Nam HC, Sung PS, Song DS, et al. Control of intracranial disease is associated with improved survival in patients with brain metastasis from hepatocellular carcinoma. *Int J Clin Oncol* 2019;24(6):666–76.
201. Okuda T, Hayashi N, Takahashi M, et al. Clinical outcomes of brain metastases from hepatocellular carcinoma: A multicenter retrospective study and a literature review. *Int J Clin Oncol* 2018;23(6):1095–100.
202. Choi SB, Kim H, Kim SH, et al. Solitary extrahepatic intraabdominal metastasis from hepatocellular carcinoma after liver transplantation. *Yonsei Med J* 2011;52(1):199–203.
203. Alexandrescu ST, Croitoru AE, Grigorie RT, et al. Aggressive surgical approach in patients with adrenal-only metastases from hepatocellular carcinoma enables higher survival rates than standard systemic therapy. *Hepatobiliary Pancreat Dis Int* 2021;20(1):28–33.
204. Torbenson MS. Morphologic subtypes of hepatocellular carcinoma. *Gastroenterol Clin North Am* 2017;46(2):365–91.
205. Murtha-Lemekhova A, Fuchs J, Schulz E, et al. Scirrhous hepatocellular carcinoma: Systematic review and pooled data analysis of clinical, radiological, and histopathological features. *J Hepatocell Carcinoma* 2021;8:1269–79.
206. Edmondson HA, Steiner PE. Primary carcinoma of the liver: A study of 100 cases among 48,900 necropsies. *Cancer* 1954;7(3):462–503.
207. Zhou L, Rui J-A, Wang S-B, et al. Factors predictive for long-term survival of male patients with hepatocellular carcinoma after curative resection. *J Surg Oncol* 2017;95:298–303.
208. Decaens T, Roudot-Thoraval F, Badran H, et al. Impact of tumor differentiation to select patients before liver transplantation for hepatocellular carcinoma. *Liver Int* 2011;31(6):792–801.
209. Kong J, Wang T, Shen S, et al. A nomogram predicting the prognosis of young adult patients diagnosed with hepatocellular carcinoma: A population-based analysis. *PLoS One* 2019;14(7):e0219654.
210. Luo Y, Ren F, Liu Y, et al. Clinicopathological and prognostic significance of high Ki-67 labeling index in hepatocellular carcinoma patients: A meta-analysis. *Int J Clin Exp Med* 2015;8(7):10235–47.
211. Isik B, Gonultas F, Sahin T, et al. Microvascular venous invasion in hepatocellular carcinoma: Why do recurrences occur? *J Gastrointest Cancer* 2020;51(4):1133–6.
212. Calderaro J, Petitprez F, Becht E, et al. Intra-tumoral tertiary lymphoid structures are associated with a low risk of early recurrence of hepatocellular carcinoma. *J Hepatol* 2019;70(1):58–65.

213. Llovet JM, Zucman-Rossi J, Pikarsky E, et al. Hepatocellular carcinoma. *Nat Rev Dis Primers* 2016;2:16018.

214. Zucman-Rossi J, Villanueva A, Nault J-C, et al. Genetic landscape and biomarkers of hepatocellular carcinoma. *Gastroenterol* 2015;149(5):1226–39e4.

215. The Cancer Genome Atlas Research Network. Comprehensive and integrative genomic characterization of hepatocellular carcinoma. *Cell* 2017;169:1327–41.

216. Schulze K, Nault J-C, Villanueva A. Genetic profiling of hepatocellular carcinoma using next-generation sequencing. *J Hepatol* 2016;65(5):1031–42.

217. Sung W-K, Zheng H, Li S, et al. Genome-wide survey of recurrent HBV integration in hepatocellular carcinoma. *Nat Genet* 2012;44(7):765–9.

218. Desert R, Rohart F, Canal F, et al. Human hepatocellular carcinomas with a periportal phenotype have the lowest potential for early recurrence after curative resection. *Hepatol* 2017;66(5):1502–18.

219. Tornesello ML, Buonaguro L, Tatangelo F, et al. Mutations in TP53, CTNNB1 and PIK3CA genes in hepatocellular carcinoma associated with hepatitis B and hepatitis C virus infections. *Genomics* 2013;102:74–83.

220. Alizadeh AA, Aranda V, Bardelli A, et al. Toward understanding and exploiting tumor heterogeneity. *Nat Med* 2015;21(8):846–53.

221. Talhao JG, Dagher I, Lino T, et al. Treatment of tumor recurrence after resection of hepatocellular carcinoma. Analysis of 97 consecutive patients. *Eur J Surg Oncol* 2007;33(6):746–51.

222. Cheng A-L, Qin S, Ikeda M, et al. Updated efficacy and safety data from IMbrave150: Atezolizumab plus bevacizumab vs. sorafenib for unresectable hepatocellular carcinoma. *J Hepatology* 2022;76:862–73.

223. Abou-Alfa GK, Lau G, Kudo M, et al. Tremelimumab plus durvalumab in Unresectable Hepatocellular Carcinoma. *NEJM Evid* 2022;1(8):EVIDoa2100070.

224. Ren Z, Xu J, Bai Y, et al. Sintilimab plus a bevacizumab biosimilar (IBI305) versus sorafenib in unresectable hepatocellular carcinoma (ORIENT-32): A randomised, open-label, phase 2–3 study. *Lancet Oncol* 2021;22:977–90.

225. Peng Z-W, Zhang Y-J, Chen M-S, et al. Radiofrequency ablation with or without transcatheter arterial chemoembolization in the treatment of hepatocellular carcinoma: A prospective randomized trial. *J Clin Oncol* 2013;31:426–32.

226. Dhondt E, Lambert B, Hermie L, et al. 90 Y Radioembolization versus drug-eluting bead chemoembolization for unresectable hepatocellular carcinoma: Results from the TRACE phase II randomized controlled trial. *Radiol* 2022;303:699–710.

227. Kudo M, Ueshima K, Ikeda M, et al. Final results of TACTICS: A randomized, prospective trial comparing transarterial chemoembolization plus sorafenib to transarterial chemoembolization alone in patients with unresectable hepatocellular carcinoma. *Liver Cancer* 2022;11:354–67.

228. Li Q-J, He M-K, Chen H-W, et al. Hepatic arterial infusion of oxaliplatin, fluorouracil, and leucovorin versus transarteri248al chemoembolization for large hepatocellular carcinoma: A randomized phase III trial. *J Clin Oncol* 2022;40:150–60.

229. Zhu AX, Kang Y-K, Yen C-J, et al. Ramucirumab after sorafenib in patients with advanced hepatocellular carcinoma and increased α-fetoprotein concentrations (REACH-2): A randomised, double-blind, placebo-controlled, phase 3 trial. *Lancet Oncol* 2019;20:282–96.

230. Abou-Alfa GK, Meyer T, Cheng A-L, et al. Cabozantinib in patients with advanced and progressing hepatocellular carcinoma. *N Engl J Med* 2018;379:54–63.

6 Biliary tract cancer

6.1 INTRODUCTION

Biliary tree cancers (BTCs) are a spectrum of invasive tumors from gallbladder carcinoma (GBC) to cholangiocarcinomas (CCAs). The latter is in turn divided by anatomic location into intrahepatic cholangiocarcinoma (iCCA) up to the second-order bile ducts, peri-hilar cholangiocarcinoma (pCCA) and distal cholangiocarcinoma (dCCA) from the distal epithelium of the cystic duct [1–3]. Each of them is associated with different risk factors (RFs), and presents different clinical features and prognoses [4, 5].

The 2020 WHO/ICD11 classification [6] has complicated the interpretation of previous studies [7], increasing the uncertainty about prognostic factors (PFs) and RFs, because many pCCAs have become iCCAs [8], but diagnostics, migrations and the burden of chronic liver disease have changed too [9].

6.1.1 EPIDEMIOLOGY

Globally, BTCs are 3% of malignancies and 10–15% of hepato-biliary tumors [10], with incidence of 0.3–6/100,000 [2, 11]. An evaluation of the WHO database documented that the overall mortality for iCCA ranged between 0.2–2.5/100,000, and was higher than p/dCCA [11]. A report from the GLOBOCAN 2020 showed an estimated 115,949 new cases and 84,695 deaths from GBC worldwide [12]. Differently from the other CCAs, GBCs are included in the European registry, and their incidence age-adjusted standardized rate (ASR) in 2022 was 1.8/100,000, with 7,851 new cases, a mortality ASR of 1.2/100,000 and 5,150 cancer deaths [13].

The incidence of BTCs has wide geographic variations, with peaks in Asia [14]. The highest rates in 2010–2014 have been registered in Europe (France, Spain, Austria, UK), Australia, and Hong Kong, while the lowest were in South America and Eastern Europe [11].

BTC incidences appear to increase with a higher rate among <50 years old [15], particularly iCCA [16], whereas GBCs appear reducing [17]. Mortality increased too [11], particularly among males and in some regions (Asia vs. Western countries) [13]. In the last decades, iCCA generally increased [4, 17–20], while d/pCCA are decreasing [4, 18, 21]. This iCCAs increase may be linked to the improvement of diagnostics, but also to the changing prevalence of RFs, the obesity pandemic, metabolic syndrome, and nonalcoholic fatty liver disease (NAFLD) [5]. For GBC in Europe, the estimated incidence by year 2040 is increasing with an additional 31.6% of new cases [13].

6.1.2 STAGING OF METASTATIC DISEASE

Regardless of the localization in the biliary tree, investigations should include medical history, assessment of comorbidities and signs of hepatitis and cirrhosis, primary sclerosing cholangitis (PSC) or autoimmune disease.

Some laboratory tests are recommended, such as liver function, alpha-fetoprotein (AFP), carbohydrate antigen 19-9 (CA 19-9) and IgG4.

Imaging consists of multiphasic chest-abdomen CT, which is necessary for diagnosis and staging. CT and MRI are useful for differential diagnosis between iCCA and hepatocellular carcinoma (HCC), when a liver nodule >2 cm occurs [22]. In the case of suspected CCA, MRI-cholangiopancreatography is preferred for primary tumor (PT) diagnosis and detection of liver metastases (LMs).

 DOI: 10.1201/9781032703350-6

Histologic classification and pathologic diagnosis should be performed on surgical samples or extensive core biopsy. Biopsy should include nonneoplastic liver tissue to assess the underlying disease, and is mandatory before any nonsurgical upfront treatment since a molecular profiling is needed. Regarding molecular testing, although activating mutations are more frequent in iCCAs, all patients with unresectable or metastatic biliary tree cancer (mBTC) who might receive second-line treatment, require evaluation of targetable alterations, such as IDH and BRAF mutations, HER2 overexpression, FGFR2 and NTRK fusion genes, and deficit of MMR system, either by immuno-histochemistry or preferably by NGS or liquid biopsy.

The 8th TNM/AJCC 2017 system is the reference for staging, while WHO classification and LI-RADS criteria are recommended for imaging evaluation.

6.1.3 PROGNOSIS OF METASTATIC DISEASE

Five-year survival was 15.2% for all BTCs, ranging from 8.5% (iCCA) to 34.5% (ampullary tumors), with lower rates for patients with distant metastases (3%) compared with locally advanced (LA) disease (19.1–31.5%) [19].

6.2 ANALYSIS OF PROGNOSTIC VARIABLES IN EARLY METASTATIC DISEASE

A systematic review of prospective trials that studied upfront therapies in patients with mBTCs resulted in the evaluation of 88 studies, published from 1993 to 2022. One study enrolled also pancreatic tumors, and was excluded.

Sixteen trials, one phase III and 15 phase II, whose results were reported in 17 articles [23–39], were selected because an analysis of PFs was carried out. Eight reported the complete results of a multivariate analysis (MVA). The current chapter focuses on the results of the PFs that have been reported in at least one of the 16 studies and the number of studies that found or did not a relationship between PFs and overall survival (OS) (Table S1).

In addition, the results of the PFs analysis performed on 66 metastatic iCCA patients undergoing chemotherapy with cisplatin and gemcitabine in the ABC-01, ABC-02, and ABC-03 trials are reported among the high-level evidence selected trials [40].

6.3 PATIENT-RELATED PROGNOSTIC FACTORS

6.3.1 PERFORMANCE STATUS

An observational study of the European ENSCCA registry found that a deteriorated ECOG PS was an unfavorable PF, though the study sample included all stages. OS reduction was detected for each PS subgroup compared to patients with good PS [41].

A prospective study and a retrospective series did not report any prognostic relationship for PS [42, 43], while four retrospective analyses confirmed the poor prognosis of deteriorated PS [44–47]. Of four retrospective studies including patients with metastatic iCCA, three showed a relationship between poor PS and reduced OS [48–50], while another was negative [51]. A short OS of patients with an ECOG PS 2–3 was reported by two retrospective series of metastatic p/dCCA patients [52, 53], as the better outcome of ECOG PS 0 of mGBC patients emerged in another study [54].

6.3.1.1 Selected studies

Eight trials investigated PS, and six demonstrated a significant relationship with OS, with a reduction of OS as PS deteriorated (Table 6.1). Six studies published HR and therefore were included in a meta-analysis, which allowed to calculate a global effect size (ES) (HR 2.65, CI 0.70–10.11; Q = 24.62, p-value = 0.0002; I^2 = 79.7%) (Figure 6.1).

TABLE S1
Prognostic factors analyzed in selected clinical trials of patients with metastatic biliary tree cancer receiving upfront treatment

Variable	No. trials	Prognostic relationship	No prognostic relationship
Patient-related			
Performance status	8	6	2
Age	9	1	8
Sex	7	1	6
Anthropometric			
Body weight	1	0	1
Body surface area	1	0	1
Body mass index	1	0	1
Lab			
Hemoglobin	3	2	1
White blood count	2	0	2
Neutrophil count	2	1	1
Derived neutrophil-lymphocyte ratio	1	1	0
Platelet count	2	1	1
Albumin	1	0	1
Bilirubin	3	0	3
Alkalyne phosphatase	2	0	2
Aspartate transaminase	2	0	2
Alanine transaminase	2	0	2
Lactic dehydrogenase	1	1	0
Markers			
CA 19-9	6	1	5
CEA	4	1	3
CA 125	1	1	0
Tumor-related			
Tumor burden			
Tumor size	2	0	2
T4 vs. T1–3	1	1	0
Disease status	5	2	3
No. sites metastases	1	0	1
Multifocality	1	0	1
Location	9	3	6
Timing of metastasis	1	0	1
Site of metastasis			
Liver metastases	1	0	1
Peritoneal metastases	1	0	1
Pathology			
Microscopic (histotype)	1	0	1
Grade	1	0	1
Previous treatments			
Primary tumor resection	2	0	2
Biliary stent	2	0	2

TABLE 6.1
Prognostic relationships of performance status in selected studies of patients with unresectable or metastatic biliary tree cancer receiving upfront treatment

Study [ref]	Phase	No. pts	Scale	Comparison	Prognostic relationship	Effect size
Indian 2004 [25]	II	30	Zubrod	≥2 vs. 0–1	Yes	HR 1.22 (0.30–4.00)
Canadian 2005 [26]	II	45	ECOG	NR	No	NR
Korean 2005 [27]	II	23	ECOG	2 vs. 0–1	Yes	OS 5.2 vs. 17.3 m
Japanese 2006 [28]	II	42	ECOG	continuous	Yes	HR 50.00 (3.85–100)
Japanese 2009 [29]	II	61	ECOG	1 vs. 0	Yes	HR 2.52 (1.44–4.42)
ABC-02 2010 [23, 24]	III	358	ECOG	1 vs. 0	Yes	HR 1.29 (1.04–1.61)
		182		2 vs. 0	Yes	HR 2.35 (1.68–3.28)
Hungarian 2013 [32]	II	17	ECOG	1 vs. 0	Yes	HR 3.23 (0.92–11.11)
		23		2 vs. 0	Yes	HR 14.29 (2.22–100)
BINGO 2014 [35]	II	141	WHO	1+ vs. 0	No	HR 1.37 (0.89–2.12)

Legend: ECOG, Eastern Cooperative Oncology Group. HR, hazard ratio. m, months. NR, not reported. OS, overall survival. WHO, World Health Organization.

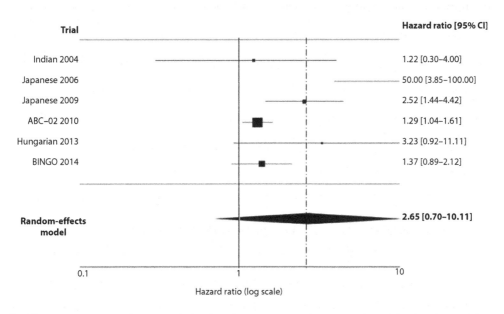

FIGURE 6.1 Forest plot of meta-analysis of performance status in prospective trials of patients with unresectable or metastatic biliary tree cancer

The pooled analysis of the 66 metastatic iCCA patients enrolled in ABC trials did not document a significant effect on the prognosis of ECOG PS 1 vs. 0, while a shorter OS was reported for ECOG PS 2 vs. 0 [40].

6.3.2 DEMOGRAPHIC

6.3.2.1 Age

A meta-analysis reported a poor outcome with increasing age in pCCA patients, but cut-offs varied from 58 to 70 years [55]. Of other eight studies [42–47, 56, 57], with similar cut-offs, only one documented a worse outcome for elderly patients [44]. No role for age >60–65 was reported from three studies enrolling advanced iCCA patients [48, 51, 58], and in other two with metastatic p/dCCA [52, 53], whereas two of four studies evaluating mGBCs [54, 59–61] documented reduced OS [54, 59].

A cohort of 847 BTC patients from the CITY trial documented longer OS for younger patients, who also presented more advanced disease and received more adjuvant and palliative therapies, but also showed different molecular profiles [62].

6.3.2.2   Sex

Among the CCAs, iCCAs have a male predominance, while GBCs have a predilection for females [63]. An unfavorable trend of poor outcomes for males was reported [41, 64]. Despite the frequent negative findings of the studies [42–44, 46], some authors suggested better OS for males [47, 57], and others for females [45, 65].

One population-based study in patients with advanced iCCA documented a prognostic relationship [58], while three retrospective studies found no differences [48, 50, 51]. In both pCCA [53] and GBC patients [54, 59–61], sex did not influence OS.

6.3.2.3   Other demographic variables

Geographic variations in CCA are partly associated with the distribution of RFs. Two SEER analyses evaluated iCCA patients and found only in one case reduced OS in Blacks vs. Whites [58, 65], while a third SEER analysis of GBC patients did not show differences between Whites and non-Whites [59], as a retrospective comparison of Caucasian vs. Asian vs. African-American mGBC patients [54].

Two studies from the SEER database also investigated marital status, ruling out its role in the prognosis of patients with metastatic iCCA [58, 65].

6.3.2.4   Selected trials

Nine studies assessed age, as resumed in Table 6.2. Only a post-hoc analysis of one study showed a poor prognosis with increasing age [34].

Seven studies investigated sex, without documenting any relationship in six (Table 6.3).

TABLE 6.2
Prognostic relationships of age in selected studies of patients with unresectable or metastatic biliary tree cancer receiving upfront treatment

Study [ref]	Phase	No. pts	Comparison	Prognostic relationship	Effect size
Indian 2004 [25]	II	30	> vs. <50	No	HR 1.33 (0.56–3.68)
Canadian 2005 [26]	II	45	NR	No	NR
Korean 2005 [27]	II	23	> vs. ≤60	No	OS 5.7 vs. 17.3 m
Japanese 2006 [28]	II	42	> vs. ≤69	No	HR 1.59 (0.27–9.09)
Japanese 2009 [29]	II	61	> vs. ≤64	No	NR
ABC-02 2010 [23, 24]	III	410	>70 vs. <60	No	HR 1.13 (0.86–1.48)
			60–70 vs. <60	No	HR 1.00 (0.80–1.25)
Hungarian 2013 [32]	II	34	NR	No	NR
AIO 2014 [34]	II	97	continuous	Yes	HR 1.04 (1.01–1.08)
MSKCC 2020 [39]	II	38	continuous	No	HR 1.00 (0.95–1.04)

Legend: HR, hazard ratio. m, months. NR, not reported. OS, overall survival.

TABLE 6.3

Prognostic relationships of sex in selected studies of patients with unresectable or metastatic biliary tree cancer receiving upfront treatment

Study [ref]	Phase	No. pts	Comparison	Prognostic relationship	Effect size
Indian 2004 [25]	II	30	M vs. F	No	HR 0.94 (0.36–2.59)
Canadian 2005 [26]	II	45	M vs. F	No	NR
Korean 2005 [27]	II	23	M vs. F	No	NR
Japanese 2006 [28]	II	42	M vs. F	Yes	HR 0.12 (0.02–0.64)
Japanese 2009 [29]	II	61	M vs. F	No	NR
ABC-02 2010 [23, 24]	III	322	M vs. F	No	HR 1.28 (1.01–1.60)
Hungarian 2013 [32]	II	34	M vs. F	No	NR

Legend: F, females. HR, hazard ratio. M, males. NR, not reported.

The pooled analysis of the three ABC trials excluded a prognostic role for age and sex in iCCAs [40].

6.3.3 ANTHROPOMETRIC

Body mass index (BMI) could play a prognostic role on the iCCAs, as suggested by the association of a 5-point BMI increase with increased risk of recurrence in a cirrhosis-independent manner [66].

High BMI, in particular obesity [67, 68], correlated with an increasing risk of GBC among women [67, 69, 70], but a retrospective analysis failed to find a prognostic role of obesity [43].

Beyond obesity, a role in the prognosis of BTC may be played by body composition [71]. In BTC patients sarcopenia was associated with poor OS and increased postoperative complications [72].

6.3.3.1 Selected trials

Some trials studied BMI [32], weight and body surface area [26], without finding significant prognostic relationships.

6.3.4 CLINIC

The overall number of comorbid conditions, measured by the Charlson Comorbidity Index, was not associated with tumor prognosis [43, 51].

The role of the comorbidities on mBTC prognosis remains poorly investigated, despite the high prevalence of diabetes mellitus (DM) [41] and NAFLD [73]. Similarly, the evidence is limited about the effect on OS from predisposing conditions. Molecular biology studies suggest a worse outcome for fluke-associated [74], while another study documented increased mortality from GBC in patients with DM [75]. If the presence of cholangitis in patients with pCCA was not associated with the prognosis [53], cirrhosis [48, 51] and HCV-related hepatopathy [51] did not affect the outcome of metastatic iCCAs, while two studies report divergent conclusions on HBV [48, 51].

6.3.4.1 Flukes

Fluke infection is associated with 5–6 times higher risk of CCA or more, especially in males [76, 77]. These are often right lobe iCCA [78], with a mass-forming and cholangiolar macroscopic appearance.

The endemic fluke-associated CCAs report a poor prognosis compared with non-fluke-associated and a different molecular landscape [74], although in some studies there is only a trend toward better outcomes [79].

6.3.4.2 Primary sclerosing colangitis

PSC is the most common predisposing condition for CCAs in Western countries, with a lifetime prevalence of 15–20% [80, 81], and higher incidence in the first year when 30–50% of diagnoses are made [82]. It is frequently associated with iCCA [83], whose prevalence has been calculated to be 8.3% [84], regardless of cirrhosis [85]. The age of onset of CCA is approximately 5 years after the diagnosis of PSC. Contrary to what is expected, in PSC-related CCA pathogenesis inflammation is not a major component [86].

There is a lack of recent evidence on the outcome of CCA arising on PSC, which appears associated with poor prognosis [87] and unresectable disease [88].

6.3.4.3 Viruses

Although cirrhosis is related to increased CCA frequency [89] and worse outcomes [90], the risk is increased for HBV and not HCV [91].

HBV-related iCCA tends to occur in younger patients, and males, and it is unclear whether it presents favorable outcomes [92, 93] or not [48], with a meta-analysis of eight studies suggesting better prognosis and clinicopathologic characteristics [94].

Though isolated case reports and small series have been described, probably around 6.6% of iCCAs are EBV-related [95]. These tumors occur often in young females, frequently appearing as lymphoepithelioma-like histotypes. The composition of the tumor microenvironment, with higher density of CD20 and CD8 lymphocytes, and overexpression of PD-1/PD-L1, correlates with higher 2-year survival rates [95].

6.3.5 LABORATORY

6.3.5.1 Hematology

Anemia and neutrophilia did not find prognostic effects in mBTCs [47, 50]. Platelet count was prognostic only in a study enrolling GBC patients [54], and not in those investigating iCCA [50] or CCA [47].

The effect of the tumor on the activation of a systemic inflammatory response (SIR) is suggested by the neutrophil-to-lymphocyte ratio (NLR). A meta-analysis of 32 studies documented an independent relationship of NLR with OS [96], but the relationship was limited to iCCAs. The NLR prognostic effect in metastatic disease is unclear, with a negative prognostic role for an NLR higher than 3–5 in some studies [43, 44, 56, 57] but not in others [46, 47]. Other five studies confirmed the prognostic negative effect of NLR in patients with advanced iCCA [51], pCCA [53] or GBC [54, 60, 61]. Platelet-to-lymphocyte ratio (PLR) >121 was associated with poor prognosis [44], but not other cut-offs [56, 57], nor in studies of iCCA [51] or GBC [60, 61].

6.3.5.2 Chemistry

A retrospective study of iCCA patients at any stage from Fudan University documented that increased bilirubin, gamma-glutamyl-transferase, and alkaline phosphatase (ALP) were associated with poor OS, as was low serum albumin [97]. Of the other nine retrospective studies, four confirmed the negative prognostic effect of hypoalbuminemia with a cut-off of 3.3–3.6 [56], including three on iCCA [48, 50, 51], while three did not [44, 47, 57]. In the two studies that evaluated serum albumin in GBC patients, no relationship with OS emerged [54, 61], but in one, increased pre-albumin correlated with better outcomes [61]. Liver transaminases did not present a prognostic relationship in BTC patients [57], with similar results for iCCA [48, 50] and GBC [54, 60]. Five studies did not suggest any prognostic role for high bilirubin [42, 43, 47, 56, 57], which was associated with poor prognosis in one of two studies of iCCA [48, 51] and one of two on GBC [54, 60]. High serum ALP was related to high rates of 6-month mortality [98], while it did not affect OS in another study [47]; three studies of iCCA patients were also negative, and only one of GBC reported poor OS for high baseline ALP [54]. The relationship of LDH with OS was reported in three studies, with conflicting results, from the lack of any prognostic effect in iCCA [97] and GBC patients [60], to a poor outcome of iCCAs with a serum LDH >220 U/L [50].

Other SIR-related parameters have been explored, with a negative effect on the outcome for C-reactive protein >1 mg/dL in iCCAs [50], but not in other studies [43, 44, 47], and a poor prognosis in both iCCAs [49] and pCCAs [53] for the increased modified Glasgow prognostic score.

6.3.5.3 Tumor markers

CA 19-9 and preoperative carcinoembryonic antigen (CEA) reinforce the prognostic role of the TNM stage [99]. In a report of the ENSCCA registry, a CA 19-9 increase reduced median OS [41]. Specifically, 59.1% of patients had an elevation of CA 19-9, more frequently in locally advanced and metastatic disease. Similarly, CEA increased in 30.9% of cases, more often in locally advanced or metastatic disease. Other authors confirm the usefulness of CA 19-9 in iCCA [100, 101], the increased expression in cases with cirrhosis and metastatic disease [102], while the evidence in favor of the prognostic role in GBC is less solid [103].

Despite CA 19-9 diagnostic limitations [104–106], four [42, 43, 45, 46] of eight studies [44, 47, 56, 57] in mBTC patients reported a relationship with OS, but cut-offs ranged from 37 to 500 U/mL. In none of the three studies of iCCA patients was a relationship between CA 19-9 and the outcome reported [48, 50, 51], as for GBC [61], while a study enrolling p/dCCA concluded for shorter OS of patients with a baseline CA 19-9 >37 U/mL [45].

Three of four studies reported a prognostic negative effect of CEA >5 ng/mL in mBTCs [43, 44, 47, 56], as well as in iCCA patients [50] and GBC [61]. Another study of GBC patients did not report a prognostic effect of CEA, but the cut-off was 3.2 ng/mL [60].

6.3.5.4 Selected trials

Among the hematologic variables, hemoglobin was evaluated in three studies, with positive results for higher cut-offs, around 12.5–13 g/dL in two studies [24, 35]. On the contrary, leukocyte count did not report prognostic effect in two trials [24, 29], whereas data on neutrophil count appear discordant [24, 35], and derived neutrophil-lymphocyte ratio (dNLR) >3 was indicative of poor prognosis in a combined analysis [107]. Only two studies evaluated the platelet count and a relationship with the outcome was evident for a cut-off of 450,000/mcL [35] but not at 150,000/mcL [29].

Biochemical variables related to liver function, such as albumin [29], ALP [29, 39], bilirubin [24, 29, 39], and transaminases [29, 39], were evaluated as continuous variables and did not show relationships with outcome [39], except a negative trend for the increasing bilirubin [24].

Six studies included oncologic markers among the possible PFs, as resumed in Table 6.4. No relationship of baseline CA 19-9 with OS was evident, except in one study [36]. Despite methodological variability, particularly for cut-off range, a combined meta-analysis of the three studies that reported the ES does not support a prognostic role for CA 19-9 (HR 1.03, CI 0.97–1.09; Q = 3.81, p-value = 0.1485; I^2 = 47.6%). Among four studies [28, 29, 36, 39], CEA <10 ng/mL was associated with increased OS in only one [36]. Their meta-analysis suggests a favorable prognostic effect for patients with low or normal CEA (HR 0.69, CI 0.58–0.82; Q = 40.85, p-value <0.0001; I^2 = 80.4%).

Pooled analysis of the three ABC trials of metastatic iCCA patients showed that elevated platelet counts were associated with poor OS in patients with liver-limited disease, while increased CEA correlated with decreased OS, contrary to CA 19-9, which lost its prognostic role after multivariate analysis [40].

TABLE 6.4

Prognostic relationships of tumor markers in selected studies of patients with unresectable or metastatic biliary tree cancer receiving upfront treatment

Study [ref]	Phase	No. pts	Comparison	Prognostic relationship	Effect size
Carbohydrate antigen 19-9 (IU/mL)					
Korean 2005 [27]	II	23	≤ vs. > 40	No	OS 17.3 vs. 7.7 m
Japanese 2006 [28]	II	42	≤ vs. > 5	No	HR 0.08 (0.01–3.50)
Japanese 2009 [29]	II	61	≤ vs. > 1,000	No	HR 0.58 (0.32–1.04)
BINGO 2014 [35]	II	150	≤ vs. > 120	No	HR 1.43 (0.95–2.15)
ABC-03 2015 [36]	II	124	≤ vs. > 10,000	Yes	HR 1.03 (1.01–1.05)
MSKCC 2020 [39]	II	42	≤ vs. >	No	HR 1.14 (0.92–1.40)
Carcinoembryonic antigen (ng/mL)					
Japanese 2006 [28]	II	42	≤ vs. > 10	No	HR 1.10 (0.23–5.16)
Japanese 2009 [29]	II	61	≤ vs. > 10	No	NR
ABC-03 2015 [36]	II	124	≤ vs. > 10	Yes	HR 1.03 (1.01–1.04)
MSKCC 2020 [39]	II	42	≤ vs. >	No	HR 1.41 (0.90–2.20)

Legend: HR, hazard ratio. m, months. NR, not reported. OS, overall survival.

6.4   TUMOR-RELATED PROGNOSTIC FACTORS

6.4.1   TUMOR BURDEN

6.4.1.1   Tumor size

Some features related to tumor burden (TB) did not maintain a prognostic role in mBTC, as two studies did not report a relationship between tumor size and OS [50, 58]. A SEER analysis of 981 metastatic iCCA patients did not find any prognostic relationship for T- or N-stage [65]. In metastatic p/dCCA, T-stage did not correlate with OS [52, 53], while mortality at three months progressively worsened for patients with stage III-IV GBC with increasing T- and N-stage [59].

Patients with advanced iCCAs presented the largest tumor sizes and multifocality since iCCAs with multiple hepatic localizations are often considered as T2b and not M1. On the other hand, iCCA patients with LMs (20%) reported shorter survival than those with a solitary tumor [108].

6.4.1.2   Disease status

The ENSCCA registry documented poor prognosis for metastatic vs. localized disease, but not for LA vs. localized, with a reducing median OS from 30.9 months in localized disease to 16.2 in LA, and 8.1 when metastases occurred, furtherly reducing to 6.1 months when at least two other organs were affected [41]. Some studies found worse outcomes for metastatic versus LA [43, 45], while others did not [42, 46, 47]. However, studies that analyzed BTCs by PT site, each reported negative prognostic relationships of metastatic vs. LA iCCA [48], pCCA [53] and GBC patients [60].

6.4.1.3   Other variables

While one study showed no difference in median OS between patients with >2 sites of metastasis versus those with ≤2 [56], three studies of metastatic iCCA confirmed the prognostic role of the number of sites of metastasis [48, 49, 51].

One study reported a negative effect for measurability by RECIST criteria [45], while study results diverged on the role of the number of metastases [51, 57, 58, 65].

6.4.1.4 Selected trials

Five trials assessed TB by analyzing disease status, with poor OS for metastatic disease in two studies (Table 6.5), but disease status did not affect OS in metastatic iCCA patients of the ABC trials [40].

Two studies, which evaluated the number of metastatic sites [27], multifocality and tumor size as a continuous variable [39], respectively, did not find prognostic relationships.

6.4.2 PRIMARY TUMOR LOCATION

Most studies have not documented prognostic differences based on the location along the biliary tree [42–44, 47, 57], with a US series reporting longer OS for iCCA [83], and a European registry for p/dCCA [41]. Some authors suggested poor outcomes for GBC vs. CCA patients [109], while others found similar outcomes of GBCs and iCCA, and better OS for p/dCCA compared with iCCA [46].

In metastatic pCCAs, the anatomic subgroups defined by the Bismuth-Corlette classification [110] did not appear to have relationships with OS. Among dCCAs, tumors of the ampulla of Vater (AVT), which account for 0.2% of gastrointestinal neoplasms, are often considered separately and have a good prognosis. The ampulla of Vater is the junction of the pancreatic duct with the common bile duct and could be interested by a pancreaticobiliary-type or intestinal-type AVT, characterized by different molecular profiles [111], with a better prognosis for the intestinal type [112].

A meta-analysis of nine retrospective studies reported that hepatic-sided T2 GBCs carry higher odds for mortality and recurrence [113], and local invasion in the gallbladder wall is one of the most important PFs, with similar 5-year survival rates between stage III and IV [114].

Various studies analyzed separately PFs by BTC site of origin, like p/dCCA [52, 115], pCCA [116, 117], and AVT [118].

6.4.2.1 Selected trials

Nine studies investigated PT sites, and are listed in Table 6.6. The more frequently reported comparison, GBCs vs. other CCAs, was evaluated by all studies. Including the five studies that reported an ES in a meta-analysis, it appeared that the overall ES was not significant (HR 2.59, CI 0.16–41.51; Q = 10.41, p-value = 0.0055; I^2 = 80.8%). The comparison between intra-hepatic and extra-hepatic bile ducts was done by one study, which concluded for similar OS [38], as well as another study specifically comparing AVTs vs. GBCs [23].

The IPDA of the three ABC trials documented a trend to prolonged median OS for the 66 iCCA patients compared with non-iCCA (HR 0.65, CI 0.36–1.19) [40].

TABLE 6.5

Prognostic relationships of disease status in selected studies of patients with unresectable or metastatic biliary tree cancer receiving upfront treatment

Study [ref]	Phase	No. pts	Comparison	Prognostic relationship	Effect size
Canadian 2005 [26]	II	45	Metastatic vs. LA	No	NR
Japanese 2006 [28]	II	42	Metastatic vs. LA	Yes	HR 8.26 (1.44–47.62)
Japanese 2009 [29]	II	61	Metastatic vs. LA	No	NR
ABC-02 2010 [23, 24]	III	410	Metastatic vs. LA	Yes	HR 1.34 (1.07–1.69)
Hungarian 2013 [32]	II	34	Metastatic vs. LA	No	NR

Legend: HR, hazard ratio. LA, locally advanced. NR, not reported.

TABLE 6.6

Prognostic relationships of primary tumor location in selected studies of patients with unresectable or metastatic biliary tree cancer receiving upfront treatment

Study [ref]	Phase	No. pts	Comparison	Prognostic relationship	Effect size
Canadian 2005 [26]	II	45	GBC vs. iCCA	Yes	HR 3.61 (1.35–9.67)
Korean 2005 [27]	II	23	GBC vs. iCCA	No	OS 7.4 vs. 7.7 m
Japanese 2006 [28]	II	42	GBC vs. iCCA	Yes	HR 11.1 (1.45–100)
Japanese 2009 [29]	II	61	GBC vs. i/p/dCCA	Yes	HR 1.88 (1.14–3.12)
ABC-02 2010 [23, 24]	III	410	GBC vs. pCCA	No	HR 1.04 (0.84–1.28)
Hungarian 2013 [32]	II	34	GBC vs. i/p/dCCA	No	NR
MSKCC 2013 [33]	II	39	GBC vs. iCCA	No	NR
BINGO 2014 [35]	II	150	GBC vs. other	No	HR 1.01 (0.61–1.69)
MDACC 2019 [38]	II	60	GBC vs. p/d vs. iCCA	No	OS 15.7 vs. 13.2 vs. NR

Legend: dCCA, distal colangiocarcinoma. GBC, gallbladder and bile duct cancer. HR, hazard ratio. iCCA, intrahepatic colangiocarcinoma. m, months. NR, not reported. OS, overall survival. pCCA, peri-hilar colangiocarcinoma.

6.4.3   TIMING OF METASTASIS

A possible prognostic role for the timing of metastasis can be inferred from other reported variables. In particular, one study showed better OS for relapsed versus unresectable disease [56], and similar results were reported by an iCCA series [49].

Similarly, another study evaluated only patients with p/dCCA documenting that an early occurrence of metachronous disease, before 2 years, was associated with poor outcome [52].

6.4.3.1   Selected trials

A study analyzed the timing of metastasis at diagnosis without finding OS differences [26]. Other two trials reported the effect on OS of primary tumor resection (PTR), therefore performed in patients with metachronous disease, documenting no relationship of PTR with OS [27, 29].

6.4.4   SITES OF METASTASIS

Data from a series of relapsed BTC patients documented local recurrence in 21.8%, hepatic in 16.8%, peritoneal in 11.8%, nodal in 10.1%, pulmonary in 9.2%, and multiple in 26.9% [119]. The pattern of metastases differs for iCCA, with the liver as the most frequent site, followed by the lung, bone, and brain [65].

LMs were more frequent in females, unmarried, with advanced T-stage, and displayed better outcomes than bone metastases [65]. Though they are associated with dismal prognosis in BTCs [57, 98], LMs do not seem to change the prognosis of iCCAs, nor does the presence of EHD [51].

Lung metastases were more frequent among patients with regional node involvement [65], and in a retrospective analysis whenever the initial pattern of recurrence included lung metastases, the outcome significantly improved [119].

Brain metastases are very rare in mBTC (0.47–1.4%), predominantly in iCCAs, with very poor prognosis [120, 121]. Notably, a SEER analysis of 12,436 iCCAs documented brain metastases at diagnosis in 112 (0.90%), the likelihood of which increased according to loco-regional stage, AFP level, and tumor size [96].

Two retrospective studies evaluated the impact of the presence of distant lymph node metastases in iCCAs, reporting conflicting findings [51, 68].

6.4.4.1 Selected trials

One trial evaluated the prognostic effect of the presence of LMs or peritoneal metastasis, with negative results for both [29].

6.4.5 PATHOLOGY

6.4.5.1 Histology

Before the 2020 WHO anatomical classification, various morphological classifications based on CCAs have been defined over time [122]. A retrospective study reported reduced OS for histotypes other than adenocarcinoma [45], while there was no difference in another study that evaluated only patients with iCCA [48].

In addition, the conventional iCCA histotype has also been subclassified according to the level of the duct in which it originates, such as small bile duct or large bile duct [123], with the former characterized by IDH mutations or FGFR2 fusions [124, 125]. Although p/dCCAs did not differ histologically from "large bile duct" iCCAs, three varieties are distinguished: papillary, tubular, and superficial spreading types. However, only some rare variants, such as those with squamous and sarcomatous differentiation, were associated with poor prognosis, while mucinous had a better outcome [126].

The lymphoepithelioma-like carcinoma is rare among iCCAs (<5%) [127]. It presents as undifferentiated carcinoma associated with significant lymphoplasmacytic infiltration, that is very similar to EBV-related tumors of other districts.

The rare mixed HCC–CCAs account for <1% of primary liver tumors [128], ranging between 0.4–14.2% [129]. They share RFs with HCC, including HBV, and could be characterized by some markers such as KIT [130]. Despite the mixed aspects, molecular studies suggest a common origin and similar PFs, with overlapping outcomes, to iCCAs.

6.4.5.2 Tumor grade

Although grading did not appear to influence OS in a study of mBTCs, the unfavorable effect of G3–G4 on OS was significant in other studies of patients with iCCA [58], p/dCCA [52], or mGBC [59].

6.4.5.3 Other pathologic variables

Morphologic classification of growth patterns was prognostic for CCAs. For iCCA, a morphologic classification between mass-forming, periductal infiltrating, and intraductal growth has been reported [131, 132], and mass-forming iCCA displayed longer OS [133–135], with the intraductal growth subgroup sometimes with an overlapping prognosis with the mass-forming iCCA, despite a higher frequency of poor differentiation and lymphovascular and perineural invasion [136]. In contrast, a study of Opisthorchis viverrinii infestation-related dCCAs identified the growth patterns as PF, since patients with intraductal growth reported better outcomes than those without [137].

6.4.5.4 Molecular biology

Four clusters based on genomic profiling have been identified, the first two in fluke-positive CCAs (clusters 1 and 2), with a prevalence of HER2 amplifications and TP53 mutations, and the other two in fluke-negative CCAs (clusters 3 and 4), with a prevalence of high copy-number alterations, PD-1/PD-L2 expression, IDH1/2 and BAP1 epigenetic mutations, FGFR rearrangements, and different methylation patterns [74]. Molecular profiling of iCCA has defined two transcriptomic classes, the inflammation and the proliferation class [138, 139]. Other authors have reported a molecular classification of p/dCCAs in four classes [140].

Molecular characterization has made it possible to define some actionable alterations of iCCAs, such as FGFR2 fusions and IDH1 mutations, while few data are yet available for the vast majority of CCAs.

FGFR2 translocations are present in 20–25% of patients with iCCAs [141], and are more frequent in young patients, with G1–G2 tumors. They are usually mutually exclusive with other gene mutations (FGFR, KRAS, BRAF, ERBB2). FGFR2 fusions are much more common in non-fluke-associated CCAs (11.2% vs. 0.8%) and exclusively in iCCAs [142], with only a slightly worsened prognosis.

IDH1 mutations have been reported in 15% [141]. The IDH mutant subtype exhibits distinct molecular aspects [143], predominates among iCCA than p/dCCA (13.1% vs. 0.8%), and in females (66%) [144]. Despite similar outcomes, molecular differences between mutated vs. wild-type IDH1 are marked, since TP53 alteration always reduces OS, whereas KRAS/NRAS and CDKN2A/B mutations affect outcomes only in mutated IDH1 CCAs [145].

A high microsatellite instability phenotype (MSI-H) is present in 10% of iCCA and in 5% of p/dCCA [146], predominantly in fluke-associated disease [79]. It is unclear whether the favorable prognostic effect of MSI-H is lost in stages III-IV [79] or in fluke-associated iCCA [147]. A meta-analysis of p/dCCAs reported poor outcomes for TP53 mutations, more prevalent in fluke-related CCAs (50% vs. 10%) [148]. While BRCA-associated BTCs are uncommon [149], alterations of genes involved in DNA damage response have been identified in 20%, mostly p/dCCA, and predict increased sensitivity to platinum-based chemotherapy [150].

6.4.5.5 Selected trials

Histotype [23], lymph node involvement, and grading [39] did not result in any significant relationship with OS. The degree of differentiation did not correlate with OS in patients with iCCA from the ABC studies [40].

Various analyses of EGFR were performed, without reporting a prognostic effect [30, 32], similar to KRAS mutation [31, 37]. Other studies of VEGFR2 [36], pERK and TP53 [33] did not report any effect on the outcome, while IDH1/2 mutations had a favorable effect on OS (HR 0.21, 0.06–0.75) [39].

6.4.6 PREVIOUS TREATMENTS

Conflicting results on the prognostic role of a previous PTR come from the favorable effect in the SEER database [58, 59, 65], and the negative result of a retrospective study [50].

No prognostic effect in mCCAs was shown for patients undergoing prior radiation therapy for iCCA [58] or prior adjuvant chemotherapy for GBC [60], while surgery of metastases in patients with iCCA correlated with better OS [65]. Previous stent placement did not change the outcome in two retrospective studies [47, 51].

In 61.8% of ENSCCA registry patients, best supportive care (BSC) consisted of biliary stent placement and systemic chemotherapy. While the pCCAs received more often BSC alone, OS after BSC was longer for dCCA and shorter for iCCA patients, with resection and active treatments nullifying the differences [41].

6.4.6.1 Selected trials

Six trials evaluated previous treatments, in two studies prior radiotherapy [27, 28], in two biliary stent placement [26, 29], in two PTR [27, 29], in one adjuvant chemotherapy [28], while the other two included all previous therapies, such as radical/palliative surgery and photodynamic therapy [23, 35]. None of them showed a relationship with OS. Likewise, previous treatments or the presence of biliary stent did not influence the outcome of iCCA patients in ABC trials [40].

6.5 PROGNOSTIC FACTORS IN DECISION-MAKING

Antineoplastic drugs are not recommended for patients with an ECOG PS ≥2, even though some authors suggest single-agent gemcitabine. In the other patients, defining the site of origin is necessary, given the better prognosis of iCCAs [40], but other PFs can be helpful in decision-making (Table 6.7).

6.5.1 UPFRONT TREATMENT

The combination of platinum+gemcitabine is the mainstay of upfront treatment [151], although there appeared to be no difference between gemcitabine and capecitabine [152]. On the other hand, when combined with gemcitabine, both cisplatin and S-1 reported similar activity [153].

However, it is noteworthy that the gemcitabine+cisplatin combination vs. gemcitabine in the ABC-02 trial was not superior in the subgroup of patients with ECOG PS 2, whereas efficacy appeared more pronounced in LA vs. metastatic disease and for some sites (iCCA, GBC) [151], with a pooled analysis confirming these findings [154]. On the other hand, a Japanese study found increased OS from adding S-1 to the doublet, especially in patients <70 and with p/dCCA or GBC [155]. In contrast, an intensification of the upfront regimen with FOLFIRINOX did not improve the results of gemcitabine+cisplatin, albeit some subgroups reported favorable PFS with the triplet, such as GBC, p/dCCA, and patients with high CEA levels [156].

TABLE 6.7

Prognostic and predictive variables in clinical decision-making in metastatic biliary tree cancer

A. Upfront systemic treatment

1	Location
	• iCCA: ICI+CHT and doublet favored (GCD is better than GC; GC is better than G)
	• GBC: doublet favored (GC is better than G)
	• GBC and p/dCCA: triplet favored (GCS is better than GC, FFX better than GC)
2	Performance status
	• ECOG PS 1: ICI+CHT favored (GCD is better than GC)
	• ECOG PS 2: monochemotherapy preferred (G is comparable to GC)
3	Disease status
	• LA: ICI+CHT and doublet favored (GCD is better than GC; GC is better than G)
4	Age
	• <70 years old: triplet favored (GCS is better than GC)
5	Timing metastasis
	• Metachronous: ICI+CHT favored (GCD is better than GC)

B. Treatment of refractory disease (untargetable)

1	Location
	• GBC: doublet favored (nIRI+FU is better than FU)
2	Albumin
	• Low (<35 g/L): doublet favored (FOLFOX is better than BSC)
3	Progression-free survival
	• Longer than 5.1 months: doublet favored (nIRI+FU is better than FU)
4	Performance status
	• ECOG PS 1: doublet favored (nIRI+FU is better than FU)

Legend: BSC, best supportive care. CHT, chemotherapy. dCCA, distal colangiocarcinoma. ECOG PS, Eastern Cooperative Oncology Group performance status. FFX, FOLFIRINOX. FU, fluorouracil. G, gemcitabine. GBC, gallbladder and bile duct cancer. GC, gemcitabine+cisplatin. GCD, gemcitabine+cisplatin+durvalumab. GCS, gemcitabine+cisplatin+S-1. iCCA, intrahepatic colangiocarcinoma. ICI, immune checkpoint inhibitor. LA, locally advanced. nIRI, liposomal irinotecan. pCCA, peri-hilar colangiocarcinoma.

Durvalumab further improved the results of the upfront doublet, with a focus on patients with ECOG PS 1 (patients with ECOG PS 2 had been excluded), in LA and iCCA disease, but also in patients with metachronous metastases [157].

6.5.2 TREATMENT OF REFRACTORY DISEASE

In this setting, the first step is to investigate for actionable targets.

6.5.2.1 Untargetable tumors

When patients do not have target alterations, evidence is available only for those receiving initial gemcitabine-based therapy. The most studied second-line regimens are fluoropyrimidine-based, such as FOLFOX [158] and NALIRI [159]. These studies are small, although suggest that FOLFOX may be more effective than BSC in the case of hypoalbuminemia, while irinotecan+fluorouracil was better than fluorouracil in GBCs, PFS $\geq$5.1 months, and ECOG PS 1.

6.5.2.2 Targetable tumors

In patients with IDH1-mutated iCCA, the treatment with ivosidenib significantly prolonged PFS in all subgroups [160].

TABLE 6.8
Prognostic factors evaluated in prospective trials of upfront treatment in patients with unresectable or metastatic biliary tree cancer

Suggested	Not suggested	Needing study
A. Intra-hepatic colangiocarcinoma		
Performance status	Age	BMI
Hemoglobin		Fluke-related
Albumin		HBV-related
Inflammation-related		CEA
		CA 19-9
Number of sites of metastasis	Previous treatments	Disease status
Liver-limited disease		Timing metastasis
		Grading
B. Peri-hilar and distal colangiocarcinoma		
Performance status	Age	Hemoglobin
CA 19-9	Sex	Inflammation-related
		CEA
Tumor location (ampulla)	Previous treatments	Disease status
		Number of sites of metastasis
		Timing metastasis
		Grading
C. Gallbladder carcinoma		
Performance status	Sex	Age
		Inflammation-related
		ALP
		CEA, CA 19-9
Local invasion (T-stage)	Previous treatments	Disease status
Tumor location (hepatic sided)		Number of sites of metastasis
		Timing metastasis
		Grading

In iCCA patients with FGFR2 fusions or other FGFR alterations, one study documented an objective response rate (ORR) of 14.8% for a selective pan-FGFR kinase inhibitor, BGJ398 [161], while the FIGHT-202 study reported for pemigatinib an ORR of 35%, predominantly in patients with FGFR2 fusions [162].

Other possible molecular alterations are amenable to the related targeted treatments, such as the combination of dabrafenib+trametinib in BRAF mutation [163], pertuzumab+trastuzumab in HER2 overexpression [164], or entrectinib/larotrectinib in NTRK fusion [165]. Finally, there is also favorable evidence for pembrolizumab in MSI-H [166], and a possible role for PARP-inhibitors in HRD or BRCAness.

6.6 CONCLUSION

Molecular diagnostics are candidates to provide additional guidance for decision-making [167]. An analysis of liquid biopsies from a cohort of 1,671 mBTC patients found targetable alterations in 44%, with high concordance between cfDNA and tissue for IDH1 and BRAF-V600E, confirming their clonality and that they are early driver events, whereas a low concordance was reported for FGFR2 fusions. In addition, cfDNA has documented further mutations of known target genes (KRAS, TP53), additional mechanisms of resistance to FGFR2 fusions, and allowed insight into variant allele fraction, which is associated with the level of resistance to treatments [168].

Considering the high heterogeneity of CCAs, a molecular characterization is recommended to explore personalized therapeutic options. Therefore, the role of NGS in the clinical management of BTCs is increasingly important [169].

Table 6.8 resumes current evidence for PFs by location. However, in the rapidly changing clinical landscape, an even more judicious approach to prognosis evaluation of the individual patient is a clinical challenge, as well as the re-interpretation of every clinical variable within any new molecular context that could address more personalized treatment strategies.

REFERENCES

1. Liao P, Cao L, Chen H, Pang S-Z. Analysis of metastasis and survival between extrahepatic and intrahepatic cholangiocarcinoma: A large population-based study. *Medicine* 2021;100(16):e25635.
2. Banales JM, Marin JJ, Lamarca A, et al. Cholangiocarcinoma 2020: The next horizon in mechanisms and management. *Nat Rev Gastroenterol Hepatol* 2020;17:577–88.
3. Nakanuma Y, Kakuda Y. Pathologic classification of cholangiocarcinoma: New concepts. *Best Practice Res Clin Gastroenterol* 2015;29(2):277–93.
4. Rizvi S, Khan SA, Hallemeier CL, Kelley RK, Gores GJ. Cholangiocarcinoma – Evolving concepts and therapeutic strategies. *Nat Rev Clin Oncol* 2018;15(2):95–111.
5. Clements O, Eliahoo J, Kim JU, Taylor-Robinson SD, Khan SA. Risk factors for intrahepatic and extrahepatic cholangiocarcinoma: A systematic review and meta-analysis. *J Hepatol* 2020;72(1):95–103.
6. World Health Organization (WHO). *International Classification of Diseases and Related Health Problems*. 11th Ed. https://icd/who.int/en. Accessed 9 May 2024.
7. Selvadurai S, Mann K, Mithra S, et al. Cholangiocarcinoma miscoding in hepatobiliary centres. *Eur J Surg Oncol* 2021;47(3 Pt B):635–9.
8. Khan SA, Emadossadaty S, Ladep NG, et al. Rising trends in cholangiocarcinoma: Is the ICD classification system misleading us? *J Hepatol* 2012;56(4):848–54.
9. McLean L, Patel T. Racial and ethnic variations in the epidemiology of intrahepatic cholangiocarcinoma in the United States. *Liver Int* 2006;26(9):1047–53.
10. Bergquist A, von Seth E. Epidemiology of cholangiocarcinoma. *Best Pract Res Clin Gastroenterol* 2015;29(2):221–32.
11. Bertuccio P, Malvezzi M, Carioli G, et al. Global trends in mortality from intrahepatic and extrahepatic cholangiocarcinoma. *J Hepatol* 2019;71(1):104–14.
12. Sung H, Ferlay J, Siegel RL, et al. Global cancer statistics 2020: GLOBOCAN estimates of incidence and mortality worldwide for 36 cancers in 185 countries. *CA Cancer J Clin* 2021;71(3):209–49.

13. ECIS – European Cancer Information System, available at https://ecis.jrc.ec.europa.eu, accessed October 31, 2023.
14. Barner-Rasmussen N, Pukkala E, Hadkhale K, Farkkila M. Risk factors, epidemiology and prognosis of cholangiocarcinoma in Finland. *United Eur Gastroenterol* 2021;9:1128–35.
15. Sung H, Siegel RL, Rosenberg PS, Jemal A. Emerging cancer trends among young adults in the USA: Analysis of a population-based cancer registry. *Lancet Public Health* 2019;4:e137–47.
16. Bleyer A, Barr R, Ries L, et al. *Cancer in Adolescents and Young Adults*. Cham; Springer International Publishing AG, 2017.
17. Rahman R, Ludvigsson JF, von Seth E, et al. Age trends in biliary tract cancer incidence by anatomical subtype: A Swedish cohort study. *Eur J Cancer* 2022;175:291–8.
18. Khan SA, Tavolari S, Brandi G. Cholagiocarcinoma: Epidemiology and risk factors. *Liver Int* 2019;39(Suppl 1):9–31.
19. Koshiol J, Yu B, Kabadi SM, et al. Epidemiologic patterns of biliary tract cancer in the United States: 2001–2015. *BMC Cancer* 2022;22:1178.
20. Dasgupta P, Henshaw C, Youlden DR, et al. Global trends in incidence rates of primary adult liver cancers: A systematic review and meta-analysis. *Front Oncol* 2020;10:171.
21. Weaver AJ, Stafford R, Hale J, Denning D, Sanabria JR. Geographical and temporal variation in the incidence and mortality of hepato-pancreato-biliary primary malignancies: 1990–2017. *J Surg Res* 2020;245:89–98.
22. Rimola J, Forner A, Reig M, et al. Cholangiocarcinoma in cirrhosis: Absence of contrast washout in delayed phases by magnetic resonance imaging avoids misdiagnosis of hepatocellular carcinoma. *Hepatology* 2009;50:791–8.
23. Bridgewater J, Lopes A, Palmer D, et al. Quality of life, long-term survivors and long-term outcome from the ABC-02 study. *Br J Cancer* 2016;114:965–71.
24. Bridgewater J, Lopes A, Wasan H, et al. Prognostic factors for progression-free and overall survival in advanced biliary tract cancer. *Ann Oncol* 2016;27:134–40.
25. Doval DC, Sekhon JS, Gupta SK, et al. A phase II study of gemcitabine and cisplatin in chemo-naive, unresectable gall bladder cancer. *Br J Cancer* 2004;90:1516–20.
26. Knox JJ, Hedley D, Oza A, et al. Combined gemcitabine and capecitabine in patients with advanced biliary cancer: A phase II trial. *J Clin Oncol* 2005;23:2332–8.
27. Park J-S, Oh S-Y, Kim S-H, et al. Single-agent gemcitabine in the treatment of advanced biliary tract cancers: A phase II study. *Jpn J Clin Oncol* 2005;35(2):68–73.
28. Kobayashi K, Tsuji A, Morita S, et al. A phase II study of LFP therapy 5-fluorouracil (5-FU) continuous infusion (CVI) and low-dose consecutive cisplatin (CDDP) in advanced biliary tract carcinoma. *BMC Cancer* 2006;6:121.
29. Furuse J, Okusaka T, Ohkawa S, et al. A phase II study of uracil-tegafur plus doxorubicin and prognostic factors in patients with unresectable biliary tract cancer. *Cancer Chemother Pharmacol* 2009;65(1):113–20.
30. Lubner SJ, Mahoney MR, Kolesar JL, et al. Report of a multicenter phase II trial testing a combination of biweekly bevacizumab and daily erlotinib in patients with unresectable biliary cancer: A phase II Consortium study. *J Clin Oncol* 2010;28(21):3491–7.
31. Borbath I, Ceratti A, Verslype C, et al. Combination of gemcitabine and cetuximab in patients with advanced cholangiocarcinoma: A phase II study of the Belgian Group of Digestive Oncology. *Ann Oncol* 2013;24(11):2824–9.
32. Rubovszky G, Lang I, Ganofzsky E, et al. Cetuximab, gemcitabine and capecitabine in patients with inoperable biliary tract cancer: A phase 2 study. *Eur J Cancer* 2013;49(18):3806–12.
33. Lee JK, Capanu M, O'Reilly EM, et al. A phase II study of gemcitabine and cisplatin plus sorafenib in patients with advanced biliary adenocarcinomas. *Br J Cancer* 2013;109(4):915–9.
34. Moehler M, Maderer A, Schimanski C, et al. Gemcitabine plus sorafenib versus gemcitabine alone in advanced biliary tract cancer: A double-blind placebo-controlled multicentre phase II AIO study with biomarker and serum programme. *Eur J Cancer* 2014;50(18):3125–35.
35. Malka D, Cervera P, Foulon S, et al. Gemcitabine and oxaliplatin with or without cetuximab in advanced biliary-tract cancer (BINGO): A randomised, open-label, non-comparative phase 2 trial. *Lancet Oncol* 2014;15(8):819–28.
36. Valle JW, Wasan H, Lopes A, et al. Cediranib or placebo in combination with cisplatin and gemcitabine chemotherapy for patients with advanced biliary tract cancer (ABC-03): A randomised phase 2 trial. *Lancet Oncol* 2015;16(8):967–78.

37. Chen JS, Hsu C, Chiang NJ, et al. A KRAS mutation status-stratified randomized phase II trial of gemcitabine and oxaliplatin alone or in combination with cetuximab in advanced biliary tract cancer. *Ann Oncol* 2015;26(5):943–9.

38. Shroff RT, Javle MM, Xiao L, et al. Gemcitabine, cisplatin, and nab-paclitaxel for the treatment of advanced biliary tract cancers: A phase 2 clinical trial. *JAMA Oncol* 2019;5(6):824–30.

39. Cercek A, Boerner T, Tan BR, et al. Assessment of hepatic arterial infusion of floxuridine in combination with systemic gemcitabine and oxaliplatin in patients with unresectable intrahepatic cholangiocarcinoma: A phase 2 clinical trial. *JAMA Oncol* 2020;6(1):60–7.

40. Lamarca A, Ross P, Wasan HS, et al. Advanced intrahepatic cholangiocarcinoma: Post Hoc analysis of the ABC-01, −02, and −03 clinical trials. *J Natl Cancer Inst* 2020;112(2):200–10.

41. Izquierdo-Sanchez L, Lamarca A, La Casta A, et al. Cholangiocarcinoma landscape in Europe: Diagnostic, prognostic and therapeutic insights from the ENSCCA registry. *J Hepatol* 2022;76(5):1109–21.

42. Grunnet M, Christensen IJ, Lassen U, et al. Decline in CA19-9 during chemotherapy predicts survival in four independent cohorts of patients with inoperable bile duct cancer. *Eur J Cancer* 2015;51(11):1381–8.

43. Lee BS, Lee SH, Son JH, et al. Neutrophil-lymphocyte ratio predicts survival in patients with advanced cholangiocarcinoma on chemotherapy. *Cancer Immunol Immunother* 2016;65(2):141–50.

44. Cho K-M, Park H, Oh D-Y, et al. Neutrophil-to-lymphocyte ratio, platelet-to-lymphocyte ratio, and their dynamic changes during chemotherapy is useful to predict a more accurate prognosis of advanced biliary tract cancer. *Oncotarget* 2017;8(2):2329–41.

45. Kim BJ, Hyung J, Yoo C, et al. Prognostic factors in patients with advanced biliary tract cancer treated with first-line gemcitabine plus cisplatin: Retrospective analysis of 740 patients. *Cancer Chemother Pharmacol* 2017;80(1):209–15.

46. Takahara N, Nakai Y, Isayama H, et al. CA19-9 kinetics during systemic chemotherapy in patients with advanced or recurrent biliary tract cancer. *Cancer Chemother Pharmacol* 2017;80(6):1105–12.

47. Iwaku A, Kinoshita A, Onoda H, et al. The Glasgow Prognostic score accurately predicts survival in patients with biliary tract cancer not indicated for surgical resection. *Med Oncol* 2014;31:787.

48. Chae H, Cho H, Yoo C, et al. Prognostic implications of hepatitis B virus infection in intrahepatic cholangiocarcinoma treated with first-line gemcitabine plus cisplatin. *Int J Biol Markers* 2018;33(4):432–8.

49. Cho H, Yoo C, Kim K, et al. Prognostic implication of inflammation-based prognostic scores in patients with intrahepatic cholangiocarcinoma treated with first-line gemcitabine plus cisplatin. *Invest New Drugs* 2018;36:496–502.

50. Ishimoto U, Kondo S, Ohba A, et al. Prognostic factors for survival in patients with advanced intrahepatic cholangiocarcinoma treated with gemcitabine plus cisplatin as first-line treatment. *Oncology* 2018;94(2):72–8.

51. Huh G, Ryu JK, Chun JW, et al. High platelet-to-lymphocyte ratio is associated with poor prognosis in patients with unresectable intrahepatic cholangiocarcinoma receiving gemcitabine plus cisplatin. *BMC Cancer* 2020;20(1):907.

52. Kim BH, Kim K, Chie EK, et al. Risk stratification and prognostic nomogram for post-recurrence overall survival in patients with recurrent extrahepatic cholangiocarcinoma. *HPB* 2017;19(5):421–8.

53. Okuno M, Ebata T, Yokoyama Y, et al. Appraisal of inflammation-based prognostic scores in patients with unresectable perihilar cholangiocarcinoma. *J Hepatobiliary Pancreat Sci* 2016;23(10):636–42.

54. Mady M, Prasai K, Tella SH, et al. Neutrophil to lymphocyte ratio as a prognostic marker in metastatic gallbladder cancer. *HPB* 2020;22(10):1490–5.

55. Bird NTE, McKenna A, Dodd J, Poston G, Jones R, Malik H. Meta-analysis of prognostic factors for overall survival in patients with resected hilar cholangiocarcinoma. *Br J Surg* 2018;105(11):1408–16.

56. Ha H, Nam A-R, Bang J-H, et al. Soluble programmed death-ligand 1 (sPDL1) and neutrophil-to-lymphocyte ratio (NLR) predicts survival in advanced biliary tract cancer patients treated with palliative chemotherapy. *Oncotarget* 2016;7(47):76604–12.

57. Zhang Z, Wang D, Zhang J, et al. Comparison of the effectiveness of chemotherapy combined with immunotherapy and chemotherapy alone in advanced biliary tract cancer and construction of the nomogram for survival prediction based on the inflammatory index and controlling nutritional status score. *Cancer Immunol Immunother* 2023;72(11):3635–49.

58. Yin L, Zhao S, Zhu H, et al. Primary tumor resection improves survival in patients with multifocal intrahepatic cholangiocarcinoma based on a population study. *Sci Rep* 2021;11(1):12166.

59. Wang J, Yang Y, Pan J, et al. Competing-risk nomogram for predicting survival in patients with advanced (stage III/IV) gallbladder cancer: A SEER population-based study. *Jpn J Clin Oncol* 2022;52(4):353–61.

60. Tao Z, Li SX, Cui X, et al. The prognostic value of preoperative inflammatory indexes in gallbladder carcinoma with hepatic involvement. *Cancer Biomarkers* 2018;1:1–7.

61. Du J-H, Lu J. Circulating CEA-dNLR score predicts clinical outcome of metastatic gallbladder cancer patient. *J Clin Lab Anal* 2019;33(2):e22684.

62. Pappas L, Baiev I, Reyes S, et al. The cholangiocarcinoma in the young (CITY) study: Tumor biology, treatment patterns, and survival outcomes in adolescent young adults with cholangiocarcinoma. *JCO Precis Oncol* 2023;7:e2200594.

63. Rustagi T, Dasanu CA. Risk factors for gallbladder cancer and cholangiocarcinoma: Similarities, differences and updates. *J Gastrointest Cancer* 2012;43(2):137–47.

64. Ledenko M, Antwi SO, Arima S, et al. Sex-related disparities in outcomes of cholangiocarcinoma patients in treatment trials. *Front Oncol* 2022;12:963753.

65. Yan X, Wang P, Zhu Z, et al. Site-specific metastases of intrahepatic cholangiocarcinoma and its impact on survival: A population-based study. *Fut Oncol* 2019;15(18):2125–37.

66. Merath K, Mehta R, Hyer JM, et al. Impact of body mass index on tumor recurrence among patients undergoing curative-intent resection of intrahepatic cholangiocarcinoma- a multi-institutional international analysis. *Eur J Surg Oncol* 2019;45(6):1084–91.

67. Li Z-M, Wu Z-X, Han B, et al. The association between BMI and gallbladder cancer risk: A meta-analysis. *Oncotarget* 2016;7(28):43669–79.

68. Wang F, Wang B, Qiao L. Association between obesity and gallbladder cancer. *Front Biosci* 2012;17:2550–7.

69. Campbell PT, Newton CC, Kitahara CM, et al. Body size indicators and risk of gallbladder cancer: Pooled analysis of individual-level data from 19 prospective cohort studies. *Cancer Epidemiol Biomarkers Prev* 2017;26(4):597–606.

70. Liu H, Zhang Y, Ai M, et al. Body mass index can increase the risk of gallbladder cancer: A meta-analysis of 14 cohort studies. *Med Sci Monit Basic Res* 2016;22:146–55.

71. Watanabe J, Matsui R, Sesanuma H, et al. Body composition assessment and sarcopenia in patients with biliary tract cancer: A systematic review and meta-analysis. *Clin Nutr* 2022;41(2):321–8.

72. Yang L, He Y, Li X. Sarcopenia predicts relevant clinical outcomes in biliary tract cancer patients: A systematic review and meta-analysis. *Nutr Cancer* 2022;74(9):3274–83.

73. Dai W, Ye L, Liu A, et al. Prevalence of nonalcoholic fatty liver disease in patients with type 2 diabetes mellitus: A meta-analysis. *Medicine* 2017;96(39):e8179.

74. Jasakul A, Cutcutache I, Yong CH, et al. Whole-genome and epigenomic landscapes of etiologically distinct subtypes of cholangiocarcinoma. *Cancer Discov* 2017;7(10):1116–35.

75. Jing C, Wang Z, Fu X. Effect of diabetes mellitus on survival in patients with gallbladder cancer: A systematic review and meta-analysis. *BMC Cancer* 2020;20(1):689.

76. Watanapa P, Watanapa WB. Liver fluke-associated cholangiocarcinoma. *Br J Surg* 2002;89:962–70.

77. Lim JH. Liver flukes: The malady neglected. *Korean J Radiol* 2011;12(3):269–79.

78. Choi BI, Park JH, Kim YI, et al. Peripheral cholangiocarcinoma and clonorchiasis: CT findings. *Radiology* 1988;169(1):149–53.

79. Kuntikeo N, Padthaisong S, Loilome W, et al. Mismatch repair deficiency is a prognostic factor predicting good survival of *Opisthorchis viverrini*-associated cholangiocarcinoma at early cancer stage. *Cancers* 2023;15(19):4831.

80. Razumilava N, Gores GJ. Classification, diagnosis, and management of cholangiocarcinoma. *Clin Gastroenterol Hepatol* 2013;11(1):13–21.

81. Trivedi PJ, Crothers H, Mytton J, et al. Effects of primary sclerosing cholangitis on risks of cancer and death in people with inflammatory bowel disease, based on sex, race, and age. *Gastroenterol* 2020;159(3):915–28.

82. Barner-Rasmussen N, Pukkala E, Jussila A, Farkkila M. Epidemiology, risk of malignancy and patient survival in primary sclerosing cholangitis: A population-based study in Finland. *Scand J Gastroenterol* 2020;55(1):74–81.

83. DeOliveira ML, Cunningham SC, Cameron JL, et al. Cholangiocarcinoma: Thirty-one-year experience with 564 patients at a single institution. *Ann Surg* 2007;245(5):755–62.

84. Weismuller TJ, Trivedi PJ, Bergquist A, et al. Patient age, sex, and inflammatory bowel disease phenotype associate with course of primary sclerosing cholangitis. *Gastroenterol* 2017;152(8):1975–84.e8.

85. Welzel TM, Graubard BI, El-Serag HB, et al. Risk factors for intrahepatic and extrahepatic cholangiocarcinoma in the United States: A population-based case-control study. *Clin Gastroenterol Hepatol* 2017;5(10):1221–8.

86. Fung BM, Tabibian JH. Primary sclerosing cholangitis-associated cholangiocarcinoma: Special considerations and best practices. *Exp Rev Gastroenterol Hepatol* 2021;15(5):487–96.
87. Ahrendt SA, Pitt HA, Nakeeb A, et al. Diagnosis and management of cholangiocarcinoma in primary sclerosing cholangitis. *J Gastrointest Surg* 1999;3(4):357–67.
88. Song J, Li Y, Bowlus CL, et al. Cholangiocarcinoma in patients with primary sclerosing cholangitis (PSC): A comprehensive review. *Clin Rev Allergy Immunol* 2020;58(1):134–49.
89. Palmer WC, Patel T. Are common factors involved in the pathogenesis of primary liver cancers? A meta-analysis of risk factors for intrahepatic cholangiocarcinoma. *J Hepatol* 2012;57(1):69–76.
90. Hui C-K, Yuen M-F, Tso W-K, et al. Cholangiocarcinoma in liver cirrhosis. *J Gastroenterol Hepatol* 2003;18(3):337–41.
91. Shaib YH, El-Serag HB, Nooka AK, et al. Risk factors for intrahepatic and extrahepatic cholangiocarcinoma: A hospital-based case-control study. *Am J Gastroenterol* 2007;102(5):1016–21.
92. Luo X, Yuan L, Wang Y, et al. Survival outcomes and prognostic factors of surgical therapy for all potentially resectable intrahepatic cholangiocarcinoma: A large single-center cohort study. *J Gastrointest Surg* 2014;18:562–72.
93. Wu Z-F, Yang N, Li D-Y, et al. Characteristics of intrahepatic cholangiocarcinoma in patients with hepatitis B virus infection: Clinicopathologic study of resected tumours. *J Viral Hepatol* 2013;20(5):306–10.
94. Jeong S, Luo G, Wang Z-H, et al. Impact of viral hepatitis B status on outcomes of intrahepatic cholangiocarcinoma: A meta-analysis. *Hepatol Int* 2018;12(4):330–8.
95. Huang Y-H, Zhang CZ, Huang Q-S, et al. Clinicopathologic features, tumor immune microenvironment and genomic landscape of Epstein-Barr virus-associated intrahepatic cholangiocarcinoma. *J Hepatol* 2021;74(4):838–49.
96. Liu D, Heij LR, Czigany Z, et al. The prognostic value of neutrophil-to-lymphocyte ratio in cholangiocarcinoma: A systematic review and meta-analysis. *Sci Rep* 2022;12(1):12691.
97. Zhang C, Wang H, Ning Z, et al. Serum liver enzymes serve as prognostic factors in patients with intrahepatic cholangiocarcinoma. *Onco Targets Ther* 2017;10:1441–9.
98. Wu C-E, Huang W-K, Chou W-C, et al. Establishment of a pretreatment nomogram to predict the 6-month mortality rate of patients with advanced biliary tract cancers undergoing gemcitabine-based chemotherapy. *Cancers* 2021;13(13):3139.
99. Sasaki K, Margonis GA, Andreatos N, et al. Serum tumor markers enhance the predictive power of the AJCC and LCSGJ staging systems in resectable intrahepatic cholangiocarcinoma. *HPB* 2018;20(10):956–65.
100. Malaguarnera G, Paladina I, Giordano M, et al. Serum markers of intrahepatic cholangiocarcinoma. *Dis Markers* 2013;34:219–28.
101. Khan SA, Thomas HC, Davidson BR, Taylor-Robinson SD. Cholangiocarcinoma. *Lancet* 2005;366(9493):1303–14.
102. Shen W-F, Zhong W, Xu F, et al. Clinicopathological and prognostic analysis of 429 patients with intrahepatic cholangiocarcinoma. *World J Gastroenterol* 15(47):5976–82.
103. Sachan A, Saluja SS, Nekarakanti PK, et al. Raised CA19-9 and CEA have prognostic relevance in gallbladder carcinoma. *BMC Cancer* 2020;20(1):826.
104. Blechacz B. Cholangiocarcinoma: Current knowledge and new developments. *Gut Liver* 2017;11(1):13–26.
105. Levy C, Lymp J, Angulo P, et al. The value of serum CA 19–9 in predicting cholangiocarcinomas in patients with primary sclerosing cholangitis. *Dig Dis Sci* 2005;50(9):1734–40.
106. Patel AH, Harnios DM, Klee GG, et al. The utility of CA 19–9 in the diagnoses of cholangiocarcinoma in patients without primary sclerosing cholangitis. *Am J Gastroenterol* 2000;95(1):204–7.
107. Grenader T, Nash S, Plotkin Y, et al. Derived neutrophil lymphocyte ratio may predict benefit from cisplatin in the advanced biliary cancer: The ABC-02 and BT-22 studies. *Ann Oncol* 2015;26:1910–6.
108. Lamarca A, Santos-Laso A, Utpatel K, et al. Liver metastases of intrahepatic cholangiocarcinoma: Implications for an updated staging system. *Hepatol* 2021;73(6):2311–25.
109. Eckel F, Schmid RM. Chemotherapy in advanced biliary tract carcinoma: A pooled analysis of clinical trials. *Br J Cancer* 2007;96:896–902.
110. Bismuth H, Nakache R, Diamond T. Management strategies in resection for hilar cholangiocarcinoma. *Ann Surg* 1992;215(1):31–8.
111. Kimura W, Futakawa N, Zhao B. Neoplastic diseases of the papilla of Vater. *J Hepatobiliary Pancreat Surg* 2004;11(4):223–31.
112. Wellner UF, Shen YF, Keck T, et al. The survival outcome and prognostic factors for distal cholangiocarcinoma following surgical resection: A meta-analysis for the 5-year survival. *Surg Today* 2017;47(3):271–9.

113. Khan SM, Emile SH, Choudhry MS, Sumbal R. Tumor location and concurrent liver resection, impact survival in T2 gallbladder cancer: A meta-analysis of the literature. *Updates Surg* 2021;73(5):1717–26.
114. Edge SB, Byrd DR, Compton CC, et al. *AJCC cancer staging manual.* 7th Ed. New York; Springer, 2010.
115. Zhao F, Yang D, He J, et al. Establishment and validation of a prognostic nomogram for extrahepatic cholangiocarcinoma. *Front Oncol* 2022;12:1007538.
116. van Keulen A-M, Franssen S, van der Geest LG, et al. Nationwide treatment and outcomes of perihilar cholangiocarcinoma. *Liver Int* 2021;41:1945–53.
117. Strijker M, Belkouz A, van der Geest LG, et al. Treatment and survival of resected and unresected distal cholangiocarcinoma: A nationwide study. *Acta Oncol* 2019;58(7):1048–55.
118. Zhou Y-M, Liao S, Wei Y-Z, Wang S-J. Prognostic factors and benefits of adjuvant therapy for ampullary cancer following pancreatoduodenectomy: A systematic review and meta-analysis. *Asian J Surg* 2020;43(12):1133–41.
119. Sumiyoshi T, Uemura K, Shintakuya R, et al. Prognostic impact of lung recurrence in patients with biliary tract cancer. *Langenbecks Arch Surg* 2023;408(1):290.
120. Frega G, Garajova I, Palloni A, et al. Brain metastases from biliary tract cancer: A monocentric retrospective analysis of 450 patients. *Oncology* 2018;94:7–11.
121. D'Andrea MR, Gill CM, Umphlett M, et al. Brain metastases from biliary tract cancers: A case series and review of the literature in the genomic era. *Oncologist* 2020;25(5):447–53.
122. Nakanuma Y, Kakuda Y. Pathologic classification of cholangiocarcinoma: New concepts. *Best Pract Res Clin Gastroenterol* 2015;29(2):277–93.
123. Akita M, Fujikura K, Ajiki T, et al. Dichotomy in intrahepatic cholangiocarcinomas based on histologic similarities to hilar cholangiocarcinomas. *Mod Pathol* 2017;30:986–97.
124. Arai Y, Totoki Y, Hosoda F, et al. Fibroblast growth factor receptor 2 tyrosine kinase fusions define a unique molecular subtype of cholangiocarcinoma. *Hepatol* 2014;59(4):1427–34.
125. Kipp BR, Voss JS, Kerr SE, et al. Isocitrate dehydrogenase 1 and 2 mutations in cholangiocarcinoma. *Hum Pathol* 2012;43(10):1552–8.
126. Ebata T, Ercolani G, Alvaro D, et al. Current status on cholangiocarcinoma and gallbladder cancer. *Liver Cancer* 2017;6:59–65.
127. Huang Y-H, Zhang CZ-Y, Huang Q-S, et al. Clinicopathologic features, tumor immune microenvironment and genomic landscape of Epstein-Barr virus-associated intrahepatic cholangiocarcinoma. *J Hepatol* 2021;74:838–49.
128. Garancini M, Goffredo P, Pagni F, et al. Combined hepatocellular-cholangiocarcinoma: A population-level analysis of an uncommon primary liver tumor. *Liver Transpl* 2014;20(8):952–9.
129. Robner F, Valentin Sinn B, Horst D. Pathology of combined hepatocellular carcinoma-cholangiocarcinoma. *Cancers* 2023;15:494.
130. Xu J, Sasaki M, Harada K, et al. Intrahepatic cholangiocarcinoma arising in chronic advanced liver disease and the cholangiocarcinomatous component of hepatocellular cholangiocarcinoma share common phenotypes and cholangiocarcinogenesis. *Histopathology* 2011;59(6):1090–9.
131. Yamasaki S. Intrahepatic cholangiocarcinoma: Macroscopic type and stage classification. *J Hepatobiliary Pancreatic Surg* 2003;10(4):288–91.
132. Nakanuma Y, Sato Y, Harada K, et al. Pathological classification of intrahepatic cholangiocarcinoma based on a new concept. *World J Hepatol* 2010;2(12):419–27.
133. Yamasaki S. Intrahepatic cholangiocarcinoma: Macroscopic type and stage classification. *J Hepatobil Pancreat Surg* 2003;10(4):288–91.
134. Tawarungruang C, Khuntikeo N, Chamadol N, et al. Survival after surgery among patients with cholangiocarcinoma in Northeast Thailand according to anatomical and morphological classification. *BMC Cancer* 2021;21(1):497.
135. Shimada K, Sano T, Sakamoto Y, et al. Surgical outcomes of the mass-forming plus periductal infiltrating types of intrahepatic cholangiocarcinoma: A comparative study with the typical mass-forming type of intrahepatic cholangiocarcinoma. *World J Surg* 2007;31(10):2016–22.
136. Bagante F, Weiss M, Alexandrescu S, et al. Long-term outcomes of patients with intraductal growth sub-type of intrahepatic cholangiocarcinoma. *HPB* 2018;20(12):1189–97.
137. Kunprom W, Aphivatanasiri C, Sa-ngiamwibool P, et al. Prognostic significance of growth pattern in predicting outcome of *Opisthorchis viverrini*-associated distal cholangiocarcinoma in Thailand. *Front Publ Health* 2022;10:816028.
138. Sia D, Hoshida Y, Villanueva A, et al. Integrative molecular analysis of intrahepatic cholangiocarcinoma reveals 2 classes that have different outcomes. *Gastroenterol* 2013;144(4):829–40.

139. Andersen JB, Spee B, Blechacz BR, et al. Genomic and genetic characterization of cholangiocarcinoma identifies therapeutic targets for tyrosine kinase inhibitors. *Gastroenterol* 2012;142(4):1021–31.

140. Montal R, Sia D, Montironi C, et al. Molecular classification and therapeutic targets in extrahepatic cholangiocarcinoma. *J Hepatol* 2020;73(2):315–27.

141. Moeini A, Sia D, Bardeesy N, Mazzaferro V, Llovet JM. Molecular pathogenesis and targeted therapies for intrahepatic cholangiocarcinoma. *Clin Cancer Res* 2015;22(2):291–300.

142. Kongpetch S, Jusakul A, Lim JQ, et al. Lack of targetable FGFR2 fusions in endemic fluke-associated cholangiocarcinoma. *JCO Global Oncol* 2020;6:628–38.

143. Farshidfar F, Zheng S, Gingras M-C, et al. Integrative genomic analysis of cholangiocarcinoma identifies distinct IDH-mutant molecular profiles. *Cell Rep* 2017;18(11):2780–94.

144. Boscoe AN, Rolland C, Kelley RK. Frequency and prognostic significance of isocitrate dehydrogenase 1 mutations in cholangiocarcinoma: A systematic literature review. *J Gastrointestinal Oncol* 2019;10(4):751–65.

145. Rimini M, Fabregat-Franco C, Burgio V, et al. Molecular profile and its clinical impact of IDH1 mutated versus IDH1 wild type intrahepatic cholangiocarcinoma. *Sci Rep* 2022;12:18775.

146. Silva VWK, Askan G, Daniel TD, et al. Biliary carcinomas: Pathology and the role of DNA mismatch repair deficiency. *Chin Clin Oncol* 2016;5(5):62.

147. Limpaiboon T, Krissadarak K, Sripa B, et al. Microsatellite alterations in liver fluke related cholangiocarcinoma are associated with poor prognosis. *Cancer Lett* 2002;181(2):215–22.

148. Wang J, Wang X, Xie S, et al. p53 status and its prognostic role in extrahepatic bile duct cancer: A meta-analysis of published studies. *Dig Dis Sci* 2011;56(3):655–62.

149. Golan T, Raitses-Gurevich M, Kelley RK, et al. Overall survival and clinical characteristics of BRCA-associated cholangiocarcinoma: A multicenter retrospective study. *Oncologist* 2017;22(7):804–10.

150. Ahn DH, Bekaii-Saab T. Biliary tract cancer and genomic alterations in homologous recombinant deficiency: Exploiting synthetic lethality with PARP inhibitors. *Chin Clin Oncol* 2020;9(1):6.

151. Valle J, Wasan H, Palmer DH, et al. Cisplatin plus gemcitabine versus gemcitabine for biliary tract cancer. *N Engl J Med* 2010;362(14):1273–81.

152. Kim ST, Kang JH, Lee J, et al. Capecitabine plus oxaliplatin versus gemcitabine plus oxaliplatin as first-line therapy for advanced biliary tract cancers: A multicenter, open-label, randomized, phase III, noninferiority trial. *Ann Oncol* 2019;30(5):788–95.

153. Morizane C, Okusaka T, Mizusawa J, et al. Combination gemcitabine plus S-1 versus gemcitabine plus cisplatin for advanced/recurrent biliary tract cancer: The FUGA-BT (JCOG1113) randomized phase III clinical trial. *Ann Oncol* 2019;30:1950–8.

154. Valle JW, Furuse J, Jitlal M, et al. Cisplatin and gemcitabine for advanced biliary tract cancer: A meta-analysis of two randomised trials. *Ann Oncol* 2014;25:391–8.

155. Ioka T, Kanai M, Kobayashi S, et al. Randomized phase III study of gemcitabine, cisplatin plus S-1 versus gemcitabine, cisplatin for advanced biliary tract cancer (KHBO1401- MITSUBA). *J Hepatobiliary Pancreat Sci* 2023;30(1):102–10.

156. Phelip JM, Desrame J, Edeline J, et al. Modified FOLFIRINOX versus CISGEM chemotherapy for patients with advanced biliary tract cancer (PRODIGE 38 AMEBICA): A randomized phase II study. *J Clin Oncol* 2022;40:262–71.

157. Oh D-Y, He AR, Qin S, et al. Durvalumab plus gemcitabine and cisplatin in advanced biliary tract cancer. *NEJM Evid* 2022;1(8):1–11.

158. Lamarca A, Palmer DH, Wasan HS, et al. Second-line FOLFOX chemotherapy versus active symptom control for advanced biliary tract cancer (ABC-06): A phase 3, open-label, randomised, controlled trial. *Lancet Oncol* 2021;22(5):690–701.

159. Yoo C, Kim K-P, Jeong JH, et al. Liposomal irinotecan plus fluorouracil and leucovorin versus fluorouracil and leucovorin for metastatic biliary tract cancer after progression on gemcitabine plus cisplatin (NIFTY): A multicentre, open-label, randomised, phase 2b study. *Lancet Oncol* 2021;22(11):1560–72.

160. Abou-Alfa GK, Macarulla T, Javle MM, et al. Ivosidenib in IDH1-mutant, chemotherapy-refractory cholangiocarcinoma (ClarIDHy): A multicentre, randomised, double-blind, placebo-controlled, phase 3 study. *Lancet Oncol* 2020;21(6):796–807.

161. Javle M, Lowery M, Shroff RT, et al. Phase II study of BGJ398 in patients with FGFR-altered advanced cholangiocarcinoma. *J Clin Oncol* 2018;36:276–82.

162. Abou-Alfa GK, Sahai V, Hollebecque A, et al. Pemigatinib for previously treated, locally advanced or metastatic cholangiocarcinoma: A multicentre, open-label, phase 2 study. *Lancet Oncol* 2020;21(5):671–84.

163. Subbiah V, Lassen U, Elez E, et al. Dabrafenib plus trametinib in patients with BRAF-V600E-mutated biliary tract cancer (ROAR): A phase 2, open-label, single-arm, multicentre basket trial. *Lancet Oncol* 2020;21:1234–43.

164. Javle M, Borad MJ, Azad NS, et al. Pertuzumab and trastuzumab for HER2-positive, metastatic biliary tract cancer (MyPathway): A multicentre, open-label, phase 2a, multiple basket study. *Lancet Oncol* 2021;22:1290–300.

165. Doebele RC, Drilon A, Paz-Ares L, et al. Entrectinib in patients with advanced or metastatic NTRK fusion-positive solid tumours: Integrated analysis of three phase 1–2 trials. *Lancet Oncol* 2020;21(2):271–82.

166. Marabelle A, Le DT, Ascierto PA, et al. Efficacy of pembrolizumab in patients with noncolorectal high microsatellite instability/mismatch repair-deficient cancer: Results from the phase II KEYNOTE-158 study. *J Clin Oncol* 2020;38(1):1–10.

167. Lapitz A, Azkargorta M, Milkiewicz P, et al. Liquid biopsy-based protein biomarkers for risk prediction, early diagnosis, and prognostication of cholangiocarcinoma. *J Hepatol* 2023;79(1):93–108.

168. Berchuk JE, Facchinetti F, DiToro DF, et al. The clinical landscape of cell-free DNA alterations in 1671 patients with advanced biliary tract cancer. *Ann Oncol* 2022;33(12):1269–83.

169. Javle M, Bekaii-Saab T, Jain A, et al. Biliary cancer: Utility of next generation sequencing for clinical management. *Cancer* 2016;122(24):3838–47.

7 Neuroendocrine neoplasms

7.1 INTRODUCTION

7.1.1 EPIDEMIOLOGY

Neuroendocrine neoplasms (NENs) include a broad spectrum of malignancies that arise from neuroendocrine cells. Variable incidences have been reported, around 3–5/100,000 [1, 2], and it is estimated that gastro-entero-pancreatic neuroendocrine neoplasms (GEP-NENs) could account for half of NENs [3, 4]. In the US they remain the digestive cancer with the second highest prevalence [5], despite the low incidences, which ranges from 0.7/100,000 for pancreatic neuroendocrine neoplasms (Pan-NENs) to 1.2/100,000 for those of the small intestine (SI-NENs) [5, 6].

From 1973 to 2012 an increase in incidence of 6.4 times has been reported, with GEP-NENs accounting for an incidence of 3.56/100,000, and the increase concerning both Pan-NEN and gastrointestinal neuroendocrine neoplasms (GI-NENs) [7]. The increase of GI-NENs was more pronounced for the rectal and well-differentiated (WD) NENs [8], but gastro-entero-pancreatic neuroendocrine carcinomas (GEP-NEC) also showed a doubling incidence in the last two decades, from 0.15 to 0.36/100,000 [9].

At present, the cause of this disproportionate increasing incidence is unclear [10], although the more extensive use of endoscopy and improved imaging could play a role.

7.1.2 STAGING OF METASTATIC DISEASE

Diagnostic workup should clearly define the site of the primary tumor (PT) and histotype. CT is the pivotal examination for diagnosis and staging, besides the low predictive value in examining lymph nodes, bone, and peritoneum [11–13]. DWI-MRI allows a better diagnostic definition of the pancreas [14–16] and liver [17, 18], but also bone and brain, while CT is the gold standard for exploring the lungs.

Somatostatin receptor (SSTR)-based whole-body imaging should be part of staging/restaging procedures. The ^{68}Ga-DOTA-SSA-PET/TC is the recommended procedure [11], as it improves visualization of lungs and lymph nodes and has a high chance of identifying the origin. FDG/PET is of choice for G3 and G2 with high mitotic index (MI) NENs, generally with low SSTR expression and poor prognosis [19, 20].

Laboratory tests can support diagnosis and be helpful in follow-up: serum chromogranin-A (CGA) and various peptides, to be defined based on the endocrine syndrome, are recommended. In NEC and poorly differentiated (PD) NET, neuron-specific enolase (NSE) and lactic dehydrogenase (LDH), can be increased.

Whenever surgical specimens are not available, pathological diagnosis requires large biopsy samples, to define histotype and grading, with immunohistochemical determinations for chromogranin, synaptophysin or other proteins.

Stage, according to the TNM Classification (AJCC 8th edition 2017), and WHO grading should be reported.

7.1.3 PROGNOSIS OF METASTATIC DISEASE

In the context of NENs, the disparity of prognosis is noteworthy, since patients with low-grade NEN can survive many years, while patients with high-grade can have a median overall survival (OS) of a few months. Most GEP-NEN patients have an advanced stage at diagnosis. The Spanish national registry RGETNE reported metastases at diagnosis in 44%, and this percentage increased for SI-NENs (68%) compared to Pan-NENs (38%), even though the 5-year survival rate was 75% for both [21]. Furthermore, localized NEN patients have a recurrence risk of 13% [22]. Over time, the SEER database documented an increasing incidence, attributable largely to localized disease, and a significant outcome improvement interesting both localized and metastatic tumors. In patients with metastatic NEN (mNEN), SEER median OS of 68 months, and 28% 5-year survival rate were reported [6], with a reduced risk of death for metastatic GEP-NENs (mGEP-NENs) patients [7]. Some authors suggest that stage migration could contribute to longer OS [23].

7.2   ANALYSIS OF PROGNOSTIC VARIABLES IN EARLY METASTATIC DISEASE

A systematic review of randomized clinical trials (RCTs) that studied upfront therapies, after excluding those with endpoints measuring other than OS, resulted in the selection of 67 trials, published from 1979 to 2022, of which 20 were phase III and 47 phase II. In 16 an analysis of prognostic factors (PFs) was done [24–39]. However, as resumed in Table S1, eight studies enrolled patients receiving previous systemic antineoplastic treatments, prevalently cytotoxic (6–60% of the enrolled patients).

Regarding PFs, the trials' review found the results summarized in Table S2, which lists all the PFs that have been investigated.

7.3   PATIENT-RELATED PROGNOSTIC FACTORS

7.3.1   Performance status

Despite the large heterogeneity of clinical course of mNENs, many studies have documented an independent prognostic relationship of performance status (PS), with longer OS for patients with good PS, after pharmacologic treatments or radiopharmaceuticals.

TABLE S1
Characteristics of the selected trials

Trial [ref]	Phase	No. patients	Pre-treated patients	Treatment	Tumor location	Grading
EST-5275 1984 [24]	3	210	0	Cytotoxic	Carcinoid all sites	NR
SWOG 1987 [25]	2	66	0	Cytotoxic	Carcinoid all sites	All G
Swedish 1990 [26]	2	84	0	Cytotoxic+/-IFN	Pancreas	All G (*)
ECOG 1992 [27]	3	105	0	Cytotoxic	Pancreas	NR
ECOG-6282 2001 [28]	2	50	22	Cytotoxic	Pancreas	NR
ECOG-1281 2005 [29]	3	163	0	Cytotoxic	Carcinoid all sites	All G
EMC 2005 [30]	2	310	52	Radiomethabolic	GEP	NR
RMN 2006 [31]	2	36	21	Targeted	GEP	NR
ITMO 2007 [32]	2	40	0	Cytotoxic	All sites	All G (**)
DFCI 2008 [33]	2	107	18	Targeted	GEP	NR
PROMID 2009 [34]	3	85	0	Targeted	Midgut	G1
British 2010 [35]	2	82	0	Cytotoxic	All sites	All G
Polish 2010 [36]	2	60	34	Radiomethabolic	GEP	G1–G2
RADIANT-3 2011 [37]	3	410	206	Targeted	Pancreas	G1–G2
SWOG-0508 2017 [38]	3	402	106	Targeted	All sites	G1–G2
CAPTEM 2021 [39]	2	30	18	Cytotoxic	GEP	G3

Legend: G, grade. GEP, gastro-entero-pancreatic. IFN, Interferon. NR, not reported. (*) included benign NET. (**) High-grade 13, low-grade 27.

TABLE S2

Prognostic factors analyzed in selected clinical trials of patients with unresectable or metastatic neuroendocrine neoplasm receiving upfront treatment

Variable	No. comparisons	Prognostic relationship	No prognostic relationship
Patient-related			
Performance status	8	5	3
Age	7	2	5
Sex	7	1	6
Clinic			
Endocrine syndrome	8	1	7
MEN-1	1	1	0
Weight loss	1	1	0
Lab			
Creatinine	1	1	0
Tumor markers			
Cromogranine-A	4	3	1
NSE	2	2	0
5-HIAA	3	1	2
Other (AFP,HCG,CA 19-9)	3	0	3
Tumor-related			
Tumor burden			
Liver involvement %	2	2	0
Misurable disease	1	0	1
Multifocality	1	0	1
Location	7	0	7
Timing of metastasis			
Time diagnosis-to-therapy	1	0	1
Site of metastasis			
Liver metastases	2	0	2
Extra-hepatic metastases	1	0	1
Bone metastases	1	1	0
Pathology			
Histotype	4	1	3
Differentiation grade	3	0	3
Grading	2	1	1
Mitotic rate	2	2	0
Ki-67	2	0	2
Previous treatments			
Primary tumor resection	3	1	2

Two retrospective studies in patients with G1–G2 mNEN found a negative prognostic effect for a deteriorated PS [40, 41], as did two of three studies evaluating G3 NENs [42–44], but not the other three [45–47]. The prognostic role of PS was more pronounced for NEC patients [44, 48, 49], and for G3-NEN, among whom patients with ECOG PS 2–3 reported a very poor survival [50].

7.3.1.1 Selected trials

Eight studies evaluated PS. The most frequent comparison was between ECOG PS 2–3 vs. PS 0–1. As a result, five of eight trials documented a significant relationship between poor PS and short OS, but only one calculated effect size (ES) (Table 7.1).

TABLE 7.1

Prognostic relationships of performance status in selected studies of patients with unresectable or metastatic neuroendocrine neoplasm receiving upfront treatment

Study [ref]	Phase	No. pts	Scale	Comparison	Prognostic relationship	Effect size
EST-5275 1984 [24]	III	210	ECOG	PS ≥2 vs. PS 0–1	Yes	NR
SWOG-8017 1987 [25]	II	66	NR	PS 2–3 vs. PS 0–1	No	NR
ECOG 1992 [27]	III	105	ECOG	PS 2–3 vs. PS 0–1	Yes	OS 2.1 vs. 1.0 years
ECOG-6282 2001 [28]	II	50	ECOG	PS 2–3 vs. PS 0–1	Yes	NR
ECOG-1281 2005 [29]	III	163	ECOG	PS 2–3 vs. PS 0–1	Yes	NR
EMC 2005 [30]	II	310	KPS	KPS ≤ vs. >70	Yes	OS 48 vs. 16 months
British 2010 [35]	II	82	NR	PS ≥2 vs. PS 0–1	No	HR 2.32 (0.89–6.05)
Polish 2010 [36]	II	60	WHO	NR	No	NR

Legend: ECOG, Eastern Cooperative Oncology Group. HR, hazard ratio. KPS, Karnofsky performance score. NR, not reported. OS, overall survival. PS, performance status. WHO, World Health Organization.

7.3.2 DEMOGRAPHIC

7.3.2.1 Age

Of thirteen population-based studies, largely from SEER, eight documented worsening outcomes with the increasing age [6, 7, 51–56], three studies found poor OS for subgroups of patients >30 or >50 years [8, 57, 58], while another detected a poor prognosis for GI-NET patients with <60 years [22], and age effect was not evident in a cohort from the RGETNE [21]. Only one of three prospective case series documented a prognostic role for advanced age [59–61], while some retrospective analyses showed poor outcomes for elderly patients with GEP-NEN [47, 62] and midgut tumors [63, 64]. Similarly, the other five studies of Pan-NENs reported a significant relationship between the younger age and good prognosis [51, 52, 62, 65, 66]. Other seven retrospective studies on GEP-NEN [40, 45, 46, 67], Pan-NEN [68] or G3-NEN [42, 43] did not find any effect of age.

A study investigated a SEER cohort of GEP-NEN patients, documenting how, along 41 years, age at diagnosis increased by 9 years in patients with localized disease and remained the same for locally advanced (LA) and metastatic tumors, though an age >60 years conferred a poor prognosis [8].

7.3.2.2 Sex

Of ten population-based studies, five documented reduced OS for males [6, 8, 51, 56, 57], and five had not [22, 31, 53, 55, 58]. No relationship emerged for WD NENs in two prospective [60, 61] and six retrospective analyses [45–47, 62, 64, 67]. For G3-GEP-NEN patients, two retrospective studies found no different outcomes by sex [42, 43].

7.3.2.3 Other demographic variables

Of the nine population-based studies analyzing race, seven of which from SEER, a worse prognosis for African-Americans emerged in five [7, 51, 54, 56, 57], but not in others [6, 8, 22, 58].

Contradictory findings were reported by three population-based studies on the prognosis of married vs. unmarried patients [22, 55, 58].

7.3.2.4 Selected trials

Seven studies investigated age. Five studies defined cut-offs, with the two positive studies reporting longer OS for patients younger than 60 [24, 29] (Table 7.2).

TABLE 7.2

Prognostic relationships of age in selected studies of patients with unresectable or metastatic neuroendocrine neoplasm receiving upfront treatment

Study [ref]	Phase	No. pts	Comparison	Prognostic relationship	Effect size
EST-5275 1984 [24]	III	210	≤60 vs. >60	Yes	NR
SWOG-8017 1987 [25]	II	66	NR	No	NR
ECOG 1992 [27]	III	105	<40 vs. 40–60 vs. >60	No	1.5 vs. 2.1 vs. 1.3 m
ECOG-1281 2005 [29]	III	163	≤60 vs. >60	Yes	NR
British 2010 [35]	II	82	continuous	No	HR 1.15 (0.84–1.59)
Polish 2010 [36]	II	60	NR	No	NR
CAPTEM 2021 [39]	II	30	≤60 vs. >60	No	HR 1.18 (0.33–4.20)

Legend: HR, hazard ratio. m, months. NR, not reported.

Seven trials evaluated sex. Among them, a prolonged OS [28] or a favorable trend for males [27] was reported. Finally, the EST trial suggested better outcomes for females only after doxorubicin-based chemotherapy [24].

7.3.3 ANTHROPOMETRIC

A Portuguese single-center study investigated body mass index (BMI) and weight in mGEP-NEN patients, without documenting prognostic differences, even after assessment of obesity and over-weight, waist circumference, and some clinical parameters related to metabolic syndrome, though a visceral obesity reduced progression-free survival (PFS) in PanNENs [67]. Similarly, another study of 135 LA or mNEN patients found no different outcomes for BMI >18.5 [46].

Although body composition does not affect OS in GEP-NETs, a loss of muscle mass was associated with reduced disease-specific survival (DSS) [69].

7.3.4 CLINIC

7.3.4.1 Endocrine syndrome

Approximately 30% of SI-NENs and 50% of Pan-NENs are functioning, i.e., they can sustain an endocrine syndrome. Furthermore, in some patients, there may also be secondary hormone secretion syndromes, given that 6% of Pan-NENs produce more hormones, and 4% turn to other hormone production [70].

Among patients with Pan-NEN, only one of nine studies [57] documented a negative prognostic effect by endocrine syndromes [6, 21, 40, 46, 53, 55, 60, 67], but only two enrolled exclusively mNENs [40, 60]. Other authors suggested a better prognosis [65, 66, 71]. Finally, two studies evaluated symptoms individually, reporting no relationship with OS for flushing and a favorable effect for diarrhea [61], while another did not demonstrate any effect for both [62]. In general, endocrine syndromes are more common in patients with familial syndromes, which reported better outcomes [53].

7.3.4.2 Glycemic control

Pan-NEN patients with high specific growth rate (SGR) of tumors experienced reduced OS. These patients were different from low SGR patients for the higher glycated hemoglobin levels [72] so the authors supported the hypothesis that inadequate glycemic control could be associated with more aggressive Pan-NEN [73].

7.3.4.3 Other clinical conditions

Data from NCDB documented that in midgut mNENs, comorbidities were inversely associated with OS [54, 64].

7.3.4.4 Selected trials

Eight studies evaluated the prognostic role of endocrine syndromes, which was not influential on OS, except one study that reported longer OS for patients with functioning tumors (FT) [26]. The same study suggested that the presence of multiple endocrine neoplasia-1 syndrome was a favorable PF [26].

Weight loss was associated with poor OS in mNEN patients receiving radiometabolic therapy.

7.3.5 LABORATORY

7.3.5.1 Hematology

Anemia was associated with progression and increased risk of death among Pan-NEN patients [74]. A study investigated leukocyte count, reporting an unfavorable OS trend for leukocytes >10,000/mcL or neutrophils >8,000/mcL, but not for lymphocytes <1,000/mcL [46]. Among the variables associated with leukocytes, the neutrophil-to-lymphocyte ratio (NLR) has been the most studied [75], with results not always superimposable with those of other inflammatory mediators in WD mNENs [46, 76]. Conversely, among metastatic Pan-NENs (mPan-NENs) a high NLR was associated with poor outcome [76], and other studies of mNENs suggested similar effects [46, 50, 77].

In G3 NENs NLR was not associated with prognosis [42–44], while the increased lymphocyte count was favorable PF [43].

7.3.5.2 Chemistry

The role of other systemic inflammation-related indexes remains controversial. The increased modified Glasgow prognostic score (mGPS) was associated with poor OS in G3-NENs [44] and unresectable NENs [46], while C-reactive protein correlated with poor prognosis in one [46] of three studies [43, 46, 50].

Baseline serum enzymes have been evaluated in mNEN patients. One of two studies documented a better prognosis for normal alkaline phosphatase (ALP) [42, 59], while no relationship with outcome was described for aspartate aminotransferase (AST), alanine aminotransferase (ALT) [47] and albumin [46]. Increased lactic dehydrogenase (LDH) was associated with poor prognosis of patients with mGEP-NEN [45], especially G3 [42, 43], but reported only unsignificant trends in other studies [46, 47, 50]. A possible negative prognostic effect of high LDH has been suggested in GEP-NEC patients. This subgroup is characterized by high glucose consumption, lactate production and high proliferation rates, as well as by hypoxic tumor microenvironment for poor vascularization [78, 79].

7.3.5.3 Tumor markers

CGA has prognostic and predictive effects [80, 81, 63], and correlates with tumor burden (TB) [82], but is subject to a high number of false positives (atrophic gastritis, hypergastrinaemia, renal insufficiency, proton pump inhibitors), and false negative results among PD NEN [83]. In metastatic disease, high CGA levels predicted poor prognosis in one study [59], but not other of WD mNEN [40, 62], and its role is unclear in FT [61]. No effect on OS was shown by high urinary 5-hydroxyindole-acetic acid (5HIAA) levels in midgut NENs [63].

NSE is another circulating marker of GEP-NENs [84, 85], which is elevated only in 30–50% of patients [86]. It correlates more with grading than with TB, as it increases mostly in NECs [87]. However, a retrospective analysis of WD NENs documented an independent negative

TABLE 7.3

Prognostic relationships of tumor markers in selected studies of patients with unresectable or metastatic neuroendocrine neoplasm receiving upfront treatment

Study [ref]	Phase	No. pts	Comparison	Prognostic relationship	Effect size
Chromogranin-A (ng/mL)					
British 2010 [35]	II	82	≤ vs. > 50	Yes	HR 6.77 (1.26–36.50)
RADIANT-3 2011 [37]	III	410	≤ vs. > 2ULN	Yes	HR 1.32 (1.00–1.75)
SWOG-0508 2017 [38]	III	402	≤ vs. > ULN	Yes	HR 1.99 (1.44–2.76)
Neuron-specific enolase (ng/mL)					
RADIANT-3 2011 [37]	III	410	≤ vs. > ULN	Yes	HR 2.44 (1.79–3.33)
SWOG-0508 2017 [38]	III	402	≤ vs. > ULN	Yes	HR 1.77 (1.29–2.42)
5-hydroxy-indol-acetic acid (mg/24h)					
EST-5275 1984 [24]	III	210	≤ vs. > 6	No	NR
SWOG-8017 1987 [25]	II	66	3 groups	No	NR
SWOG-0508 2017 [38]	III	402	≤ vs. > ULN	Yes	NR

Legend: HR, hazard ratio. NR, not reported. OS, overall survival. ULN, upper limit of normal.

prognostic role for NSE >15 ng/mL [40], while in Pan-NENs it predicted OS and everolimus response [84, 86].

7.3.5.4 Selected trials

A pooled analysis of the RADIANT-3 and RADIANT-4 found that a reduced NLR was associated with longer PFS, regardless of treatment [88].

CGA appears to be a reliable PF in three trials, albeit at variable cut-offs. A meta-analysis of these studies calculated a pooled ES (HR 2.04, CI 1.27–15.69; Q = 3.62, p-value = 0.1633; I^2 = 44.8%). NSE was analyzed in two studies reporting in both cases a relationship with OS [37, 38]. Of the three studies evaluating the prognostic role of urinary 5HIAA, only one found a relationship between high levels and poor OS [38] (Table 7.3).

7.4 TUMOR-RELATED PROGNOSTIC FACTORS

7.4.1 TUMOR BURDEN

Population-based studies reported shorter OS with advancing stage [7, 8, 21], and with the increasing T- and N-stage [21, 55], with one exception in Pan-NENs [58] and GI-NENs [22].

A relationship between PT size and OS is documented by some authors [8, 22] but not in other studies of midgut [54, 64] and Pan-NENs [57, 60].

A number of population-based studies have compared LA vs. localized and metastatic vs. localized disease, reporting poor OS for metastatic disease [6–8, 42, 51, 56, 57]. While two studies did not document prognostic differences between LA and metastatic NENs [46, 67], three studies found a poor outcome of M1 vs. M0 [22, 53, 55], and another of stage IV vs. stage I [47].

None of the three studies that assessed the number of metastasis sites documented an OS reduction for multiple vs. single sites [46, 55, 62].

Liver involvement (LI) was also consistently associated with poor OS, both at >25% [40, 60, 61] and >75% cut-offs [68], as well as the presence of >10 liver metastases (LMs) [62].

Furthermore, a variable such as ^{68}Ga-DOTATATE total volume was studied in Pan-NEN, which in addition to the TB also expresses various degrees of activity of the functional state of the tumor. This "metabolic" volume was associated with a reduced DSS [20, 89–91].

7.4.1.1 Selected trials

Two studies investigated the LI by NEN as an indicator of TB, using different variables, one study comparing an extensive involvement vs. moderate/none [30], and the PROMID trial quantifying a tridimensional hepatic tumor load by imaging with 10% cut-off [34]. In any case, the high LI predicted a poor prognosis.

Conversely, multifocality [24] and disease measurability [28] did not report any effect on OS.

7.4.2 PRIMARY TUMOR LOCATION

Different study selection criteria and comparisons with reference to tumor location do not allow homogeneous conclusions about tumor location as a PF. Poor outcomes have been reported for hepatic [7, 51], gastric [7, 51], duodenal [51], colic and rectal [51], esophageal [22], and sometimes pancreatic NENs [51], while generally a better prognosis has been found for SI-NENs, mostly of jejunum and appendix [7, 8, 22, 51, 54, 56, 59]. In the context of Pan-NENs, some authors found longer OS for distal body-tail tumors [55, 57]. Few data on G3-GEP-NENs document no differences [67] or detect poor outcomes for GI-NENs than those of hepato-biliary-pancreatic origin [42].

Few data are available on prognosis and treatments for esophageal NENs, which are poorly influenced by surgery [92]. From SEER database esophageal NEC incidence is increasing, and the prognosis is worse than carcinomas [93]. A series of 183 esophageal NEC patients documented some characteristics associated with unfavorable outcomes, such as location in the middle third, brain or LMs [94].

Significant shorter OS for gastric NENs was reported by SEER [7] and RGETNE [21], but only a trend to poor prognosis of foregut GEP-NENs emerged from a retrospective study [62].

The small intestine origin was independently related to better outcomes in patients from a prospective database of patients with LMs [59]. A study by the Icelandic Cancer Registry identified 113 SI-NEN patients and reported that long-term survival was doubled after incidental diagnosis and non-emergency surgery [95]. However, in some small studies, midgut and ileal tumors did not report a different prognosis than other NENs [47, 62].

Despite the increased incidence of rectal NENs, from 0.2 to 0.86/100,000 from 1973 to 2004 [96], over time the patients with rectal NEN reported a progressive OS improvement, contrary to those with a colic NEN, with a similar 5-year survival rate for metastatic disease [97].

Hepatic NENs are rare. A retrospective analysis of 41 patients with unresectable disease suggested that chemotherapy could be superior to TACE, especially for patients with Ki-67 >55%, and that a very poor outcome was evident for those with a Ki-67 >60% and an ECOG PS 2 [98].

Some retrospective studies compared pancreatic origin with other sites of NEN, suggesting poor prognosis of Pan-NENs [45, 60], but results were not confirmed [46, 47]. A SEER database evaluation of 882 patients with non-functioning Pan-NEN found better outcomes for patients with body-tail localization [52].

7.4.2.1 Selected trials

Seven studies evaluated the site of origin, reporting different comparisons, as listed in Table 7.4. Three studies compared pancreatic vs. non-pancreatic [33, 35, 39], and another one intestinal vs. pulmonary location [25]. In any case, the site of origin did not exert any effect on the outcome.

7.4.3 TIMING OF METASTASIS

A prospective database identified 172 patients with resected NEN LMs and did not report significant OS differences by the timing of metastases [99]. On the contrary, a more recent multi-institutional database of 420 NEN patients receiving radical resection of LMs, suggested that synchronous disease is associated with higher recurrence rates [100], similar to another retrospective study [62]. No difference in long-term outcomes was identified between early and late metachronous metastases [100].

TABLE 7.4

Prognostic relationships of primary tumor location in selected studies of patients with unresectable or metastatic neuroendocrine neoplasm receiving upfront treatment

Trial [ref]	Phase	No. pts	Comparison	Prognostic relationship	Effect size
EST-5275 1984 [24]	III	210	Various	No	NR
SWOG-8017 1987 [25]	II	66	GI vs. lung	No	NR
ECOG-1281 2005 [29]	III	163	Various	No	NR
DFCI 2008 [33]	II	107	Pan vs. carcinoid	No	OS not reached vs. 25 m
British 2010 [35]	II	82	Pan vs. non-Pan	No	HR 0.54 (0.26–1.11)
Polish 2010 [36]	II	60	Foregut vs. midgut	No	NR
CAPTEM 2021 [39]	II	30	Pan vs. other	No	HR 0.90 (0.12–7.14)

Legend: GI, gastro-intestinal. HR, hazard ratio. m, months. NR, not reported. OS, overall survival. Pan, pancreas.

7.4.3.1 Selected trials

One study evaluated the timing from diagnosis to enrollment (<3 vs. 3–12 vs. >12 months), without reporting a relationship with prognosis [27], and three of four studies examining primary tumor resection (PTR) did not document different OS, suggesting that metachronous disease has not a prognostic role.

7.4.4 SITE OF METASTASIS

The Swedish Cancer Registry documented that LMs occurred in 82% of mNEN, mostly in SI-NEN patients (56% vs. 10% of colic and hepatobiliary NENs). Overall, the risk of metastatic disease was higher for SI and pancreaticobiliary NEN than for all other sites [101]. A SEER analysis documented a reduced survival after the occurrence of LMs [7], affecting 61–91% of SI-NENs and 28–77% of PanNENs [102, 103]. Sometimes surgery can be curative for patients with LMs, but even after a radical liver resection the 5-year survival rate decreased to 13–54% [104, 105], while the recurrence following R0 metastasectomy is high, exceeding 70% at 3 years [106–111]. According to some authors, the resection of LMs may be appropriate even in the presence of bone metastases and low TB [112], although in patients with LMs, the extrahepatic disease (EHD) appears generally associated with a poor prognosis [99, 106]. However, the prognostic role of EHD in patients with LMs remains uncertain [54, 60]. While the Spanish RGETNE reports short survival for peritoneal and lung but not bone metastases [53], in mNEN LMs do not change OS [45, 44].

In contrast, in a study after univariate analysis, the presence of lymph node metastases reduced the risk of death [52].

From a meta-analysis of 149 studies reporting bone metastases, it appeared that bone metastases are underreported and underdiagnosed, are metachronous (60%) and osteoblastic, are best diagnosed by FDG-PET, and only 46% are symptomatic. However, their occurrence was associated with short OS, which was furtherly reduced in patients with symptoms and poor PS [113]. SEER database reported bone metastases in 115/2,003 mGEP-NEN patients, and brain metastases in 27, with median OS of 9 and 2 months respectively [114]. Another review of the SEER database and a retrospective study excluded a prognostic effect of bone metastases [53, 62].

While the same SEER analysis documents a worse prognosis for patients with lung metastases [53], a retrospective analysis of 118 WD GEP-NENs did not confirm such an association [62].

7.4.4.1 Selected trials

Two studies evaluated a generic variable "site of metastasis", without detecting prognostic effect [24, 25]. Other authors investigated the impact of LMs on OS, which was not significant [25, 36], as well as the occurrence of EHD [36]. Conversely, bone metastases were associated with a reduced median OS [30].

7.4.5 PATHOLOGY

Tumor differentiation and grading have been well characterized and define a different clinical course [115]. However, in PD NEN details of histology are required.

7.4.5.1 Histology

The histotype greatly affects the prognosis of GEP-NENs, as it correlates with the behavior of tumors. Its relevance was evident in the RGETNE registry, in which the 5-year survival rate ranged from 50% of mixed pancreatic NENs to 95–100% of gastrinoma and somatostatinoma [21], even though in a retrospective analysis of advanced Pan-NEN gastrinoma reported a similar outcome to the other Pan-NENs [68]. Still, NEC patients demonstrated an even shorter OS than G3-NET [22].

Histology should well define the PD NENs, according to the WHO classification [116], and distinguish between NEC and NET G3. This classification should always be reported [117], because they are two different diseases, although it is insufficient to explain the prognostic heterogeneity of the PD NENs, with OS ranging from 5 to 34 months [48, 118].

GEP-NECs are 10–20% of all NENs and have a different distribution, mainly affecting the esophagus, pancreas, ampulla of Vater and colon while they are rare in the ileum [48]. In the context of NEC various negative PFs have been identified, such as Ki-67 >80%, elevated serum LDH and ALP levels, presence of LMs, and poor PS, which have been used to define a GI-NEC score [49]. This score grouped patients into two prognostic categories, with median OS of 19.4 vs. 5.2 months respectively. Another analysis of 85 patients with extra-pulmonary mNECs confirmed the negative prognostic role of high LDH and NLR >3 [50]. Similarly, a doubling AST serum level can be an indicator of poor prognosis [119]. The NORDIC NEC study was a retrospective analysis of 305 GI-NEC patients receiving chemotherapy. It concluded that those with a Ki-67 <55% had lower response rates but longer OS. The most important variables associated with short survival were poor PS, colorectal origin, elevated platelet count and high LDH levels [120, 121]. A retrospective series of 258 Japanese patients with unresectable or recurrent GEP-NEC receiving chemotherapy reported a better outcome for GI vs. hepato-biliary-pancreatic PT location and for patients with normal LDH [45]. Another analysis of 109 GEP-NEC patients suggested only two independent negative PFs, elevated LDH and AST [119]. Other variables as leukocytosis [121] and thrombocytosis [120] have been associated with a poor prognosis. PD GEP-NETs have a different behavior than NECs. Some authors have documented how the effect of some PFs may be different in the two subgroups: an analysis of NEC vs. G3-NET patients reported similar median OS of 13 months, but while mGPS was always associated with the outcome, only in the NEC subgroup Ki-67 and GI-NEC score had a prognostic effect [44]. Other authors suggested a further prognostic subclassification of all patients with a diagnosis of G3 GEP-NEN, taking into account a score that included ECOG PS, LDH and lymphocyte count [43].

7.4.5.2 Tumor grade

Over time, the NEN cell proliferation rate, despite the measure (Ki-67 staining, MI, grading, differentiation grade) has been associated with the outcome [122–125].

Ki-67 contributes to define a proliferation grading system based on Ki-67 rate and mitotic count (MC) (Ki-67 <2% and MC <2/10HPF vs. Ki-67 3–20% and/or MC 2–20/10HPF vs. Ki-67 >20% and/or MC >20/10HPF), with 5-year survival rates of 83.3% vs. 77.1% vs. 43.5%, respectively [118,

126]. However, the relevance of Ki-67 was continuous. Various Ki-67 cut-offs have been used, but a progressive reduction in OS was seen with increasing Ki-67 [21, 40], although sometimes only for values >20% [60] and consequently less relevant in WD mGEP-NENs [62]. In G3-NENs Ki-67 >55% correlated with poor outcome in one study [44], but not in others [43, 50]. Similar prognostic differences have been shown for the differentiation, with higher 5-year survival rates for WD vs. PD NENs (83.3% vs. 39.1%) [21].

While in population-based studies, G3 and G4 NENs were associated with reduced OS [6–8, 22, 46, 52, 53, 56–58], a significant difference also emerged between G2 and G1 [6–8, 51, 56, 57] although it was not confirmed by all authors [47, 53, 68]. Similarly, a reduced OS was evident for PD vs. WD [54, 55] and PD vs. moderately differentiated [55]. Other studies of metastatic disease also found poor prognosis for G2—G3 vs. G1 [59] or G2 vs. G1 [67], while a retrospective experience found significant differences only between G3 vs. G1 [64].

7.4.5.3 Molecular biology

The GEP-NENs are distinguished among the NENs by their diploid arrangement [126], even though chromosomal losses are reported (18 loss in SI-NENs, 1q/3p/11q loss and 10q/7q/9q gain in Pan-NENs). The mutation rate is low in SI-NENs [127], prevalently in the CDKN1B gene (8–10% [128]), and elevated in Pan-NENs, in which MEN1 is mutated in 35–50% [129], ATRX in 10% [130], DAXX in 20%. The analysis of the genomic profiles identified two profiles of SI-NENs, those producing serotonin and those producing various amines [131], while other two entities were reported for Pan-NETs [132], whose behavior varies according to the positivity of ARX and PDX1, with the more aggressive ones expressing an ARX+/PDX1– phenotype [133].

In addition, other studies suggested a possible prognostic and predictive role for transcriptome [134, 135]. A PCR-based neuroendocrine tumors liquid biopsy (NETest), a transcriptomics signature evaluating 51 genes, has been studied as predictive and PF [136]. Peptide receptor radionuclide therapy (PRRT) prediction quotient (PPQ), a blood-based assay that evaluates eight genes and accurately predicts the response of NETs to PRRT, has also been validated [137].

Even methylation profiles were different in SI-NENs [138] and Pan-NENs [139, 140]. However, the predictive significance of O^6-methylguanine-DNA-methyltransferase (MGMT) promoter methylation remains doubtful, even though a meta-analysis of 11 studies documented a marked increase of ORRs after alkylating agents in NEN patients with MGMT promoter methylation (or low MGMT expression) [141].

A systematic review of 41 studies of the molecular characteristics of GEP-NECs reported that TP53 alterations were most frequent regardless of site, but MSI-H and other alterations were present in 10% of gastric and colorectal NECs. On the contrary, in mixed adeno-neuroendocrine carcinoma (MANECs) the molecular alterations are those of the adenocarcinomatous component [142].

7.4.5.4 Selected trials

Four studies analyzed the histotype, defining different histotype-related variables, but only one study documented a relationship with poor OS for patients with gastrinoma/insulinoma/VIPoma [30].

Whether the degree of differentiation did not correlate with prognosis in three studies [25, 35, 39], in one of two trials that evaluated tumor grading, the median OS of low vs. high-grade NENs was 40 vs. 5 months [32]. No differences were reported by the other study that distinguished three different grades [35]. No relationship with OS occurred even for Ki-67 at 9% and 25% cut-offs [35]. On the other hand, the two studies that analyzed the MI reported a significantly improved OS for <1 mitosis/HPF [25] and for 1 vs. >5 mitoses/10HPF [35].

The CAPTEM trial analyzed MGMT as a predictive variable in patients receiving a temozolomide-based regimen and did not find any relationship with OS for its loss of expression or promoter methylation [39, 143]. An analysis of RADIANT-3 excluded a prognostic role for serum levels of VEGFR1, VEGFR2, VEGF-A, and bFGF [37].

7.4.6 PREVIOUS TREATMENTS

7.4.6.1 Primary tumor resection

Palliative PTR is recommended in FTs or SI-NENs with obstruction or bleeding. However, some guidelines investigated PTR reporting a possible OS improvement for all SI-NENs [144], while the benefit described for Pan-NENs has to be counterbalanced with the high morbidity of the surgical procedure.

Although in population-based studies PTR is associated with better outcomes [6, 22, 52, 54, 55, 57, 58] mainly in patients with resectable disease, even in prospective case series of mPan-NEN eligible for PTR [60] or FTs [61], PTR is a favorable PF. In contrast, less consistent were the findings of two retrospective trials of midgut mNETs [63, 64] and one on mGEP-NEN [62], in which PTR was associated with better OS and other retrospective studies that did not document any relevance for PTR [45, 47, 68].

A systematic review selected 13 studies that evaluated the prognostic role of PTR in mGEP-NENs. A meta-analysis of 6 of the 13 studies demonstrated a longer OS for both Pan-NEN and SI-NEN after PTR. Furthermore, heterogeneity and publication bias were not significant, so the authors suggested considering PTR in patients with low TB and good PS [145]. Another study of the NCDB that included 6,088 mNENs without any resection of metastases has suggested prolonged OS for all GEP-NEN after PTR and defined organ-specific PFs in patients undergoing PTR [146].

Other studies have reported retrospective analyses in cohorts of patients with mSI-NEN, with favorable disease-specific mortality despite differences in PS and grading [147], and even in patients without symptoms and with unresectable metastases [63, 148, 149]. However, a cohort study of 363 mSI-NEN patients of the Uppsala University Hospital reported that those receiving upfront prophylactic surgery had a similar median OS, 7.9 vs. 7.6 years [150]. Therefore, the NANTS guidelines suggest that surgical procedures in SI-NEN should be taken into account in patients with a good PS and a limited LI (<50–70%) [151].

A systematic review of three cohort studies supported a possible benefit of PTR in unresectable mPan-NENs [152], and a meta-analysis identifying 10 studies of PTR in unresectable Pan-NEN, concluded that the effect of PTR was favorable and not explained by LI or grading, nor by heterogeneity or publication bias [153].

However, the PTR in the case of G3 remains highly debated. In a retrospective study on 201 G3 GEP-NEN/MANEC, PTR was associated with longer OS among patients with localized disease and some selected stage IV [154].

7.4.6.2 Debulking surgery

Debulking surgery, involving 80–90% removal of metastases, improved OS in some studies [111, 155]. An effect was also reported when removing 70% [156], which was comparable to 100% in terms of OS [157]. Also, studies evaluating ablative procedures concomitant to surgery suggest a positive effect on OS [107, 158].

While one population-based study on SEER found no differences in outcomes related to surgery of metastases [22], two studies reported a benefit from LMs surgery [59, 61].

7.4.6.3 Selected trials

Three studies evaluated patients with PTR versus those who did not receive a PTR, without documenting any significant relationship of PTR with OS in two [29, 36], and longer OS of patients with PTR in the PROMID trial [34].

7.5 PROGNOSTIC FACTORS IN DECISION-MAKING

Histotype and grading influence the treatment decisions more than any other variable (Table 7.5). Therefore, a diagnosis of NEC must be reported, since the approach tends to be conservative also in localized disease, even though their management is uncertain, due to many studies being small case series and the current definition of NEC vs. G3-NET is of 2017 [159].

TABLE 7.5
Prognostic and predictive variables in clinical decision-making in metastatic neuroendocrine tumor

A. Upfront treatment

1	Endocrine syndrome (refractory to medical treatment)
	• Regional treatment of metastases (included debulking if Ki-67 <10%) can contribute to control refractory endocrine syndrome
2	Grading
	• G1-G2 (Ki-67 <10%): aggressive regional treatment of metastases can improve outcomes
	• Ki-67 <2%: LANR favored (LANR more active than placebo)
3	Tumor burden
	• Low (resectable liver metastases, no EHD): aggressive regional treatment of metastases can improve outcomes
	• Low: OCT-LAR favored (OCT-LAR is better than placebo in HL <10%)
	• Low: LANR favored (LANR is better than placebo in hepatic tumor volume <25%)
4	Primary tumor resection
	• No PTR: LANR favored (LANR is better than placebo; OCT-LAR is similar to placebo)
5	Tumor growth rate
	• Low: aggressive regional treatment of metastases can improve outcomes
	• Low (longer time from diagnosis to treatment): SSRA are more active
6	Serum chromogranin
	• Normal: OCT-LAR favored (OCT-LAR is better than placebo; LANR is similar to placebo)

B. Treatment of refractory disease
Pancreatic (after SSRA progression)

1	Performance status
	• ECOG PS 1: EVE or SUN favored (EVE/SUN are better than placebo)
2	Serum chromogranin
	• Chromogranin <2ULN: SURU is similar to placebo
3	Endocrine syndrome
	• Present: SUN is similar to placebo
4	Sex
	• Males: EVE or SUN favored (EVE/SUN are better than placebo)

Midgut (after SSRA progression and PRRT)

1	Sex
	• Males: SURU favored (SURU is better than placebo)
2	Age
	• >65 years old: EVE favored (EVE is better than placebo)
3	Serum markers
	• Low (CGA <2ULN): SURU favored (SURU is better than placebo)
	• Low (NSE <ULN): EVE favored (EVE is better than placebo)
4	Previous treatments
	• No previous treatments: SURU favored (SURU is better than placebo)
	• Previous SSRA: EVE favored (EVE is better than placebo)

Legend: CGA, chromogranin A. ECOG PS, Eastern Cooperative Oncology Group Performance Status. EHD, extra-hepatic disease. EVE, everolimus. HL, hepatic tumor load. LANR, lanreotide. NSE, neuron-specific enolase. OCT-LAR, octreotide long-acting release. PRRT, Peptide Receptor Radionuclide Therapy. PTR, primary tumor resection. SSRA, somatostatin analogues. SUN, sunitinib. SURU, surufatinib. ULN, upper limit of normal.

In patients with NEC, the different prognosis and sensitivity to the same regimens of small cell lung cancer were evident from retrospective data, in which the etoposide+platinum (EP) regimen was associated with similar OS but significantly higher PFS for G3 [160]. A recent phase III trial comparison of irinotecan+platinum (IP) vs. EP, closed early because it did not document differences, though suggesting a more pronounced EP activity in pancreatic NECs [161]. Evidence for second-line, sunitinib [162], or chemotherapy (FOLFIRI or XELOX), remains limited.

The first decision in a patient with mNET is to define the treatment approach. In this context, in the first months after diagnosis, follow-up and surgical evaluation are necessary to rule out the indication for orthotopic liver transplantation (OLT) and help define the best strategy for regional treatment of metastases, but also the usefulness of palliative surgery. At present, access to OLT for patients with NET remains limited, mostly to patients with unresectable liver-limited disease, but according to some authors it should be reserved for patients with <60 years, long disease stability, LI <50%, and NET G1–G2 with Ki-67 <10%, preferably functioning.

An aggressive approach may be justified based on grading (G1–G2), TB, slow tumor growth, and absence of EHD. However, palliative surgery may be necessary for locally symptomatic NETs or endocrine syndromes that cannot be controlled with medical therapy, although debulking surgery remains contraindicated for Ki-67 >10%.

Depending on the site of origin, the role of PTR changes. Poor data are available about PTR in Pan-NET patients. Even though a meta-analysis suggests an improvement of OS, studies are heterogeneous and retrospective, therefore it could be considered if symptoms occur and based on other factors (good PS, G1–G2, LI, and EHD) [163]. For patients with GI-NET, no improvement from PTR has been reported in RCTs, consequently, PTR should be reserved for symptomatic patients, or those who risk becoming symptomatic soon [150].

Based on two studies, including midgut NENs and midgut/Pan-NETs, octreotide and lanreotide demonstrated longer PFS and are considered the upfront treatments in symptomatic and asymptomatic patients. The SSA activity is more pronounced in the midgut than pancreatic NETs, but their role according to PS was poorly studied. Though indicated in all G1–G2 NETs, studies report superior PFS in midgut, Ki-67 ≤2% [164], in cases with LI <10%, PTR [165]. There remains a favorable trend for slow-growing tumors (time to definitive deterioration >4–5 years). However, SSAs have been poorly studied after chemotherapy in non-White patients [164] and KPS <80% [165].

For Pan-NETs, in the setting of disease progression after SSAs, the first approach is a systemic treatment using at least three drugs to be sequenced, such as everolimus (EVE), anti-VEGFR (sunitinib or surufatinib), and alkylating (streptozotocin or temozolomide). Apart from the different toxicity profiles of the three options, patient preferences, and local licensing regulations, there are no studies that would make one sequence preferable over another. While EVE has the largest study and is effective in all subgroups examined [37], for tyrosine kinase inhibitors (TKIs) sunitinib is less active in FTs [166], while surufatinib works less in treatment-naive patients, males, and CGA <2ULN [167]. About the alkylating chemotherapy regimen there are no documented predictive factors, excluded MC [143], nor differences in RCTs [27, 168]. For PRRT there are only retrospective data suggesting better efficacy in VIPoma, gastrinoma, and insulinoma [30].

For GI-NETs, studies evaluated midgut tumors, although sometimes included all extra-pancreatic sites [169, 170]. Unless there are specific contraindications, the treatment of choice after progression to SSAs is PRRT, which reported longer PFS than long-acting octreotide 60 mg in all subgroups, while OS improvement was maintained only in the subgroup with poor PS, despite cross-over in 31.6% [171]. Some options are available for patients with PRRT refractory disease, such as EVE and VEGFRi. Although RADIANT4 enrolled GI and bronchial NETs, EVE reported poor activity in some subgroups (males, White, CGA <2ULN, NSE >ULN, treatment-naive). If sunitinib was ineffective in the nonfunctioning, surufatinib did not improve outcomes of patients >65 years old, with previous SSA treatment. The limited activity suggests the use of chemotherapy and interferon only upon failure of all the reported options.

TABLE 7.6

Prognostic factors evaluated in prospective trials of upfront treatment in patients with unresectable or metastatic neuroendocrine neoplasm

Suggested	Not suggested	Needing study
A Neuroendocrine tumor		
Performance status		Age
Cromogranin-A		Sex
Neurono-specific enolase		Endocrine syndrome/MEN
		Co-morbidities (midgut)
		NLR/inflammation-related
Disease status	No. sites of metastasis	Location (midgut better)
Liver involvement (volume %)	Timing of metastasis	Extra-hepatic metastasis
Ki-67	Liver metastasis	NETest
Tumor grading		
PTR		
B Neuroendocrine carcinoma		
Performance status		Age
LDH		Sex
Neurono-specific enolase		NLR and PLR
		Liver enzymes
Liver metastasis	Disease status	Liver involvement (volume %)
Ki-67 and mitotic rate		Location
		PTR

7.6 CONCLUSION

Few PFs are reliable in mNENs, as summarized in Table 7.6. Given the heterogeneity of features and the number of classifications over time, evidence on PFs is very limited.

If the weight of MI/MC is higher in WD NENs and Ki-67 in PD tumors, it can be argued that G3 NETs, and G2 with Ki-67 >20%, can be considered orphan diseases of PFs. Dedicated observational studies are urgently needed, as Ki-67 itself is not always associated with prognosis.

On the other hand, for NEC patients the GI-NEC score allows better prognostic stratification. However, given the low impact of treatments, in these patients, it seems more relevant to exclude the presence of MSI-H and eligibility for immunotherapy trials and to take into account lymphocyte counts and systemic inflammatory indices.

In WD NENs, it is important to have more evidence-based trials on the best attitude toward the primary tumor even in non-functioning tumors, given the possible favorable effects of surgical treatment and regional therapies. Similarly, the availability of dedicated studies on LMs in WD-NENs remains limited. To date, low TB and good PS guide the clinical decision, but a standard cut-off for LI is lacking. In such patients however, a standardized TB-related PF is necessary, such as ^{68}Ga-DOTATATE total volume, but it will also be useful a better understanding of the relationships with the outcome of LDH, NSE and NLR, especially in Pan-NETs, as well as timing of LMs.

REFERENCES

1. Modlin IM, Oberg K, Chung DC, et al. Gastroenteropancreatic neuroendocrine tumours. *Lancet Oncol* 2008;9(1):61–72.
2. Huguet I, Grossman AB, O'Toole D. Changes in the epidemiology of neuroendocrine tumours. *Neuroendocrinol* 2017;104(2):105–11.

3. Boyar Cetinkaya R, Aagnes B, Thiis-Evensen E, et al. Trends in incidence of neuroendocrine neoplasms in Norway: A report of 16,075 cases from 1993 through 2010. *Neuroendocrinol* 2017;104(1):1–10.

4. Miller HC, Drymousis P, Flora R, et al. Role of Ki-67 proliferation index in the assessment of patients with neuroendocrine neoplasias regarding the stage of disease. *World J Surg* 38(6):1353–61.

5. Dasari A, Shen C, Halperin D, et al. Trends in the incidence, prevalence, and survival outcomes in patients with neuroendocrine tumors in the United States. *JAMA Oncol* 2017;3(10):1335–42.

6. Sonbol MB, Mazza GL, Mi L, et al. Survival and incidence patterns of pancreatic neuroendocrine tumors over the last 2 decades: A SEER database analysis. *Oncologist* 2022,27:573–8.

7. Dasari A, Shen C, Halperin D, et al. Trends in the incidence, prevalence, and survival outcomes in patients with neuroendocrine tumors in the United states. *JAMA Oncol* 2017;3(10):1335–42.

8. Xu Z, Wang L, Dai S, et al. Epidemiologic trends of and factors associated with overall survival for patients with gastroenteropancreatic neuroendocrine tumors in the United states. *JAMA Netw Open* 2021;4(9):e2124750.

9. Korse CM, Taal BG, van Velthuysen M-LF, Visser O. Incidence and survival of neuroendocrine tumours in the Netherlands according to histological grade: Experience of two decades of cancer registry. *Eur J Cancer* 2013;49(8):1975–83.

10. Chauhan A, Kohn E, Del Rivero J. Neuroendocrine tumors – Less well known, often misunderstood, and rapidly growing in incidence. *JAMA Oncol* 2019;6(1):21–2.

11. Sundin A, Arnold R, Baudin E, et al. ENETS consensus guidelines for the standards of care in neuroendocrine tumors: Radiological, nuclear medicine & hybrid imaging. *Neuroendocrinol* 2017;105(3):212–44.

12. Gabriel M, Decristoforo C, Kendler D, et al. 68Ga-DOTA-Tyr3-octreotide PET in neuroendocrine tumors: Comparison with somatostatin receptor scintigraphy and CT. *J Nucl Med* 2007;48(4):508–18.

13. Procacci C, Carbognin G, Accordini S, et al. Nonfunctioning endocrine tumors of the pancreas: Possibilities of spiral CT characterization. *Eur Radiol* 2001;11(7):1175–83.

14. Putzer D, Gabriel M, Henninger B, et al. Bone metastases in patients with neuroendocrine tumor: 68Ga-DOTA-Tyr3-octreotide PET in comparison to CT and bone scintigraphy. *J Nucl Med* 2009;50(8):1214–21.

15. Schmid-Tannwald C, Schmid-Tannwald C, Morelli JN, et al. Comparison of abdominal MRI with diffusion-weighted imaging to 68Ga-DOTATATE PET/CT in detection of neuroendocrine tumors of the pancreas. *Eur J Nucl Med Mol Imaging* 2013;40(6):897–907.

16. Brenner R, Metens T, Bali M, et al. Pancreatic neuroendocrine tumor: Added value of fusion of T2-weighted imaging and high b-value diffusion-weighted imaging for tumor detection. *Eur J Radiol* 2012;81(5):e746–9.

17. Ronot M, Clift AK, Baum RP, et al. Morphological and functional imaging for detecting and assessing the resectability of neuroendocrine liver metastases. *Neuroendocrinol* 2018;106(1):74–88.

18. Dromain C, de Baere T, Lumbroso J, et al. Detection of liver metastases from endocrine tumors: A prospective comparison of somatostatin receptor scintigraphy, computed tomography, and magnetic resonance imaging. *J Clin Oncol* 2005;23(1):70–8.

19. Binderup T, Knigge U, Loft A, et al. 18F-fluorodeoxyglucose positron emission tomography predicts survival of patients with neuroendocrine tumors. *Clin Cancer Res* 2010;16(3):978–85.

20. Has Simsek D, Kuyumcu S, Turkmen C, et al. Can complementary 68Ga-DOTATATE and 18F-FDG PET/CT establish the missing link between histopathology and therapeutic approach in gastroenteropancreatic neuroendocrine tumors? *J Nucl Med* 2014;55(11):1811–7.

21. Garcia Carbonero R, Capdevila J, Crespo-Herrero G, et al. Incidence, patterns of care and prognostic factors for outcome of gastroenteropancreatic neuroendocrine tumors (GEP-NETs): Results from the National Cancer Registry of Spain (RGETNE). *Ann Oncol* 2010;21:1794–803.

22. Cai W, Tan Y, Ge W, et al. Pattern and risk factors for distant metastases in gastrointestinal neuroendocrine neoplasms: A population-based study. *Cancer Med* 2018;786:2699–709.

23. Liu X, Chen B, Chen J, Su Z, Sun S. The incidence, prevalence, and survival analysis of pancreatic neuroendocrine tumors in the United States. *J Endocrinol Invest* 2023;46:1373–84.

24. Engstrom PF, Lavin PT, Moertel CG, et al. Streptozotocin plus fluorouracil versus doxorubicin therapy for metastatic carcinoid tumor. *J Clin Oncol* 1984;2(11):1255–9.

25. Bukowski RM, Johnson KG, Peterson RF, et al. A phase II trial of combination chemotherapy in patients with metastatic carcinoid tumors. A Southwest Oncology Group study. *Cancer* 1987;60:2891–5.

26. Eriksson B, Skogseid B, Lundqvist G, et al. Medical treatment and long-term survival in a prospective study of 84 patients with endocrine pancreatic tumors. *Cancer* 1990;65:1883–90.

27. Moertel CG, Lefropoulo M, Lipsitz S, et al. Streptozotocin-doxorubicin, streptozotocin-fluorouracil, or chlorozotocin in the treatment of advanced isled-cell carcinoma. *N Engl J Med* 1992;326:519–23.

28. Ramanathan RK, Cnaan A, Hahn RG, et al. Phase II trial of dacarbazine (DTIC) in advanced pancreatic islet cell carcinoma. Study of the Eastern Cooperative Oncology Group-E6282. *Ann Oncol* 2001;12:1139–43.

29. Sun W, Lipsitz S, Catalano P, et al. Phase II/III study of doxorubicin with fluorouracil compared with streptozocin with fluorouracil or dacarbazine in the treatment of advanced carcinoid tumors: Eastern Cooperative Oncology Group study E1281. *J Clin Oncol* 2005;23:4897–904.

30. Kwekkeboom DJ, de Herder WW, Kam BL, et al. Treatment with the radiolabeled somatostatin analog [^{177}Lu-DOTA^{0},Tyr^{3}]octreotate: Toxicity, efficacy, and survival. *J Clin Oncol* 2008;26:2124–30.

31. Duran I, Kortmansky J, Singh D, et al. A phase II clinical and pharmacodynamic study of temsirolimus in advanced neuroendocrine carcinomas. *Br J Cancer* 2006;95:1148–54.

32. Bajetta E, Catena L, Procopio G, et al. Are capecitabine and oxaliplatin (XELOX) suitable treatments for progressing low-grade and high-grade neuroendocrine tumours? *Cancer Chemother Pharmacol* 2007;59:637–42.

33. Kulke MH, Lenz H-J, Meropol NJ, et al. Activity of sunitinib in patients with advanced neuroendocrine tumors. *J Clin Oncol* 2008;26:3403–10.

34. Rinke A, Wittenberg M, Schade-Brittinger C, et al. Placebo-controlled, double-blind, prospective, randomized study on the effect of octreotide LAR in the control of tumor growth in patients with metastatic neuroendocrine midgut tumors (PROMID): Results of long-term survival. *Neuroendocrinol* 2017;104:26–32.

35. Turner NC, Strauss SJ, Sarker D, et al. Chemotherapy with 5-fluorouracil, cisplatin and streptozocin for neuroendocrine tumours. *Br J Cancer* 2010;102:1106–12.

36. Cwikla JB, Sankowski A, Seklecka N, et al. Efficacy of radionuclide treatment DOTATATE Y-90 in patients with progressive metastatic gastroenteropancreatic neuroendocrine carcinomas (GEP-NETs): A phase II study. *Ann Oncol* 2010;21:787–94.

37. Yao JC, Pavel M, Lombard-Bohas C, et al. Everolimus for the treatment of advanced pancreatic neuroendocrine tumors: Overall survival and circulating biomarkers from the randomized, phase III RadIANT-3 study. *J clin Oncol* 2016;34:3906–13.

38. Yao JC, Guthrie K, Moran C, et al. Phase III prospective randomized comparison trial of depot octreotide plus interferon alfa-2b versus depot octreotide plus bevacizumab in patients with advanced carcinoid tumors: SWOG S0518. *J Clin Oncol* 2017;35:1695–703.

39. Jeong H, Shin J, Jeong JH, et al. Capecitabine plus temozolomide in patients with grade 3 unresectable or metastatic gastroenteropancreatic neuroendocrine neoplasms with Ki-67 index <55%: Single-arm phase II study. *ESMO Open* 2021;6(3):1–8.

40. Ezziddin S, Attassi M, Yong-Hing CJ, et al. Predictors of long-term outcome in patients with well-differentiated gastroenteropancreatic neuroendocrine tumors after peptide receptor radionuclide therapy with ^{177}Lu-octreotide. *J Nucli Med* 2014;55:183–90.

41. Kim H-J, Lee K-H, Shim HJ, et al. Prognostic significance of the neutrophil-lymphocyte ratio and platelet-lymphocyte ratio in neuroendocrine carcinoma. *Chonn Med J* 2022;58:29–36.

42. Lin Z, Wang H, Zhang Y, et al. Development and validation of a prognostic nomogram to guide decision-making for high-grade digestive neuroendocrine neoplasms. *Oncologist* 2020;25.e659–e667.

43. Rosery V, Mika S, Schmid KW, et al. Identification of a new prognostic score for patients with high-grade metastatic GEP-NEN treated with palliative chemotherapy. *J Cancer Res Clin Oncol* 2023;149:4315–25.

44. Abdelmalak R, Lythgoe MP, Evans J, et al. Exploration of novel prognostic markers in grade 3 neuroendocrine neoplasia. *Cancers* 2021;13:4232.

45. Yamaguchi T, Machida N, Morizane C, et al. Multicenter retrospective analysis of systemic chemotherapy for advanced neuroendocrine carcinoma of the digestive system. *Cancer Sci* 2014;105:1176–81.

46. Zou J, Li Q, Kou F, et al. Prognostic value of inflammation-based markers in advanced or metastatic neuroendocrine tumours. *Curr Oncol* 2019;26(1):e30–e38.

47. Acikgoz Y, Bal O, Dogan M. Albumin-to-alkaline phosphatase ratio. Does it predict survival in grade 1 and grade 2 neuroendocrine tumors? *Pancreas* 2021;50:111–7.

48. Sorbye H, Strosberg J, Baudin E, et al. Gastroenteropancreatic high-grade neuroendocrine carcinoma. *Cancer* 2014;120:2814–23.

49. Lamarca A, Walter T, Pavel M, et al. Design and validation of the GI-NEC score to prognosticate overall survival in patients with high-grade gastrointestinal neuroendocrine carcinomas. *J Natl Cancer Inst* 2017;109(5):djw277.

50. Kim H-J, Lee KH, Shim HJ, et al. Prognostic significance of the neutrophil-lymphocyte ratio and platelet-lymphocyte ratio in neuroendocrine carcinoma. *Chonnam Med J* 2022;58:29–36.

51. Yao JC, Hassan M, Phan A, et al. One hundred years after "carcinoid": Epidemiology of and prognostic factors for neuroendocrine tumors in 35,825 cases in the United States. *J Clin Oncol* 2008;26:3063–72.

52. Keutgen XM, Nilubol N, Glanville J, et al. Resection of primary tumor site is associated with prolonged survival in metastatic nonfunctioning pancreatic neuroendocrine tumors. *Surgery* 2016;159:311–9.

53. Nunez-Valdovinos B, Carmona-Bayonas A, Jimenez-Fonseca P, et al. Neuroendocrine tumor heterogeneity adds uncertainty to the World Health Organization 2010 classification: Real-world data from the Spanish Tumor Registry (R-GETNE). *Oncologist* 2018;23:422–32.

54. Polcz M, Schlegel C, Edwards GC, et al. Primary tumor resection offers survival benefit in patients with metastatic midgut neuroendocrine tumors. *Ann Surg Oncol* 2020;27:2795–803.

55. Lu Z, Li T, Liu C, et al. Development and validation of a survival prediction model and risk stratification for pancreatic neuroendocrine neoplasms. *J Endocrinol Invest* 2023;46:927–37.

56. Wu P, He D, Chang H, Zhang X. Epidemiologic trends of and factors associated with overall survival in patients with neuroendocrine tumors over the last two decades in the United States. *Endocr Connect* 2023;12(12):e230331.

57. Liu X, Chen B, Chen J, Su Z. The incidence, prevalence, and survival analysis of pancreatic neuroendocrine tumors in the United States. *J Endocrinol Invest* 2023;46:1373–84.

58. Huttner FJ, Schneider L, Tarantino I, et al. Palliative resection of the primary tumor in 442 metastasized neuroendocrine tumors of the pancreas: A population-based, propensity score-matched survival analysis. *Langenbecks Arch Surg* 2015;400:715–23.

59. Fairweather M, Swanson R, Wang J, et al. Management of neuroendocrine tumor liver metastases: Long-term outcomes and prognostic factors from a large prospective database. *Ann Surg Oncol* 2017;24:2319–25.

60. Bertani E, Fazio N, Radice D, et al. Assessing the role of primary tumour resection in patients with synchronous unresectable liver metastases from pancreatic neuroendocrine tumour of the body and tail. A propensity score survival evaluation. *Eur J Surg Oncol* 2017;43:372–9.

61. Citterio D, Pusceddu S, Facciorusso A, et al. Primary tumour resection may improve survival in functional well-differentiated neuroendocrine tumours metastatic to the liver. *Eur J Surg Oncol* 2017;43:380–7.

62. Durante C, Boukheris H, Dromain C, et al. Prognostic factors influencing survival from metastatic (stage IV) gastroenteropancreatic well-differentiated endocrine carcinoma. *Endocr Relat Cancer* 2009;16(2):585–97.

63. Ahmed A, Turner G, King B, et al. Midgut neuroendocrine tumours with liver metastases: Results of the UKINETS study. *Endocr Relat Cancer* 2009;16(3):885–94.

64. Gangi A, Manguso N, Gong J, et al. Midgut neuroendocrine tumors with liver-only metastases: Benefit of primary tumor resection. *Ann Surg Oncol* 2020;27:4525–32.

65. Halfdanarson TR, Rabe KG, Rubin J, Petersen GM. Pancreatic neuroendocrine tumors (PNETs): Incidence, prognosis and recent trend toward improved survival. *Ann Oncol* 2008;19(10):1727–33.

66. Bilimoria KY, Talamonti MS, Tomlinson JS, et al. Prognostic score predicting survival after resection of pancreatic neuroendocrine tumors: Analysis of 3851 patients. *Ann Surg* 2008;247(3):490–500.

67. Santos AP, Rodrigues J, Henrique R, Cardoso MH, Monteiro MP. Visceral obesity is associated with shorter progression-free survival in well-differentiated gastro-entero-pancreatic neuroendocrine neoplasia. *J Clin Med* 2022;11:6026.

68. Kouvaraki MA, Ajani JA, Hoff P, et al. Fluorouracil, doxorubicin, and streptozocin in the treatment of patients with locally advanced and metastatic pancreatic endocrine carcinomas. *J Clin Oncol* 2004;22:4762–71.

69. Sebastian-Valles F, Sanchez de la Blanca Carrero N, Rodriguez-Laval V, et al. Impact of change in body composition during follow-up on the survival of GEP-NET. *Cancers* 2022;14:5189.

70. Crona J, Norlen O, Antonodimitrakis P, et al. Multiple and secondary hormone secretion in patients with metastatic pancreatic neuroendocrine tumours. *J Clin Endocrinol Metab* 2016;101(2):445–52.

71. Gao H, Liu L, Wang W, et al. Novel recurrence risk stratification of resected pancreatic neuroendocrine tumor. *Cancer Lett* 2018;412:188–93.

72. Baechle JJ, Marincola Smith P, Tan M, et al. Specific growth rate as a predictor of survival in pancreatic neuroendocrine tumors: A multi-institutional study from the United States neuroendocrine study group. *Ann Surg Oncol* 2020;27:3915–23.

73. Garcia-Jimenez C, Garcia-Martinez JM, Chocarro-Calvo A, De la Vieja A. A new link between diabetes and cancer: Enhanced WNT/β-catenin signaling by high glucose. *J Mol Endocrinol* 2013;52(1):R51–R66.

74. Halperin R, Ahron-Hananel G, Badarna M, et al. Plasma hemoglobin and red blood cell mass levels as dynamic prognostic markers for progression and survival in pancreatic neuroendocrine tumors. *Horm Metab Res* 2021;53(12):810–7.

75. Salman T, Kazaz SN, Varol U, et al. Prognostic value of the pretreatment neutrophil-to-lymphocyte ratio and platelet-to-lymphocyte ratio for patients with neuroendocrine tumors: An Izmir Oncology Group study. *Chemotherapy* 2016;61(6):281–6.

76. Pusceddu S, Barretta F, Trama A, et al. A classification prognostic score to predict OS in stage IV well-differentiated neuroendocrine tumors. *Endocr Relat Cancer* 2018;25(6):607–18.

77. Cao L-L, Lu J, Lin J-X, et al. A novel predictive model based on preoperative blood neutrophil-to-lymphocyte ratio for survival prognosis in patients with gastric neuroendocrine neoplasms. *Oncotarget* 2017;7(27):42045–58.

78. Freis P, Graillot E, Rousset P, et al. Prognostic factors in neuroendocrine carcinoma: Biological markers are more useful than histomorphological markers. *Sci Rep* 2017;7:40609.

79. Carideo L, Prosperi D, Panzuto F, et al. Role of combined [68Ga]Ga-DOTA-SST analogues and [18F] FDG PET/CT in the management of GEP-NENs: A systematic review. *J Clin Med* 2019;8(7):1032.

80. Marotta V, Zatelli MC, Sciammarella C, et al. Chromogranin A as circulating marker for diagnosis and management of neuroendocrine neoplasms: More flaws than fame. *Endocr Relat Cancer* 2018;25(1):R11–29.

81. Janson ET, Holmberg L, Stridsberg M, et al. Carcinoid tumors: Analysis of prognostic factors and survival in 301 patients from a referral center. *Ann Oncol* 1997;8(7):685–90.

82. Zatelli MC, Torta M, Leon A, et al. Chromogranin A as a marker of neuroendocrine neoplasia: An Italian multicenter study. *Endocr Relat Cancer* 2007;14(2):473–82.

83. Chan DL, Clarke SJ, Diakos CI, et al. Prognostic and predictive biomarkers in neuroendocrine tumours. *Crit Rev Oncol Hematol* 2017;113:268–82.

84. Yao JC, Pavel M, Phan AT, et al. Chromogranin A and neuron-specific enolase as prognostic markers in patients with advanced pNET treated with everolimus. *J Clin Endocrinol Metab* 2011;96(12):3741–9.

85. Modlin IM, Oberg K, Taylor A, et al. Neuroendocrine tumor biomarkers: Current status and perspectives. *Neuroendocrinol* 2014;100(4):265–77.

86. van Adrichem RCS, Kamp K, Vandamme T, et al. Serum neuron-specific enolase level is an independent predictor of overall survival in patients with gastroenteropancreatic neuroendocrine tumors. *Ann Oncol* 2016;27(4):746–7.

87. Korse CM, Taal BG, Vincent A, et al. Choice of tumour markers in patients with neuroendocrine tumours is dependent on the histological grade. A marker study of Chromogranin A, Neuron specific enolase, Progastrin-releasing peptide and cytokeratin fragments. *Eur J Cancer* 2012;48(5):662–71.

88. Chan DL, Yao JC, Carnaghi C, et al. Markers of systemic inflammation in neuroendocrine tumors: A pooled analysis of the RADIANT-3 and RADIANT-4 studies. *Pancreas* 2021;50(2):130–7.

89. Deppen SA, Liu E, Blume JD, et al. Safety and Efficacy of 68Ga-DOTATATE PET/CT for diagnosis, staging, and treatment management of neuroendocrine tumors. *J Nucl Med* 2016;57(5):708–14.

90. Tirosh A, Papadakis GZ, Millo C, et al. Prognostic utility of total 68Ga-DOTATATE-avid tumor volume in patients with neuroendocrine tumors. *Gastroenterol* 2018;154(4):998–1008.

91. Ambrosini V, Campana D, Polverari G, et al. Prognostic value of 68Ga-DOTANOC PET/CT SUVmax in patients with neuroendocrine tumors of the pancreas. *J Nucl Med* 2015;56(12):1843–8.

92. Deng H-Y, Li G, Luo J, et al. The role of surgery in treating resectable limited disease of esophageal neuroendocrine carcinoma. *World J Surg* 2018;42(8):2428–36.

93. Cai W, Tan Y, Ge W, Ding K, Hu H. Pattern and risk factors for distant metastases in gastrointestinal neuroendocrine neoplasms: A population-based study. *Cancer Med* 2018;7(6):2399–709.

94. Chen C, Hu H, Zheng Z, et al. Clinical characteristics, prognostic factors, and survival trends in esophageal neuroendocrine carcinomas: A population-based study. *Cancer Med* 2022;11(24):4935–45.

95. Snorradottir S, Asgeirsdottir A, Rognvaldsson S, et al. Incidence and prognosis of patients with small intestinal neuroendocrine tumors in a population based nationwide study. *Cancer Epidemiol* 2022;79:102197.

96. Caplin M, Sundin A, Nillson O, et al. ENETS Consensus Guidelines for the management of patients with digestive neuroendocrine neoplasms: Colorectal neuroendocrine neoplasms. *Neuroendocrinol* 2012;95:88–97.

97. Ford MM. Neuroendocrine tumors of the colon and rectum. *Dis Colon Rectum* 2017;60(10):1018–21.

98. Li S, Niu M, Deng W, et al. Efficacy of chemotherapy versus transcatheter arterial chemoembolization in patients with advanced primary hepatic neuroendocrine carcinoma and an analysis of the prognostic factors: A retrospective study. *Cancer Manag Res* 2021;13:9085–93.

99. Glazer ES, Tseng JF, Al-Refaie W, et al. Long-term survival after surgical management of neuroendocrine hepatic metastases. *HBP* 2010;12(6):427–33.

100. Zhang X-F, Beal EW, Weiss M, et al. Timing of disease occurrence and hepatic resection on long-term outcome of patients with neuroendocrine liver metastasis. *J Surg Oncol* 2018;117(2):171–81.

101. Riihimaki M, Hemminki A, Sundquist K, et al. The epidemiology of metastases in neuroendocrine tumors. *Int J Cancer* 2016;139(12):2679–86.

102. Panzuto F, Boninsegna L, Fazio N, et al. Metastatic and locally advanced pancreatic endocrine carcinomas: Analysis of factors associated with disease progression. *J Clin Oncol* 2011;29(17):2372–7.
103. Pavel M, O'Toole D, Costa F, et al. ENETS consensus guidelines update for the management of distant metastatic disease of intestinal, pancreatic, bronchial neuroendocrine neoplasms (NEN) and NEN of unknown primary site. *Neuroendocrinol* 2016;103(2):172–85.
104. Frilling A, Modlin IM, Kidd M, et al. Recommendations for management of patients with neuroendocrine liver metastases. *Lancet Oncol* 2014;15:e8–21.
105. Rindi G, D'Adda T, Froio E, et al. Prognostic factors in gastrointestinal endocrine tumors. *Endocr Pathol* 2007;18(3):145–9.
106. Saxena A, Chua TC, Perera M, et al. Surgical resection of hepatic metastases from neuroendocrine neoplasms: A systematic review. *Surg Oncol* 2012;21(3):e131–41.
107. Mayo SC, de Jong MC, Pulitano C, et al. Surgical management of hepatic neuroendocrine tumor metastasis: Results from an international multi-institutional analysis. *Ann Surg Oncol* 2010;17:3129–36.
108. Zhang X-F, Beal EW, Chakedis J, et al. Early recurrence of neuroendocrine liver metastasis after curative hepatectomy: Risk factors, prognosis, and treatment. *J Gastrotest Surg* 2017;21(11):1821–30.
109. Xiang J-X, Zhang X-F, Weiss M, et al. Early recurrence of well-differentiated (G1) neuroendocrine liver metastasis after curative-intent surgery: Risk factors and outcome. *J Surg Oncol* 2018;118(7):1096–104.
110. Spolverato G, Bagante F, Aldrighetti L, et al. Management and outcomes of patients with recurrent neuroendocrine liver metastasis after curative surgery: An international multi-institutional analysis. *J Surg Oncol* 2017;116(3):298–306.
111. Sarmiento JM, Heywood G, Rubin J, et al. Surgical treatment of neuroendocrine metastases to the liver: A plea for resection to increase survival. *J Am Coll Surg* 2003;197(1):29–37.
112. Croome KP, Burns JM, Que FG, Nagorney DM. Hepatic resection for metastatic neuroendocrine cancer in patients with bone metastases. *Ann Surg Oncol* 2016;23(11):3693–8.
113. Garcia-Torralba E, Spada F, Lim KHJ, et al. Knowns and unknowns of bone metastases in patients with neuroendocrine neoplasms: A systematic review and meta-analysis. *Cancer Treat Rev* 2021;94:102168.
114. Zheng Z, Chen C, Jiang L, et al. Incidence and risk factors of gastrointestinal neuroendocrine neoplasm metastasis in liver, lung, bone, and brain: A population-based study. *Cancer Med* 2019;8(17):7288–98.
115. Rindi G, Arnold R, Bosman FT, et al. Nomenclature and classification of neuroendocrine neoplasms of the digestive system. In: Bosman FT, Carneiro F, Hruban RH, Theise ND, editors. *WHO Classification of Tumours of the Digestive System*. 4th Ed. Lyon; International Agency for Research on Cancer, 2010:13–40.
116. Klimstra DS, Klöppel G, La Rosa S, Rindi G. Classification of neuroendocrine neoplasms of the digestive system. In: *WHO Classification of Tumours*, 5th Ed. Digestive system tumours. Lyon; IARC, 2019:16–9.
117. Craig Z, Swain J, Batman E, et al. NET-02 trial protocol: A multicentre, randomised, parallel group, open-label, phase II, single-stage selection trial of liposomal irinotecan (nal-IRI) and 5-fluorouracil (5-FU)/folinic acid or docetaxel as second-line therapy in patients with progressive poorly differentiated extrapulmonary neuroendocrine carcinoma (NEC). *BMJ Open* 2020;10(2):e034527.
118. Basturk O, Yang Z, Tang LH, et al. The high-grade (WHO G3) pancreatic neuroendocrine tumor category is morphologically and biologically heterogenous and includes both well differentiated and poorly differentiated neoplasms. *Am J Surg Pathol* 2015;39(5):683–90.
119. Freis P, Graillot E, Rousset P, et al. Prognostic factors in neuroendocrine carcinoma: Biological markers are more useful than histomorphological markers. *Sci Rep* 2017;7:40609.
120. Sorbye H, Welin S, Langer SW, et al. Predictive and prognostic factors for treatment and survival in 305 patients with advanced gastrointestinal neuroendocrine carcinoma (WHO G3): The NORDIC NEC study. *Ann Oncol* 2013;24(1):152–60.
121. Haider K, Shahid RK, Finch D, et al. Extrapulmonary small cell cancer. A Canadian province's experience. *Cancer* 2006;107:2262–9.
122. Nagtegaal ID, Odze RD, Klimstra D, et al. The 2019 WHO classification of tumours of the digestive system. *Histopathol* 2020;76(2):182–8.
123. Ekeblad S, Skogseid B, Dunder K, et al. Prognostic factors and survival in 324 patients with pancreatic endocrine tumor treated at a single institution. *Clin Cancer Res* 2008;14(23):7798–803.
124. Martin-Perez E, Capdevila J, Castellano D, et al. Prognostic factors and long-term outcome of pancreatic neuroendocrine neoplasms: Ki-67 index shows a greater impact on survival than disease stage. The large experience of the Spanish National Tumor Registry (RGETNE). *Neuroendocrinol* 2013;98(2):156–68.
125. Hochwald SN, Zee S, Conlon KC, et al. Prognostic factors in pancreatic endocrine neoplasms: An analysis of 136 cases with a proposal for low-grade and intermediate-grade groups. *J Clin Oncol* 2002;20(11):2633–42.

126. Simbolo M, Vicentini C, Mafficini A, et al. Mutational and copy number asset of primary sporadic neuroendocrine tumors of the small intestine. *Virchows Arch* 2018;473(6):709–17.

127. Banck MS, Kanwar R, Kulkarni AA, et al. The genomic landscape of small intestine neuroendocrine tumors. *J Clin Invest* 2013;123(6):2502–8.

128. Francis JM, Kiezun A, Ramos AH, et al. Somatic mutation of CDKN1B in small intestine neuroendocrine tumors. *Nat Genet* 2013;45(12):1483–6.

129. Jiao Y, Shi C, Edil BH, et al. DAXX/ATRX, MEN1, and mTOR pathway genes are frequently altered in pancreatic neuroendocrine tumors. *Science* 2011;331(6021):1199–203.

130. Scarpa A, Chang DK, Nones K, et al. Whole-genome landscape of pancreatic neuroendocrine tumours. *Nature* 2017;543:65–71.

131. Kidd M, Modlin IM, Drozdov I. Gene network-based analysis identifies two potential subtypes of small intestinal neuroendocrine tumors. *BMC Genomics* 2014;15(1):595.

132. Duerr E-M, Mizukami Y, Ng A, et al. Defining molecular classifications and targets in gastroenteropancreatic neuroendocrine tumors through DNA microarray analysis. *Endocr Relat Cancer* 2008;15(1):243–56.

133. Cejas P, Drier Y, Dreijerink KMA, et al. Enhancer signatures stratify and predict outcomes of nonfunctional pancreatic neuroendocrine tumors. *Nat Med* 2019;25(8):1260–5.

134. Andersson E, Arvidsson Y, Sward C, et al. Expression profiling of small intestinal neuroendocrine tumors identifies subgroups with clinical relevance, prognostic markers and therapeutic targets. *Mod Pathol* 2016;29:616–29.

135. Puliani G, Di Vito V, Feola T, et al. NETest: A systematic review focusing on the prognostic and predictive role. *Neuroendocrinol* 2022;112(6):523–36.

136. Oberg K, Califano A, Strosberg JR, et al. A meta-analysis of the accuracy of a neuroendocrine tumor mRNA genomic biomarker (NETest) in blood. *Ann Oncol* 2020;31(2):202–12.

137. Bodei L, Kidd MS, Singh A, et al. PRRT genomic signature in blood for prediction of ^{177}Lu-octreotate efficacy. *Eur J Nucl Med Mol Imaging* 2018;45(7):1155–69.

138. Karpathakis A, Dibra H, Pipinikas C, et al. Prognostic impact of novel molecular subtypes of small intestinal neuroendocrine tumor. *Clin Cancer Res* 2016;22(1):250–8.

139. Mafficini A, Scarpa A. Genomic landscape of pancreatic neuroendocrine tumours: The International Cancer Genome Consortium. *J Endocrinol* 2018;236(3):R161–7.

140. Roldo C, Missiaglia E, Hagan JP, et al. MicroRNA expression abnormalities in pancreatic endocrine and acinar tumors are associated with distinctive pathologic features and clinical behavior. *J Clin Oncol* 2006;24(29):4677–84.

141. Qi Z, Tan H. Association between MGMT status and response to alkylating agents in patients with neuroendocrine neoplasms: A systematic review and meta-analysis. *Biosci Rep* 2020;40(3):BSR20194127.

142. Girardi DM, Silva ACB, Rego JFM, et al. Unraveling molecular pathways of poorly differentiated neuroendocrine carcinomas of the gastroenteropancreatic system: A systematic review. *Cancer Treat Rev* 2017;56:28–35.

143. Cives M, Ghayouri M, Morse B, et al. Analysis of potential response predictors to capecitabine/temozolomide in metastatic pancreatic neuroendocrine tumors. *Endocr-Relat Cancer* 2016;23:759–67.

144. Niederle B, Pape U-F, Costa F, et al. ENETS consensus guidelines update for neuroendocrine neoplasms of the jejunum and ileum. *Neuroendocrinology* 2016;103(2):125–38.

145. Almond LM, Hodson J, Ford SJ, et al. Role of palliative resection of the primary tumour in advanced pancreatic and small intestinal neuroendocrine tumours: A systematic review and meta-analysis. *Eur J Surg Oncol* 2017;43(10):1808–15.

146. Tierney JF, Chivukula SV, Wang X, et al. Resection of primary tumor may prolong survival in metastatic gastroenteropancreatic neuroendocrine tumors. *Surgery* 2019;165(3):644–51.

147. Levy S, Arthur JD, Banks M, et al. Primary tumor resection is associated with improved disease-specific mortality in patients with stage IV small intestinal neuroendocrine tumors (NETs): A comparison of upfront surgical resection versus a watch and wait strategy in two specialist NET centers. *Ann Surg Oncol* 2022;29:7822–32.

148. Hellman P, Lundstrom T, Ohrvall U, et al. Effect of surgery on the outcome of midgut carcinoid disease with lymph node and liver metastases. *World J Surg* 2002;26(8):991–7.

149. Givi B, Pommier SJ, Thompson AK, Diggs BS, Pommier RF. Operative resection of primary carcinoid neoplasms in patients with liver metastases yields significantly better survival. *Surgery* 2006;140(6):891–7.

150. Daskalakis K, Karakatsanis A, Hessman O, et al. Association of a prophylactic surgical approach to stage IV small intestinal neuroendocrine tumors with survival. *JAMA Oncol* 2018;4(2):183–9.

151. Howe JR, Cardona K, Fraker DL, et al. The surgical management of small bowel neuroendocrine tumors: Consensus guidelines of the North American neuroendocrine tumor society. *Pancreas* 2017;46(6):715–31.

152. Capurso G, Bettini R, Rinzivillo M, Bononsegna L, et al. Role of resection of the primary pancreatic neuroendocrine tumour only in patients with unresectable metastatic liver disease: A systematic review. *Neuroendocrinology* 2011;93(4):223–9.

153. Zhou B, Zhan C, Ding Y, et al. Role of palliative resection of the primary pancreatic neuroendocrine tumor in patients with unresectable metastatic liver disease: A systematic review and meta-analysis. *Onco Targ Ther* 2018;11:975–82.

154. Pommergaard H-C, Nielsen K, Sorbye H, et al. Surgery of the primary tumour in 201 patients with high-grade gastroenteropancreatic neuroendocrine and mixed neuroendocrine-non-neuroendocrine neoplasms. *J Neuroendocrinol* 2021;33(5):e12967.

155. Ejaz A, Reames BN, Maithel S, et al. Cytoreductive debulking surgery among patients with neuroendocrine liver metastasis: A multi-institutional analysis. *HPB* 2018;20(3):277–84.

156. Scott AT, Breheny PJ, Keck KJ, et al. Effective cytoreduction can be achieved in patients with numerous neuroendocrine tumor liver metastases (NETLMs). *Surgery* 2019;165(1):166–75.

157. Morgan RE, Pommier SJ, Pommier RF. Expanded criteria for debulking of liver metastasis also apply to pancreatic neuroendocrine tumors. *Surgery* 2018;163(1):218–25.

158. Taner T, Atwell TD, Zhang L, et al. Adjunctive radiofrequency ablation of metastatic neuroendocrine cancer to the liver complements surgical resection. *HPB* 2013;15:190–5.

159. Lloyd RV, Osamura RY, Kloppel G, et al. *WHO Classification of Tumors of Endocrine Organs*. 4th Ed., Lyon, France, 2017, volume 10:209–40.

160. Mitry E, Baudin E, Ducreux M, et al. Treatment of poorly differentiated neuroendocrine tumours with etoposide and cisplatin. *Br J Cancer* 1999;81(8):1351–5.

161. Morizane C, Machida N, Homma Y, et al. Effectiveness of etoposide and cisplatin vs irinotecan and cisplatin therapy for patients with advanced neuroendocrine carcinoma of the digestive system. The TOPIC-NeC phase 3 randomized clinical trial. *JAMA Oncol* 2022;8(10):1447–55.

162. Pellat A, Dreyer C, Couffignal C, et al. Clinical and biomarker evaluations of sunitinib in patients with grade 3 digestive neuroendocrine neoplasms. *Neuroendocrinol* 2018;107(1):24–31.

163. Partelli S, Cirocchi R, Rancoita PMV, et al. A systematic review and meta-analysis on the role of palliative primary resection for pancreatic neuroendocrine neoplasm with liver metastases. *HPB* 2018;20:197–203.

164. Caplin ME, Pavel M, Cwikla JB, et al. Lanreotide in metastatic enteropancreatic neuroendocrine tumors. *N Engl J Med* 2014;371:224–33.

165. Rinke A, Muller H-H, Schade-Brittinger C, et al. Placebo-controlled, double-blind, prospective, randomized study on the effect of octreotide LAR in the control of tumor growth in patients with metastatic neuroendocrine midgut tumors: A report from the PROMID study group. *J Clin Oncol* 2009;27:4656–63.

166. Raymond E, Dahan L, Raoul J-L, et al. Sunitinib malate for the treatment of pancreatic neuroendocrine tumors. *N Engl J Med* 2011;364:501–13.

167. Xu J, Shen L, Bai C, et al. Surufatinib in advanced pancreatic neuroendocrine tumours (SANET-p): A randomised, double-blind, placebo-controlled, phase 3 study. *Lancet Oncol* 2020;21:1489–99.

168. Kunz PL, Graham NT, Catalano PJ, et al. Randomized study of temozolomide or temozolomide and capecitabine in patients with advanced pancreatic neuroendocrine tumors (ECOG-ACRIN E2211). *J Clin Oncol* 2023;41:1359–69.

169. Yao JC, Fazio N, Singh S, et al. Everolimus for the treatment of advanced, non-functional neuroendocrine tumours of the lung or gastrointestinal tract (RADIANT-4): A randomised, placebo-controlled, phase 3 study. *Lancet* 2016;387:968–77.

170. Xu J, Shen L, Zhou Z, et al. Surufatinib in advanced extrapancreatic neuroendocrine tumours (SANET-ep): A randomised, double-blind, placebo-controlled, phase 3 study. *Lancet Oncol* 2020;21:1500–12.

171. Strosberg JR, Caplin ME, Kunz PL, et al. 177Lu-Dotatate plus long-acting octreotide versus high-dose long-acting octreotide in patients with midgut neuroendocrine tumours (NETTER-1): Final overall survival and long-term safety results from an open-label, randomised, controlled, phase 3 trial. *Lancet Oncol* 2021;22:1753–63.

8 Gastro-intestinal stromal tumors

8.1 INTRODUCTION

8.1.1 EPIDEMIOLOGY

Worldwide gastrointestinal stromal tumor (GIST) incidence varies around 1.0–1.5/100,000 person-years (range 0.4–2.2). It can be assumed that in Europe is between 1.0 and 1.77/100,000 person-years [1–11].

The lowest incidence rates have been shown in Shanxi and the highest in Shanghai, Hong Kong, Taiwan, and Norway [12]. However, two Chinese registries of 430 million subjects reported an incidence of 0.40/100,000 person-years in 2016, much lower than other provinces [13]. The incidence data is more homogeneous in other areas, such as North America (0.68–0.70/100,000 person-years) [14–18] and Korea (1.6/100,000 person-years) [19].

The Dutch PALGA registry has documented an increasing incidence from 2.1 to 17.7 per million inhabitants from 1995 to 2018, which only partly can be attributed to the diagnostic anti-CD117 antibody [1, 3, 6]. Another report by the Netherlands Cancer Registry (NCR) documented an increased incidence of localized disease, from 3.1 to 7.0/1,000,000 person-years from 2001 to 2012, against a stable incidence of metastatic GISTs around 1.3/1,000,000 person-years [20].

A systematic review documented that the median age at diagnosis was 60, gastric localization prevailed (55.6%), followed by small bowel (31.8%), colorectal (6%), and esophagus (0.7%) [12], similar to other authors [21]. However, the median age of incidence is also affected by geographic variations, ranging from 55.2 years in China [13] to 65–67 years in Europe and Japan [1, 20, 22–25].

8.1.2 STAGING OF METASTATIC DISEASE

Diagnostics vary according to upper or lower gastrointestinal site and tumor size [26]. EUS+biopsy is the standard approach for upper GISTs, whereas for lower GISTs EUS is often nondiagnostic because of extra-mucosal growth, making excisional biopsy necessary. For lesions ≥2 cm, biopsy and/or excision are key diagnostic investigations.

For diagnostics, MRI is preferred as the first investigation over abdominal CT, and for lower tumors, it is often necessary in conjunction with excisional biopsy. Indeed, especially in rectal GISTs, regardless of size and mitotic index (MI), the risk of progression to clinically significant GISTs is high. In metastatic disease, biopsy of metastases is the best approach and is mandatory before starting systemic treatment.

Pathologic diagnosis is based on morphology and immunohistochemistry [27, 28]. Mitotic count (MC) has prognostic value and should be expressed as the number of mitoses in a 5 mm^2 area.

KIT and PDGFRA mutations should be routinely sought in all GISTs, except for small (<2 cm) localized upper GISTs. Mutational analysis also has prognostic and predictive value. In KIT/PFGDR negative GISTs, succinate dehydrogenase (SDH) immunohistochemistry may be required for diagnosis, and if negative, a diagnosis of neurofibromatosis-1 (NF1) should be excluded (quadruple negative GISTs, with wild-type KIT/PDGFRA/BRAF/SDH) [29], but also BRAF and NTRK have therapeutic implications [30].

DOI: 10.1201/9781032703350-8

The eighth UICC-TNM system is rarely used for staging, and the more used classifications refer to mutated KIT GISTs, such as the Armed Forces Institute of Pathology classification, which incorporates MC, size, and location [31, 32]. For risk stratification, a nomogram has been developed too [33]. However, MI and size are continuous variables regardless of classification [34].

For staging, abdominal CT is the investigation of choice, although MRI may be a viable option. [18]FDG-PET is useful when early assessment of response to imatinib is of particular interest or when considering surgical resection of metastases [35]. PET responses have been observed as early as 24–48 hours after imatinib initiation and correlate with symptom control, typically precede tumor shrinkage by several weeks and are associated with prolonged progression-free survival (PFS) [35].

8.1.3 PROGNOSIS OF METASTATIC DISEASE

In the NCR 5-year survival rates of patients with metastatic vs. localized tumor were 48.2% versus 88.8%, but 5-year survival rates increased from 71.0% to 81.4% from 2001 to 2012, and better outcomes were reported for females [20]. In 15–50%, GIST occurs as a metastatic disease at diagnosis, mainly to the liver [6, 25, 36, 37], and usually after radical excision of localized disease, a tumor relapse affects 40–50% of patients over 2–10 years [38, 39], with 35% of patients receiving adjuvant imatinib experiencing a relapse [40, 41].

If the prognostic factors (PFs) have been extensively studied in localized GIST, few data are available on metastatic GIST. However, prognosis greatly depends on the sensitivity to imatinib, which in turn changes based on the mutational profile. Despite the frequent GIST recurrence [42], the median OS of metastatic GIST tripled after imatinib introduction [43, 44].

Prognostic assessment of metastatic GIST patients is complicated by some limitations of OS as an outcome measure. OS should be replaced by disease-specific survival (DSS) because a high incidence of second primary tumors (SPT) affects GIST patients. Indeed, since the first description of the high incidence of gastric epithelial cancer in patients with gastric GIST [45], various articles have documented multiple primary tumors in 14–43% of GIST patients [46–53]. In a large GIST registry, after 48 months of follow-up subsequent malignancies occurred in 31.9%, mostly gastrointestinal tumors (138/836), gynecological (61/836), breast (26/836), with SPT reducing 5-year survival rates from 83.4% to 62.8%, but the 5-year DSS was similar (90.8% vs. 90.9%). Therefore, the analysis concluded that 34.2% of deaths were not related to GIST [54].

8.2   ANALYSIS OF PROGNOSTIC VARIABLES IN EARLY METASTATIC DISEASE

A systematic review of prospective randomized clinical trials (RCTs) that studied upfront therapies of patients with unresectable or metastatic GIST (mGIST) resulted in the selection of 22 studies, published from 2001 to 2022. In four trials, PFs were assessed, and a Cox multivariate analysis (MVA) was reported [55–58]. Despite the limitations related to the selection and analysis of the variables, this review led to the results of all PFs that have been reported in at least one study and the number of studies that found or did not find a relationship between the PFs and OS (DSS was rarely reported) (Table S1).

8.3   PATIENT-RELATED PROGNOSTIC FACTORS

8.3.1   PERFORMANCE STATUS

Various retrospective studies have found that among the PFs in patients with mGIST, even in the imatinib era, performance status (PS) remains a variable closely related to survival.

The Meta-GIST analysis evaluated 1,640 patients with mGIST, all receiving imatinib within two clinical trials, and found a significant detrimental effect of a deteriorating PS on OS, regardless of

TABLE S1

Prognostic factors analyzed in selected trials of patients with unresectable or metastatic gastrointestinal stromal tumors receiving upfront treatment

Variable	No. trials	Prognostic relationship	No prognostic relationship
Patient-related			
Performance status	4	4	0
Demographic			
Age	2	2	0
Sex	4	4	0
Anthropometric			
Clinic			
Lab			
Hemoglobin	3	3	0
Leukocyte count	1	1	0
Granulocyte count	2	2	0
Neutrophil count	2	2	0
Lymphocyte count	1	1	0
Platelet count	2	2	0
Albumin	2	2	0
Bilirubin	1	1	0
Alkalyne phosphatase	1	0	1
Creatinine	1	0	1
Tumor-related			
Tumor burden			
Tumor size	4	4	0
Disease status	1	1	0
Location	2	0	2
Timing of metastasis	2	0	2
Sites of metastasis	2	0	2
Pathology			
KIT mutations	2	2	0
Previous treatments			
Previous surgery	2	1	1
Previous radiotherapy	2	1	1
Previous chemotherapy	2	2	0

mutational status [59]. Three of four retrospective studies confirmed an unfavorable prognostic role for ECOG PS 2–3 vs. ECOG PS 0–1 [60–63].

A Spanish survey compared 64 vs. 70 mGIST patients who had received imatinib for more or less than five years, intending to identify predictors of long-term response. It emerged that the responders had 11-year PFS and complete remission in 34%. In addition to carrying KIT mutations at exon-11, the 64 long-term survivors had low tumor burden (TB), in most cases ECOG PS 0, and none having ECOG PS 2–3. After MVA by logistic regression, ECOG PS was the independent variable associated with the longest OS [64].

8.3.1.1 Selected trials

The four selected studies agree in reporting poor outcomes for patients with a compromised PS compared to those with a good PS. PS was evaluated according to different scales. Generally, the comparisons reported a poor outcome for the worse PS, as summarized in Table 8.1.

TABLE 8.1

Prognostic relationships of performance status in selected studies of patients with unresectable or metastatic gastrointestinal stromal tumors receiving upfront treatment

Study [ref]	Phase	No. pts	Scale	Comparison	Prognostic relationship	Effect size
Intergroup 2004	III	819	WHO	PS 1 vs. PS 0	Yes	HR 1.48 (1.25–1.75)
[55]		528		PS 2 vs. PS 0		HR 1.74 (1.42–2.40)
		471		PS 3 vs. PS 0		HR 3.04 (2.09–4.42)
BRF14 2007 [56]	III	47	ECOG	PS 1 vs. PS 0	Yes	HR 1.35 (0.84–2.16)
		35		PS 2–3 vs. PS 0		HR 3.67 (1.80–7.58)
B2222 2008 [57]	II	147	ECOG	PS 2–3 vs. PS 0–1	Yes	HR 1.70 (p = 0.003)
S0033 2008 [58]	III	694	Zubrod	PS 2–3 vs. PS 0–1	Yes	HR 2.31 (1.69–3.14)

Legend: ECOG, Eastern Cooperative Oncology Group. HR, hazard ratio. PS, performance status. WHO, World Health Organization.

8.3.2 DEMOGRAPHIC

8.3.2.1 Age

Despite the changing median age of onset and the different age cut-offs used in the studies, various population-based analyses including mGIST patients agree on the negative prognostic effect of advanced age. Notably, four studies of different case series from the SEER database and other registries such as the German Clinical Cancer Registry and the Life Raft Group Registry, confirm this association, although they do not report separate analyses for patients with metastatic disease [65–70]. The finding was also shown by a retrospective analysis of the Knight Cancer registry [71] and some retrospective studies [37, 63, 72, 73], while others did not find outcome changes by age [61, 62, 74–77]. The age effect is continuous, as demonstrated by an analysis of the SEER database which reported a shorter OS in every age group vs. <50 [66], and could be explained by more frequent SPTs [54], as well as poor PS, increased Charlson Comorbidity Index, hypoalbuminemia [78]. In mGIST patients, imatinib showed significantly higher toxicity-related discontinuation rates (32.7% vs. 5.1%) in the elderly, with similar PFS and lower OS [78]. A retrospective evaluation of a cohort of elderly patients >75 investigated the reasons for imatinib dose reduction or discontinuation and excluded that pharmacokinetics or comorbidities interfered with treatment tolerance, while a deteriorated PS was the only variable associated with poor OS [79].

8.3.2.2 Sex

Although the incidence is similar between males and females [25], sometimes slightly higher in males [22], the prognosis differs significantly in favor of females at every stage [80–82]. This finding was confirmed by four of six population-based studies [15, 66, 68, 69], by the Meta-GIST analysis [59] and one retrospective study [74], but not by other authors [37, 61–63, 67, 71–73, 75, 76].

Analyzing the subgroup of young patients of the Ulmer GIST registry, the DSS difference was significant between males and females. The longer DSS of young patients was more pronounced in favor of young than elderly females (5-year DSS 100% vs. 83.2%), although a difference by age was also present among males [54]. It has been hypothesized that these differences by sex are attributable to the effect of sex hormones. Possible reasons of molecular epidemiology have also been hypothesized. In fact, many studies report an excess of gastric GIST in the age group <40 years in the female sex [83–87], and this could influence a higher frequency of SDH-mutated GISTs among females, but the incidence is very low to explain such differences.

8.3.2.3   Other demographic variables

Only an article revealed an unfavorable prognostic relationship for African Americans [15], which has not been confirmed furtherly [66].

Some SEER analyses reported a poor prognosis of unmarried patients [66, 70, 88].

8.3.2.4   Selected trials

Two studies analyzed age and reported OS reductions with increasing age. The Intergroup study analyzed age groups comparing them with <40 years old, and reporting shorter OS for patients >70 years and in the 50–60 years group [55]. The SWOG S0033 study analyzed the effect of age considering the progressive risk for each additional decade and reporting a worsening OS per decade [58].

The four selected studies agree on the better prognosis of females, with an effect size being very similar in the two larger studies, and the pooled analysis of three trials suggesting a favorable trend for females (HR 0.79, CI 0.54–1.13; Q = 4.06, p-value = 0.1311; I^2 = 50.8%) (Table 8.2).

8.3.3   ANTHROPOMETRIC

Although data on mGIST are lacking and obesity was regarded as a favorable PF in localized tumors, malnutrition is common among GIST patients, but prognosis is not affected by BMI [89, 90].

8.3.4   CLINIC

Generally, the clinical presentation of GISTs is unspecific, with vague abdominal discomfort, and this can explain the diagnostic delay. Due to its extraluminal growth, the GIST could reach very large sizes without causing symptoms. Symptoms at diagnosis, obstructive or hemorrhagic, are associated with larger tumor sizes [6] and are very rare when the tumor diameter is <5 cm [91]. A retrospective study did not find a relationship between the primary tumor-related symptoms and the outcome [77], whereas another series of resected GISTs reported poor relapse-free survival for patients with gastrointestinal bleeding [92].

8.3.5   LABORATORY

8.3.5.1   Hematology

Gastrointestinal bleeding occurs in 40% of GIST at diagnosis, and among mGIST patients, therefore the resulting anemia could affect prognosis [61, 93–95]. Some studies have documented a prognostic role of anemia in mGIST [61, 96], but others have ruled it out [60, 63]. However, anemia may

---

TABLE 8.2

Prognostic relationships of sex in selected studies of patients with unresectable or metastatic gastrointestinal stromal tumors receiving upfront treatment

Study [ref]	Phase	No. pts	Comparison	Prognostic relationship	Effect size
Intergroup 2004 [55]	III	946	M vs. F	Yes	HR 0.83 (0.70–0.97)
BRF14 2007 [56]	III	58	M vs. F	Yes	HR 0.48 (0.29–0.80)
B2222 2008 [57]	II	147	M vs. F	Yes	HR 0.49 (p = 0.0093)
S0033 2008 [58]	III	694	M vs. F	Yes	HR 0.78 (0.65–0.94)

Legend: F, females. HR, hazard ratio. M, males.

TABLE 8.3

Prognostic relationships of laboratory variables in selected studies of patients with unresectable or metastatic gastrointestinal stromal tumors receiving upfront treatment

Study [ref]	Phase	No. pts	Comparison	Prognostic relationship	Effect size
Red blood cells					
BRF14 2007 [56]	III	58	Hb: <11.5/13.0 vs. ≥	Yes	HR 1.53 (1.00–2.34)
B2222 2008 [57]	II	147	Hb CTC: ≥G1 vs. <	Yes	HR 1.65
S0033 2008 [58]	III	694	Hb (cut-off NR): > vs. <	Yes	HR 0.16 (0.07–0.32)
White blood cells					
BRF14 2007 [56]	III	58	Granu count > vs. < 7500	Yes	HR 2.10 (1.12–3.96)
			Lymph count > vs. < 1000	Yes	HR 0,42 (0.21–0.81)
B2222 2008 [57]	II	147	Neutro count > vs. < 4500	Yes	HR 2.25
			Granu count > vs. < 5000	Yes	HR 1.65
S0033 2008 [58]	III	694	WBC count > vs. <	Yes	HR 2.45 (1.86–3.24)
			Neutro count > vs. <	Yes	HR 1.59 (1.21–2.10)
Platelets					
B2222 2008 [57]	II	147	PLT count > vs. < 275	Yes	HR 1.66
S0033 2008 [58]	III	694	PLT count > vs. <	Yes	HR 1.44 (1.10–1.89)
Chemistry					
BRF14 2007 [56]	III	58	ALP: ≥ vs. < 100 U/L	No	HR 1.50 (0.98–2.30)
B2222 2008 [57]	II	147	Albumin CTC: ≥G1 vs. <	Yes	HR 2.35
S0033 2008 [58]	III	694	Albumin: ≥ vs. <3.5 g/dL	Yes	HR 0.67 (0.51–0.87)
			Bilirubin: > vs. <	Yes	HR 1.29 (1.01–1.66)

Legend: ALP, alkaline phosphatase. CTC G, Common Toxicity Criteria Grade. Granu, granulocytes. Hb, hemoglobin. HR, hazard ratio. Lymph, lymphocytes. Neutro, neutrophils. NR, not reported. PLT, platelets. WBC, White blood cells.

be a result of the systemic inflammatory response, whose unfavorable prognostic effect is likely in mGIST, as can be speculated from the report of increased neutrophil count being associated with poor outcomes [59, 61, 63, 96]. Few data were reported in mGIST, but available studies documented a relationship between NLR and PLR with prognosis [94, 97].

8.3.5.2 Chemistry

In addition to being included in various inflammation-related measures, albumin has been studied per se, and a reduction in its concentrations has been related to a poor prognosis [59–61].

8.3.5.3 Selected trials

Three of the selected studies investigated the effect of laboratory tests on the prognosis of patients with mGIST receiving imatinib, and often documented a significant and independent effect of inflammation-related variables, such as leukocyte and neutrophil counts, lymphocyte count, platelet count, but also hemoglobin, albumin, and bilirubin (Table 8.3).

8.4 TUMOR-RELATED PROGNOSTIC FACTORS

8.4.1 Tumor burden

A SEER database analysis reported that the AJCC stage was not associated with prognosis, while the classification into localized, regional, or metastatic disease, and primary tumor size >10 centimeters predicted OS [66]. The relationship between poor outcome and increasing primary tumor size was confirmed by other database analyses [67, 68, 70], MetaGIST [59], prospective cohorts [71, 96] and retrospective studies [60, 61, 63, 73]. In contrast, other small studies were negative [62, 72, 75]. However, it should be considered that this variable is subject to change also as a function of the improvement of diagnostic tests, as suggested by a Polish study of 430 mGIST patients, that documented a progressive reduction from 2001 to 2012 of the baseline size of the primary tumor from 90 to 58 mm [60].

Prognostic relationships were also not reported for T-stage [71] and N-stage [77], but the presence of distant metastases correlated with worse outcomes [68, 69], similar to the comparison between metastatic and locally advanced [15] or between metastatic vs. localized [66, 67, 70].

Not all studies have reported a prognostic effect from the number of metastases [74, 77, 98]. A cohort of 115 patients showed that oligometastatic disease (presence of <3 metastases) was associated with a 10-year survival of 71% vs. 20% [61], while a retrospective Korean cohort showed that the oligometastatic disease was associated only with a trend of longer survival (5-year survival 91.7% vs. 55.3%; p-value = 0.080) [76]. Still, a retrospective Spanish survey of 64 long-survivors mGIST recorded a low number of metastases [64].

Multifocal disease did not change prognosis [72], while the percentage of liver involvement [77] and some imaging features [99] remain poorly studied.

8.4.1.1 Selected trials

Some TB assessments were common in the four studies. All studies documented a significant relationship between the increasing size and the poor prognosis. Only one study evaluated prognosis based on comparing locally advanced vs. metastatic disease, and reported longer survival for locally advanced tumors [56]. TB-related findings of the selected trials are listed in Table 8.4.

8.4.2 PRIMARY TUMOR LOCATION

Multiple locations have been compared in the studies. Broadly speaking, in population-based studies, a trend toward better OS was observed for gastric GISTs [66, 67, 70], whereas poor outcomes were reported for some locations of the colon (ascending and sigma) [67], the cardias, the esophagus [66–68] and small intestine [15, 67, 69]. Other studies did not document differences by site [37, 60, 61, 63, 71, 76, 77], but they invariably detect better outcomes for gastric GISTs [62, 75]. In

---

TABLE 8.4
Prognostic relationships of tumor burden-related variables in selected studies of patients with unresectable or metastatic gastrointestinal stromal tumors receiving upfront treatment

Study [ref]	Phase	No. pts	Comparison	Prognostic relationship	Effect size
Tumor diameter (cm)					
Intergroup 2004 [55]	III	946	continuous (*)	Yes	HR 1.03 (1.02–1.04)
BRF14 2007 [56]	III	58	continuous	Yes	HR 1.002 (1.000–1.004)
S0033 2008 [58]	III	694	continuous (*)	Yes	HR 1.04 (1.03–1.06)
Tumor size (cm^2)					
B2222 2008 [57]	II	147	> vs. <39.1 cm^2	Yes	HR 2.31 (p = 0.0063)
Disease status					
BRF14 2007 [56]	III	58	Metastatic vs. LA	Yes	HR 1.96 (1.16–3.23)

Legend: (*), Increased risk of death for each cm of tumor diameter. HR, hazard ratio. LA, locally advanced.

particular, in a retrospective Asian series of 188 mGIST patients, those with extra-gastric and extra-small intestine sites of origin (colorectal GISTs in 50%) reported a poor outcome (median OS of 16.9 vs. 62–72 months) [62].

An analysis of 83 esophageal GIST patients documented that the PFs after resection were similar to other sites, and a poor OS was evident for elderly patients, while only an unfavorable trend for tumor size and MI [100].

The good prognosis of gastric GISTs has been attributed to different molecular biology (SDH-related tumors; KIT exon-11 mutations occurring in 89% and decreasing distally) [101]. However, compared with the cardias, all the other gastric sites, except the small curve, displayed a better prognosis [66].

From a review of 448 colorectal GIST patients, some authors have built a specific prognostic model. After MVA, a poor DSS was associated to older age, right-sidedness, poorly differentiated tumors, stage III/IV AJCC, no surgery, and tumor diameter >65 millimeters [102]. In addition, rectal origin at the time of primary tumor resection (PTR) was associated with a higher rate of metachronous liver metastases (LMs) [103].

8.4.2.1 Selected trials

The Intergroup study did not provide significant site definitions, as it evaluated small intestine, gastric and other sites versus "abdominal" origin [55], while the S0033 study considered only the small intestine origin [58]. In both cases, they did not demonstrate a prognostic effect for primary tumor location.

8.4.3 Timing of metastases

Of six studies that assessed the timing of metastases, one found poor prognosis for synchronous vs. metachronous LMs, but no difference based on timing of extra-hepatic disease (EHD) [77], and another study found OS reduction for synchronous metastases but only after univariate analysis [73], while other authors have not documented OS differences by timing of metastasis [37, 61, 63, 76].

On the other hand, patients with metachronous disease reported better outcomes for longer disease-free intervals (DFIs). DFI of 24 months after resection is a reliable surrogate outcome measure because it predicted 10-year PFS (73% vs. 19%) and 10-year OS [71]. From a clinical point of view, this cut-off suggests an indolent disease, which could benefit from more aggressive treatments.

8.4.3.1 Selected trials

Two studies evaluated the timing from diagnosis to imatinib, without finding OS differences, both when time ranges were defined [55] or when it was considered as a continuous variable [58].

8.4.4 Sites of metastases

The most frequent sites of metastasis are the liver (50–60%) and peritoneum (20–40%) [104]. While some authors associate the presence of LMs with OS reduction [60], others did not document prognostic change based on liver or liver-limited sites of metastases [61, 63, 74, 75, 98]. To date, few data are available about the poor outcomes of peritoneal metastases [37]. Given the rarity, little is known about the prognostic relevance of other metastatic sites.

A study reported PFS and OS of mGIST patients with LMs vs. EHD and concluded that after 39 months imatinib treatment eliminated any outcome difference [105].

8.4.4.1 Selected trials

One study compared lung metastases vs. other sites not documenting prognostic changes [58], while another did not detect a poor prognosis in the presence of LMs and peritoneal metastases [56].

8.4.5 PATHOLOGY

8.4.5.1 Histology

GISTs are the most frequent gastrointestinal mesenchymal malignancies, originating from the interstitial cells of Cajal in the myenteric plexus. Mutations in genes required for neural and synapse development could explain some GIST [106]. The main regulatory signal for these cells is determined by KIT [107], and sometimes ETS translocation variant 1 (ETV1) [108].

Molecular profile defines GIST and its prognosis, while morphology and immunohistochemistry are still relevant for diagnosis.

8.4.5.2 Tumor grade

Some authors have documented reduced OS for patients with GIII vs. GI/GII tumors [66], but other studies did not find differences between GII and GI [71, 77]. Similarly, shorter OS have been registered for patients with poorly differentiated GISTs [67].

Another variable often unsuccessfully assessed in patients with mGIST, is the number of mitoses [61, 66, 70], which is PF [96], even when assessed in metastasis and $\geq$5/50HPF [98].

8.4.5.3 Other pathologic variables

The relationship of imatinib with the immune system is still poorly understood, but it is known that imatinib therapy reduces IDO expression, and activates CD8+ lymphocytes and apoptosis of GIST-infiltrating T-reg cells. It also inhibits the KIT expression of dendritic cells, facilitating their communication with NKs and the production of interferon-gamma [109]. The intratumoral T-reg/NK ratio could therefore be indicative of the response to imatinib [110].

8.4.5.4 Molecular biology

GISTs are sustained by the mutation of a tyrosine kinase, such as KIT in 75%, or PDGFR-A in 15–20% [111–115]. The remaining 5–15% have been defined as wild-type GISTs (wt-GISTs), but are heterogeneous populations characterized by multiple gene mutations. In 30% of wt-GISTs, a mutation in the SDH gene has been found [86, 116], and is typical of gastric GISTs with indolent behavior, sometimes falling within the clinical picture of Carney Stratakis syndrome [117]. Other genetic alterations at the origin of wt-GISTs are infrequent and may involve NF1 [118], NTRK, BRAF [119], RAS, FGFRA, and PIK3CA [120]. Although mutational status has not yet been included in any classification, some genotypes have distinct natural histories [121], such as wt-GISTs, GISTs with KIT exon-11 deletions at codons 557–558, which are associated with a high risk of recurrence [122], GISTs with PDGFRA D842V mutation, with good prognosis but resistance to imatinib [78], and GISTs with a SDH deficit, for which a questionable efficacy of known tyrosine kinase inhibitors (TKIs) has been reported [123].

Further molecular alterations are expressions of pathologic activation of cellular pathways, which may be associated with poor prognosis, such as PTEN downregulation [124], alterations of histone methylation [125], or other alterations of KIT itself (exon-9 duplications, exon-11 deletions) [122].

Many studies have analyzed the prognostic impact of the driver mutation, reporting poor prognosis for exon-9 vs. exon-11 KIT mutations [59, 73, 96], wild-type vs. exon-11 [59, 60], PDGFR-A vs. wild-type [60], or other mutations within exon-11 [96]. In contrast, other authors have not found survival differences of patients with different KIT driver mutations [61, 63, 71, 74]. However, the introduction of new drugs after imatinib has also downgraded the negative prognostic relevance of some mutations, which became molecular targets.

8.4.5.5 Selected trials

The prognostic impact of KIT mutations was also evaluated in RCTs. As expected from the different sensitivity to imatinib, the Intergroup trial documented a good prognosis for exon-11 KIT mutation compared to other GISTs (exon-9 vs. exon-11: HR 1.87, CI 1.36–2.57; wild-type vs. exon-11:

HR 2.10, CI 1.57–2.81; others vs. exon-11: HR 2.68, CI 1.68–4.28) [55]. Similar conclusions were reported by the S0033 trial (other vs. exon-11: HR 0.40, p-value = 0.0004) [58].

8.4.6 Previous treatments

8.4.6.1 Primary tumor resection

Though population-based studies include large case series only partly consisting of patients with mGIST, they are expected to document an advantage for PTR [15, 66, 70]. Indeed, to date, there is a lack of prospective studies elucidating the usefulness of PTR in asymptomatic mGIST, while some retrospective studies have not found benefit from PTR [77].

8.4.6.2 Extensive surgery

Surgery of LMs in the pre-imatinib era resulted in 30% of long-survivors [126, 127]. After the introduction of imatinib, the outcome improvement has been questioned, and some authors claimed that also the pre-imatinib cytoreductive surgery has not been shown to improve prognosis.

Data from the NCR reported lower 5-year survival rates for patients with mGIST receiving systemic therapy alone than for those undergoing surgery and systemic therapy (39.7% vs. 77.4%) [20], but a multivariate propensity score-matched analysis demonstrated that the number of metastases and TB were lower in the resected patients. However, the study still detected an improved outcome from surgery, regardless of TB [128]. A review of 11 studies, including 240 mGIST patients undergoing resection of LMs, was also favorable to surgery [129], while a retrospective Korean evaluation of 102 mGIST patients with liver-limited disease suggested that the effect of the surgery was not significant after MVA (5-year survival 85.7% vs. 59.6%; p-value = 0.095) [76]. In contrast, other studies did not document any improvement from surgery or radiofrequency ablation of metastases [37, 72, 75], and from nonradical (R2) removal of metastases [74, 98], even on residual disease after imatinib [130]. Data of the Knight Cancer Registry demonstrated that resection of the recurrent/metastatic GIST did not affect OS [71].

A prospective observational EORTC trial, reported longer median OS after R0/R1 resection (8.7 vs. 5.3 years), with a more marked difference in the group that had post-imatinib remission at the time of liver resection [74]. Other retrospective studies documented a significant effect of surgical cytoreduction after imatinib when surgery removes all residual disease [60, 61, 73] or >75% of the disease [63]. A US retrospective study documented that cytoreductive surgery outside of mGISTs with unifocal progressive disease did not provide any outcome improvement over medical therapy alone. Indeed, in patients receiving imatinib, the study reported a negative prognostic effect of multifocal progressive disease [98].

8.4.6.3 Other previous treatments

While in an analysis of the SEER database, prior radiation therapy was found to be detrimental [15], the effect on prognosis of prior adjuvant therapy is unclear [71, 72].

8.4.6.4 Selected trials

The two studies that analyzed the impact of previous treatments on the prognosis of mGIST patients reported in one case a significant favorable effect on OS for prior surgery, radiotherapy, and chemotherapy [55], while in the other only for chemotherapy [58].

8.5 PROGNOSTIC FACTORS IN DECISION-MAKING

Medical therapy depends on the detected driver mutation. It is continued until progression, and the last TKI or imatinib may be recommended beyond progression. However, some PFs can be considered in decision-making (Table 8.5).

TABLE 8.5

Prognostic and predictive variables in clinical decision-making in metastatic gastrointestinal stromal tumors

A. Upfront treatment

1	Mutation	
	• KIT exon-9 mutation: IMA 800 favored (IMA 800 is better than IMA 400)	
	• PDGFRA-D842V mutation: AVA favored	
2	Pattern of progression to imatinib	
	• Unifocal: local treatment should be considered	
	• Residual disease: local treatment could be considered	

B. Treatment of refractory disease

1	Mutation	
	• KIT exon-9 mutation: SUN favored (SUN is better than RIP)	
	• PDGFRA-D842V mutation: AVA favored (AVA is better than REG)	
2	Imatinib treatment duration	
	• ≤6 months: SUN favored (SUN is better than placebo)	
3	Location	
	• Gastric: PIM favored (PIM is better than placebo)	
4	Previous treatments	
	• 2 lines: REG favored (REG is better than AVA in PDGFRA wild-type)	
	• ≥3 lines: REG or RIP favored (REG/RIP are better than placebo)	

Legend: AVA, avapritinib. IMA, imatinib. PIM, pimitespib. REG, regorafenib. RIP, ripretinib. SUN, sunitinib.

8.5.1 Upfront treatment

Except for wild-type or PDGFRA-D842V mutated GISTs, imatinib is the standard treatment at 400 mg/die for patients with mGIST, and for patients who relapsed after adjuvant imatinib [55, 57, 58, 131]. Treatment should be continued indefinitely, unless toxicity/intolerance occurs, as imatinib discontinuation is usually followed by rapid progression. In case of progression to the standard dose, it could be increased to 800 mg/die, whereas imatinib 800 mg/die is the standard initial dose for patients with exon-9 KIT mutation [59], for whom it led to a longer OS in the Intergroup study [132]. Though none of the patient characteristics and possible PFs were studied in the imatinib trials considering the imatinib activity in mGIST, it should be remembered that the trials compared imatinib dose levels [55, 58, 133] or continuous vs. intermittent schedules [56], and did not compare imatinib with placebo.

Avapritinib is the upfront therapy for PDGFRA-D842V mutated mGIST [134], while SDH-deficient GISTs are not responsive to imatinib, but may respond to sunitinib or regorafenib, and NTRK-rearranged forms are sensitive to NTRK inhibitors [135].

8.5.2 Treatment of refractory disease

In case of confirmed progression, the standard second-line regimen is sunitinib [136, 137]. Progression on imatinib most often occurs within 24 months [58, 132], and secondary mutations of KIT are frequently detected [138–140]. They are mostly located in exon 17 and exon 13, and their frequency varies with the site of origin of GIST and occurs in carriers of exon-11 mutations (46–61%) more than in exon-9 (0–15%). This difference could be related to the longer duration of therapy with imatinib in exon-11 mutation carriers, and to the selective pressure of imatinib.

Second-line sunitinib vs. placebo documented an increased PFS in all subgroups, although less pronounced among patients with imatinib duration <6 months [136]. In contrast, a recent comparison of ripretinib vs. sunitinib did not report any difference in PFS, except a superiority for sunitinib in the exon-9 mutation carriers [141]. The different molecular origin implies a different pharmacological approach and various possible molecular strategies [142], and the longer OS after sunitinib of patients with exon-9 vs. exon-11 mutation supports this hypothesis. Secondary mutations also influence the efficacy of sunitinib: patients with secondary mutations of KIT at exon-13 or exon-14 have a better outcome compared to exon-17 and exon-18. However, the intra- and inter-lesional genetic heterogeneity of imatinib-resistant GISTs must be considered, and biopsy may not detect it.

BRAF-mutated GISTs benefit of BRAF-inhibitors (including BRAF-MEK inhibitors combination) [143]. The indication is off-label and is justified by biological plausibility.

Regorafenib is the standard third-line after imatinib and sunitinib [144].

Ripretinib, whose dual mechanism of action allows an effective inhibition of a wide range of KIT and PDGFRA mutations, is the fourth-line treatment [145].

Rechallenge with imatinib, when initially a response has occurred, or continuation of TT beyond progression are an option. In the absence of feasible alternatives, rechallenge with imatinib was shown to be better than placebo in all subgroups examined in the RIGHT trial [146]. Similar was the result of regorafenib, which, however, has been poorly studied in patients with disease refractory to imatinib within 6 months: in the 22 patients enrolled, regorafenib was not superior to placebo [144]. However, in the comparison with avapritinib, regorafenib was similar in activity, although PFS was significantly longer when excluding the 13 patients with PDGFRA-D842V [147]. Aside from the rechallenge data [146], continuing the latest TT beyond progression is particularly appropriate in slow-growing GISTs, but data on other TKIs after imatinib are poor [148, 149].

MGMT expression suggests a possible response to alkylating drugs in wt-GISTs [150].

After imatinib, studies have generally considered PFS as an endpoint, even when evaluating subgroups.

8.6 CONCLUSION

The diagnosis of increasingly smaller and better molecularly defined GISTs, as well as the availability of new targeted therapies could render obsolete the reported results on PFs, which are summarized in Table 8.6.

The current expanding knowledge about patients with wild-type GISTs and the fragmentation of molecular alterations in GISTs, especially in disease with secondary resistance to imatinib, dictate new classifications related to the predominant signal pathway that can guide treatment planning.

TABLE 8.6

Prognostic factors evaluated in prospective trials of upfront treatment in patients with unresectable or metastatic gastrointestinal stromal tumor

Suggested	Not suggested	Needing study
Performance status		Hemoglobin
Age		Neutrophil count
Sex		Platelet count
Albumin		
Tumor diameter	Site of metastasis	Tumor state
Location		Number metastases
Imatinib resistance		Timing metastasis (DFI >24m)
		Primary tumor resection
		Surgery of metastasis

In this context, it is important to have a good understanding of the variables that contribute to TT response, beyond the type of mutation. Studies to date suggest that PS, sex, and indirectly age, might influence the response to TT, but the effects of TT on TME are little known. Furthermore, the negative role of hepatic involvement, especially if early, should be contextualized in the various molecular subgroups, but also in relation to SIR, TME composition, and changes after TT. This could allow defining subgroups of patients with LMs who might benefit from more aggressive regional treatments.

REFERENCES

1. Verschoor AJ, Bovée JVMG, Overbeek LIH, et al. The incidence, mutational status, risk classification and referral pattern of gastro-intestinal stromal tumours in the Netherlands: A nationwide pathology registry (PALGA) study. *Virchows Arch* 2018;472(2):221–9.
2. Tryggvason G, Gislason HG, Magnusson MK, Jonasson JG. Gastrointestinal stromal tumors in Iceland, 1990–2003: The icelandic GIST study, a population-based incidence and pathologic risk stratification study. *Int J Cancer* 2005;117(2):289–93.
3. Goettsch WG, Bos SD, Breekveldt-Postma N, et al. Incidence of gastrointestinal stromal tumours is underestimated: Results of a nation-wide study. *Eur J Cancer* 2005;41(18):2868–72.
4. Cassier PA, Ducimetiere F, Lurkin A, et al. A prospective epidemiological study of new incident GISTs during two consecutive years in Rhone Alpes region: Incidence and molecular distribution of GIST in a European region. *Br J Cancer* 2010;103(2):165–70.
5. Ahmed I, Welch NT, Parsons SL. Gastrointestinal stromal tumours (GIST) –17 years experience from Mid Trent Region (United Kingdom). *Eur J Surg Oncol* 2008;34(4):445–9.
6. Nilsson B, Bumming P, Meis-Kindblom JM, et al. Gastrointestinal stromal tumors: The incidence, prevalence, clinical course, and prognostication in the preimatinib mesylate era. *Cancer* 2005;103(4):821–9.
7. Rubio J, Marcos-Gragera R, Ortiz MR, et al. Population-based incidence and survival of gastrointestinal stromal tumours (GIST) in Girona, Spain. *Eur J Cancer* 2007;43(1):144–8.
8. Rubio-Casadevall J, Borras JL, Carmona C, et al. Temporal trends of incidence and survival of sarcoma of digestive tract including gastrointestinal stromal tumours (GIST) in two areas of the north-east of Spain in the period 1981–2005: A population-based study. *Clin Transl Oncol* 2014;16(7):660–7.
9. Mucciarini C, Rossi G, Bertolini F, et al. Incidence and clinicopathological features of gastrointestinal stromal tumors. A population-based study. *BMC Cancer* 2007;7:230.
10. Monges G, Bisot-Locard S, Blay J-Y, et al. The estimated incidence of gastrointestinal stromal tumors in France. Results of PROGIST study conducted among pathologists. *Bull Cancer* 2010;97(3):E16–22.
11. Steigen SE, Eide TJ. Trends in incidence and survival of mesenchymal neoplasm of the digestive tract within a defined population of northern Norway. *APMIS* 2006;114(3):192–200.
12. Soreide K, Sandvik OM, Soreide JA, et al. Global epidemiology of gastrointestinal stromal tumours (GIST): A systematic review of population-based cohort studies. *Cancer Epidemiol* 2016;40:39–46.
13. Xu L, Ma Y, Wang S, et al. Incidence of gastrointestinal stromal tumor in Chinese urban population: A national population-based study. *Cancer Med* 2020;10:737–44.
14. Yan BM, Kaplan GG, Urbanski S, et al. Epidemiology of gastrointestinal stromal tumors in a defined Canadian Health Region: A population-based study. *Int J Surg Pathol* 2008;16(3):241–50.
15. Tran T, Davila JA, El-Serag HB. The epidemiology of malignant gastrointestinal stromal tumors: An analysis of 1,458 cases from 1992 to 2000. *Am J Gastroenterol* 2005;100(1):162–8.
16. Perez EA, Livingstone AS, Franceschi D, et al. Current incidence and outcomes of gastrointestinal mesenchymal tumors including gastrointestinal stromal tumors. *J Am Coll Surg* 2006;202(4):623–9.
17. Patel N, Benipal B. Incidence of gastrointestinal stromal tumors in the United states from 2001–2015: A United States cancer statistics analysis of 50 states. *Cureus* 2019;11(2):e4120.
18. Ma GL, Murphy JD, Martinez ME, Sicklick JK. Epidemiology of gastrointestinal stromal tumors in the era of histology codes: Results of a population-based study. *Cancer Epidemiol Biomarkers Prev* 2015;24(1):298–302.
19. Cho M-Y, Sohn JH, Kim JM, et al. Current trends in the epidemiological and pathological characteristics of gastrointestinal stromal tumors in Korea, 2003–2004. *J Korean Med Sci* 2010;25(6):853–62.
20. van der Graaf WTA, Tielen R, Bonenkamp JJ, et al. Nationwide trends in the incidence and outcome of patients with gastrointestinal stromal tumour in the imatinib era. *Br J Surg* 2018;105:1020–7.

21. Nishida T, Yoshinaga S, Takahashi T, Naito Y. Recent progress and challenges in the diagnosis and treatment of gastrointestinal stromal tumors. *Cancers* 2021;13:3158.
22. Ahmed M. Recent advances in the management of gastrointestinal stromal tumor. *World J Clin Cases* 2020;8(15):3142–55.
23. Yamamoto H, Oda Y. Gastrointestinal stromal tumor: Recent advances in pathology and genetics. *Pathol Int* 2015;65(1):9–18.
24. Parab TM, DeRogatis MJ, Boaz AM, et al. Gastrointestinal stromal tumors: A comprehensive review. *J Gastrointest Oncol* 2019;10(1):144–54.
25. von Mehren M, Joensuu H. Gastrointestinal stromal tumors. *J Clin Oncol* 2018;36:136–43.
26. Scarpa M, Bertin M, Ruffolo C, et al. A systematic review on the clinical diagnosis of gastrointestinal stromal tumors. *J Surg Oncol* 2008;98(5):384–92.
27. Rubin BP, Blanke CD, Demetri GD, et al. Protocol for the examination of specimens from patients with gastrointestinal stromal tumor. *Arch Pathol Lab Med* 2010;134:165–70.
28. Novelli M, Rossi S, Rodriguez-Justo M, et al. DOG1 and CD117 are the antibodies of choice in the diagnosis of gastrointestinal stromal tumours. *Histopathol* 2010;57:259–70.
29. Gasparotto D, Rossi S, Polano M, et al. Quadruple-negative GIST is a sentinel for unrecognized neuro-fibromatosis type 1 syndrome. *Clin Cancer Res* 2017;23(1):273–82.
30. Brenca M, Rossi S, Polano M, et al. Transcriptome sequencing identifies eTV6-NTRK3 as a gene fusion involved in GIST. *J Pathol* 2016;238(4):543–9.
31. Miettinen M, Lasota J. Gastrointestinal stromal tumors: Pathology and prognosis at different sites. *Semin Diagn Pathol* 2006;23(2):70–83.
32. Miettinen M, Lasota J. Gastrointestinal stromal tumors: Review on morphology, molecular pathology, prognosis, and differential diagnosis. *Arch Pathol Lab Med* 2006;130(10):1466–78.
33. Gold JS, Gonen M, Gutierrez A, et al. Development and validation of a prognostic nomogram for recurrence-free survival after complete surgical resection of localised primary gastrointestinal stromal tumour: A retrospective analysis. *Lancet Oncol* 2009;10(11):1045–52.
34. Rossi S, Miceli R, Messerini L. Natural history of imatinib-naive GISTs: A retrospective analysis of 929 cases with long-term follow-up and development of a survival nomogram based on mitotic index and size as continuous variables. *Am J Surg Pathol* 2011;35:1646–56.
35. Stroobants S, Goeminne J, Seegers M, et al. 18FDG-Positron emission tomography for the early prediction of response in advanced soft tissue sarcoma treated with imatinib mesylate (Glivec). *Eur J Cancer* 2003;39(14):2012–20.
36. Miettinen M, Lasota J. Gastrointestinal stromal tumors. *Gastroenterol Clin North Am* 2013;42(2):399–415.
37. Shi Y-N, Li Y, Wang L-P, et al. Gastrointestinal stromal tumor (GIST) with liver metastases. An 18-year experience from the GIST cooperation group in North China. *Medicine* 2017;96:e8240.
38. DeMatteo RP, Lewis JJ, Leung D, et al. Two hundred gastrointestinal stromal tumors: Recurrence patterns and prognostic factors for survival. *Ann Surg* 2000;231(1):51–8.
39. Joensuu H. Risk stratification of patients diagnosed with gastrointestinal stromal tumor. *Hum Pathol* 2008;39(10):1411–9.
40. Joensuu H, Eriksson M, Hall KS, et al. One vs three years of adjuvant imatinib for operable gastrointestinal stromal tumor: A randomized trial. *JAMA* 2012;307(12):1265–72.
41. Blesius A, Cassier PA, Bertucci F, et al. Neoadjuvant imatinib in patients with locally advanced non metastatic GIST in the prospective BRF14 trial. *BMC Cancer* 2011;11:72.
42. Antonescu CR, Besmer P, Guo T, et al. Acquired resistance to imatinib in gastrointestinal stromal tumor occurs through secondary gene mutation. *Clin Cancer Res* 2005;11(11):4182–90.
43. Keung EZ, Raut CP, Rutkowski P. The landmark series: systemic therapy for resectable gastrointestinal stromal tumors. *Ann Surg Oncol* 2020;27(10):3659–71.
44. Vassos N, Agaimy A, Hohenberger W, Croner RS. Management of liver metastases of gastrointestinal stromal tumors (GIST). *Ann Hepatol* 2015;14(4):531–9.
45. Maiorana A, Fante R, Cesinaro AM, Fano RA. Synchronous occurrence of epithelial and stromal tumors in the stomach: A report of 6 cased. *Arch Pathol Lab Med* 2000;124(5):682–6.
46. Agaimy A, Wunsch PH, Sobin LH, Lasota J, Miettinen M. Occurrence of other malignancies in patients with gastrointestinal stromal tumors. *Semin Diagn Pathol* 2006;23(2):120–9.
47. Liszka L, Zielinska-Pajak E, Pajak J, et al. Coexistence of gastrointestinal stromal tumors with other neoplasms. *J Gastroenterol* 2007;42(8):641–9.
48. Ferreira SS, Werutsky G, Garcia Toneto M, et al. Synchronous gastrointestinal stromal tumors (GIST) and other primary cancers: Case series of a single institution experience. *Int J Surg* 2010;8(4):314–7.

49. Goncalves R, Linhares E, Albagli R, et al. Occurrence of other tumors in patients with GIST. *Surg Oncol* 2010;19(4):e140–3.
50. Sevinc A, Seker M, Bilici A, et al. Co-existence of gastrointestinal stromal tumors with other primary neoplasms. *Hepatogastroenterol* 2011;58(107–108):824–30.
51. Pandurengan RK, Dumont AG, Araujo DM, et al. Survival of patients with multiple primary malignancies: A study of 783 patients with gastrointestinal stromal tumor. *Ann Oncol* 2010;21(10):2107–11.
52. Vassos N, Agaimy A, Hohenberger W, Croner RS. Coexistence of gastrointestinal stromal tumors (GIST) and malignant neoplasms of different origin: Prognostic implications. *Int J Surg* 2014;12(5):371–7.
53. Rubio-Casadevall J, Borras JL, Carmona-Garcia MC, et al. Correlation between mutational status and survival and second cancer risk assessment in patients with gastrointestinal stromal tumors: A population-based study. *World J Surg Oncol* 2015;13:47.
54. Kramer K, Wolf S, Mayer B, et al. Frequence, spectrum and prognostic impact of additional malignancies in patients with gastrointestinal stromal tumors. *Neoplasia* 2015;17(1):134–40.
55. Verweij J, Casali PG, Zalcberg J, et al. Progression-free survival in gastrointestinal stromal tumours with high-dose imatinib: Randomised trial. *Lancet* 2004;364:1127–34.
56. Patrikidou A, Domont J, Chabaud S, et al. Long-term outcome of molecular subgroups of GIST patients treated with standard-dose imatinib in the BRF14 trial of the French Sarcoma Group. *Eur J Cancer* 2016;52:173–80.
57. Blanke CD, Demetri GD, von Mehren M, et al. Long-term results from a randomized phase II trial of standard- versus higher-dose imatinib mesylate for patients with unresectable or metastatic gastrointestinal stromal tumors expressing KIT. *J Clin Oncol* 2008;26:620–5.
58. Blanke CD, Rankin C, Demetri GD, et al. Phase III randomized, Intergroup trial assessing imatinib mesylate at two dose levels in patients with unresectable or metastatic gastrointestinal stromal tumors expressing the kit receptor tyrosine kinase: S0033. *J Clin Oncol* 2008;26:626–32.
59. Gastrointestinal Stromal Tumor Meta-Analysis Group (MetaGIST). Comparison of two doses of imatinib for the treatment of unresectable or metastatic gastrointestinal stromal tumors: A meta-analysis of 1,640 patients. *J Clin Oncol* 2010;28:1247–53.
60. Rutkowski P, Andrzejuk J, Bylina E, et al. What are the current outcomes of advanced gastrointestinal stromal tumors: Who are the long-term survivors treated initially with imatinib? *Med Oncol* 2013;30:765.
61. Hompland I, Bruland OS, Holmebakk T, et al. Prediction of long-term survival in patients with metastatic gastrointestinal stromal tumor: Analysis of a large, single-institution cohort. *Acta Oncol* 2017;56:1317–23.
62. Hung KD, Van QL, Hoang GN, et al. Imatinib mesylate for patients with unresectable or recurrent gastrointestinal stromal tumors: 10-year experience from Vietnam. *Cancer Control* 2019;26:1–7.
63. An HJ, Ryu M-H, Ryoo B-Y, et al. The effects of surgical cytoreduction prior to imatinib therapy on the prognosis of patients with advanced GIST. *Ann Surg Oncol* 2013;20(13):4212–8.
64. Serrano C, Garcia-del-Muro X, Valverde C, et al. Clinicopathological and molecular characterization of metastatic gastrointestinal stromal tumors with prolonged benefit to frontline imatinib. *Oncologist* 2019;24:680–7.
65. Tran T, Davila JA, El-Serag HB. The epidemiology of malignant gastrointestinal stromal tumors: An analysis of 1,458 cases from 1992 to 2000. *Am J Gastroenterol* 2005;100(1):162–8.
66. Liu M, Song C, Zhang P, et al. A nomogram for predicting cancer-specific survival of patients with gastrointestinal stromal tumors. *Med Sci Monit* 2020;26:e922378.
67. Khan J, Ullah A, Waheed A, et al. Gastrointestinal stromal tumors (GIST): A population-based study using the SEER database, including management and recent advances in targeted therapy. *Cancers* 2022;14:3689.
68. Abdalla TSA, Pieper L, Kist M, et al. Gastrointestinal stromal tumors of the upper GI tract: Population-based analysis of epidemiology, treatment and outcome based on data from the German Clinical Cancer Registry Group. *J Cancer Res Clin Oncol* 2023;149:7461–9.
69. Call J, Wojtkowiak J, Evans D, et al. Gastrointestinal stromal tumor patients with molecular testing exhibit superior survival compared to patients without testing: Results from the Life Raft Group (LRG) registry. *Cancer Invest* 2023;41(5);474–86.
70. Wang S, Wang Y, Luo J, et al. Development and validation of a prognostic nomogram for gastrointestinal stromal tumors in the post-imatinib era: A study based on the SEER database and a Chinese cohort. *Cancer Med* 2023;12:15970–82.
71. Sutton TL, Walker BS, Billingsley KG, et al. Disease-free interval is associated with oncologic outcomes in patients with recurrent gastrointestinal stromal tumor. *Ann Surg Oncol* 2021;28:7912–20.

72. Brudvik KW, Patel SH, Roland CL, et al. Survival after resection of gastrointestinal stromal tumor and sarcoma liver metastases in 146 patients. *J Gastrointest Surg* 2015;19(8):1476–83.

73. Kim JH, Ryu M-H, Yoo C, et al. Long-term survival outcome with tyrosine kinase inhibitors and surgical intervention in patients with metastatic or recurrent gastrointestinal stromal tumors: A 14-year, single-center experience. *Cancer Med* 2019;8:1034–43.

74. Bauer S, Rutkowski P, Hohenberger P, et al. Long-term follow-up of patients with GIST undergoing metastasectomy in the era of imatinib – Analysis of prognostic factors (EorTC-STBSG collaborative study). *Eur J Surg Oncol* 2014;40:412–9.

75. Ogata K, Kimura A, Nakazawa N, et al. Long-term imatinib treatment for patients with unresectable or recurrent gastrointestinal stromal tumors. *Digestion* 2018;97:20–5.

76. Xiao B, Peng J, Tang J, et al. Liver surgery prolongs the survival of patients with gastrointestinal stromal tumor liver metastasis: A retrospective study from a single center. *Cancer Manage Res* 2018;10:6121–7.

77. Kraft A, Croitoru A, Gheorghe C, et al. Liver resection for metastases from gastrointestinal stromal tumors: Does it improve long-term survival? *Chirurgia* 2021;116:438–50.

78. Farag S, van Coevorden F, Sneekes E, et al. Elderly patients with gastrointestinal stromal tumours (GIST) receive less treatment irrespective of performance score or comorbidity – A retrospective multi-centre study in a large cohort of GIST patients. *Eur J Cancer* 2017;86:318–25.

79. Italiano A, Saada E, Cioffi A, et al. Treatment of advanced gastrointestinal stromal tumors in patients over 75 years old: Clinical and pharmacological implications. *Target Oncol* 2013;8(4):295–300.

80. Chen Z, Lin R-M, Bai Y-K, Zhang Y. Establishment and verification of prognostic nomograms for patients with gastrointestinal stromal tumors: A SEER-based study. *BioMed Res Int* 2019;2019:8293261.

81. Singer S, Rubin BP, Lux ML, et al. Prognostic value of KIT mutation type, mitotic activity, and histologic subtype in gastrointestinal stromal tumors. *J Clin Oncol* 2002;20:3898–905.

82. Fujimoto Y, Nakanishi Y, Yoshimura K, Shimoda T. Clinicopathologic study of primary malignant gastrointestinal stromal tumor of the stomach, with special reference to prognostic factors: Analysis of results in 140 surgically resected patients. *Gastric Cancer* 2003;6(1):39–48.

83. Dwight T, Benn DE, Clarkson A, et al. Loss of SDHA expression identifies SDHA mutations in succinate dehydrogenase-deficient gastrointestinal stromal tumors. *Am J Pathol* 2013;37(2):226–33.

84. Miettinen M, Lasota J. Succinate dehydrogenase deficient gastrointestinal stromal tumors (GISTs) – A review. *Int J Biochem Cell Biol* 2014;53C:514–9.

85. Miettinen M, Sarlomo-Rikala M, McCue P, et al. Mapping of succinate dehydrogenase losses in 2258 epithelial neoplasms. *Appl Immunohistochem Mol Morphol* 2014;22(1):31–6.

86. Miettinen M, Wang Z-F, Sarlomo-Rikala M, et al. Succinate dehydrogenase-deficient GISTs: A clinico-pathologic, immunohistochemical, and molecular genetic study of 66 gastric GISTs with predilection to young age. *Am J Surg Pathol* 2011;35(11):1712–21.

87. Wardelmann E. Translational research and diagnosis in GIST. *Pathologe* 2012;33:273–7.

88. Rong J, Chen S, Song C, et al. The prognostic value of gender in gastric gastrointestinal stromal tumors: A propensity score matching analysis. *Biol Sex Differ* 2020;11:43.

89. Zemla P, Stelmach A, Jablonska B, et al. A retrospective study of postoperative outcomes in 98 patients diagnosed with gastrointestinal stromal tumor (GIST) of the upper, middle, and lower gastrointestinal tract between 2009 and 2019 at a single center in Poland. *Med Sci Monit* 2021;27:e932809.

90. Ding P, Guo H, Yang P, et al. Association between the nutritional risk and the survival rate in newly diagnosed GIST patients. *Front Nutr* 2021;8:743475.

91. Miettinen M, Lasota J. Gastrointestinal stromal tumors – Definition, clinica, histological, immunohistochemical, and molecular genetic features and differential diagnosis. *Virchows Arch* 2001;438(1):1–12.

92. Lv A, Li Z, Tian X, et al. SKP2 high expression, KIT exon 11 deletions, and gastrointestinal bleeding as predictors of poor prognosis in primary gastrointestinal stromal tumors. *PLoS ONE* 2013;8(5):e62951.

93. Yang Z, Wang F, Liu S, Guan W. Comparative clinical features and short-term outcomes of gastric and small intestinal gastrointestinal stromal tumours: A retrospective study. *Sci Rep* 2019;9(1):10033.

94. Rutkowski P, Teterycz P, Klimczak A, et al. Blood neutrophil-to-lymphocyte ratio is associated with prognosis in advanced gastrointestinal stromal tumors treated with imatinib. *Tumori* 2018;104(6):415–22.

95. Italiano A, Cioffi A, Coco P, et al. Patterns of care, prognosis, and survival in patients with metastatic gastrointestinal stromal tumors (GIST) refractory to first-line imatinib and second-line sunitinib. *Ann Surg Oncol* 2012;19(5):1551–9.

96. Lee CK, Goldstein D, Gibbs E, et al. Development and validation of prognostic nomograms for metastatic gastrointestinal stromal tumour treated with imatinib. *Eur J Cancer* 2015;51:853–60.

97. Chang Y-R, Huang W-K, Wang S-Y, et al. A nomogram predicting progression free survival in patients with gastrointestinal stromal tumor receiving sunitinib: Incorporating pre-treatment and post-treatment parameters. *Cancers* 2021;13:2587.

98. Fairweather M, Balachandran VP, Li GZ, et al. Cytoreductive surgery for metastatic gastrointestinal stromal tumors treated with tyrosine kinase inhibitors: A two institutional analysis. *Ann Surg* 2018;268(2):296–302.

99. Fu J, Fang M-J, Dong D, et al. Heterogeneity of metastatic gastrointestinal stromal tumor on texture analysis: DWI texture as potential biomarker of overall survival. *Eur J Radiol* 2020;125:108825.

100. Mohammadi M, Ijzerman NS, Hohenberger P, et al. Clinicopathological features and treatment outcome of oesophageal gastrointestinal stromal tumour (GIST): A large, retrospective multicenter european study. *Eur J Surg Oncol* 2021;47:2173–81.

101. Sharma AK, de la Torre J, Ijzerman NS, et al. Location of gastrointestinal stromal tumor (GIST) in the stomach predicts tumor mutation profile and drug sensitivity. *Clin Cancer Res* 2021;27(19):5334–42.

102. Li Y, Zhang Y, Fu Y, et al. Development and validation of a prognostic model to predict the prognosis of patients with colorectal gastrointestinal stromal tumor: A large international population-based cohort study. *Front Oncol* 2022;12:1004662.

103. Zhou G, Xiao K, Gong G, et al. A novel nomogram for predicting liver metastasis in patients with gastrointestinal stromal tumor: A SEER-based study. *BMC Surg* 2020;20:298.

104. McDonnell MJ, Punnoose S, Viswanath YKS, et al. Gastrointestinal stromal tumours (GISTs): An insight into clinical practice with review of literature. *Frontline Gastroenterol* 2017;8(1):19–25.

105. Zhu J, Yang Y, Zhou L, et al. A long-term follow-up of the imatinib mesylate treatment for the patients with recurrent gastrointestinal stromal tumor (GIST): The livermetastasis and the outcome. *BMC Cancer* 2010;10:199.

106. Wang C-J, Zhang Z-Z, Xu J, et al. SLITRK3 expression correlation to gastrointestinal stromal tumor risk rating and prognosis. *World J Gastroenterol* 2015;21(27):8398–407.

107. Ran L, Chen Y, Sher J, et al. FOXF1 defines the core-regulatory circuitry in gastrointestinal stromal tumor. *Cancer Discov* 2018;8(2):234–51.

108. Chi P, Chen Y, Zhang L, et al. ETV1 is a lineage survival factor that cooperates with KIT in gastrointestinal stromal tumours. *Nature* 2010;467(7317):849–53.

109. Delahaye NF, Rusakiewicz S, Martins I, et al. Alternatively spliced NKp30 isoforms affect the prognosis of gastrointestinal stromal tumors. *Nat Med* 2011;17(6):700–7.

110. Arshad J, Costa PA, Barreto-Coelho P, et al. Immunotherapy strategies for gastrointestinal stromal tumor. *Cancers* 2021;13:3525.

111. Corless CL, Fletcher JA, Heinrich MC. Biology of gastrointestinal stromal tumors. *J Clin Oncol* 2004,22(18):3813–25.

112. Klug LR, Khosroyani HM, Kent JD, Heinrich MC. New treatment strategies for advanced-stage gastrointestinal stromal tumours. *Nat Rev Clin Oncol* 2022;19(5):328–41.

113. Hirota S, Isozaki K, Moriyama Y, et al. Gain-of-function mutations of c-kit in human gastrointestinal stromal tumors. *Science* 1998;279(5350):577–80.

114. Heinrich MC, Corless CL, Duensing A, et al. PDGFRA activating mutations in gastrointestinal stromal tumors. *Science* 2003;299(5607):708–10.

115. Joensuu H. Gastrointestinal stromal tumor (GIST). *Ann Oncol* 2006;17:x280–6.

116. Janeway KA, Kim SY, Lodish M, et al. Defects in succinate dehydrogenase in gastrointestinal stromal tumors lacking KIT and PDGFRA mutations. *Proc Natl Acad Sci U S A*;108(1):314–8.

117. Pasini B, McWhinney SR, Nei T, et al. Clinical and molecular genetics of patients with the Carney-Stratakis syndrome and germline mutations of the genes coding for the succinate dehydrogenase subunits SDHB, SDHC, and SDHD. *Eur J Hum Genet* 2008;16(1):79–88.

118. Miettinen M, Fetsch JF, Sobin LH, Lasota J. Gastrointestinal stromal tumors in patients with neurofibromatosis 1: A clinicopathologic and molecular genetic study of 45 cases. *Am J Surg Pathol* 2006;30(1):90–6.

119. Agaimy A, Terracciano LM, Dirnhofer S, et al. V600E BRAF mutations are alternative early molecular events in a subset of KIT/PDGFRA wild-type gastrointestinal stromal tumours. *J Clin Pathol* 2009;62(7):613–6.

120. Mathias-Machado MC, Fonseca de Jesus VH, de Carvalho Oliveira LJ, et al. Current molecular profile of gastrointestinal stromal tumors and systemic therapeutic implications. *Cancers* 2022;14:5330.

121. Rossi S, Gasparotto D, Miceli R, et al. KIT, PDGFRA, and BRAF mutational spectrum impacts on the natural history of imatinib-naive localized GIST: A population-based study. *Am J Surg Pathol* 2015;39(7):922–30.

122. Wozniak A, Rutkowski P, Schoffski P, et al. Tumor genotype is an independent prognostic factor in primary gastrointestinal stromal tumors of gastric origin: A European multicenter analysis based on ConticaGIST. *Clin Cancer Res* 2014;20(23):6105–16.

123. Janeway KA, Albritton KH, Van Den Abbeele A, et al. Sunitinib treatment in pediatric patients with advanced GIST following failure of imatinib. *Pediatr Blood Cancer* 2009;52(7):767–71.

124. Feng X, Li H, Fourquet J, et al. Refining prognosis in localized gastrointestinal stromal tumor: Clinical significance of phosphatase and tensin homolog low expression and gene loss. *JCO Precis Oncol* 2022;6:e2200129.

125. Huang KK, McPherson JR, Tay ST, et al. SETD2 histone modifier loss in aggressive GI stromal tumours. *Gut* 2015;65(12):1960–72.

126. DeMatteo RP, Shah A, Fong Y, et al. Results of hepatic resection for sarcoma metastatic to liver. *Ann Surg* 2001;234(4):540–7.

127. Nunobe S, Sano T, Shimada K, et al. Surgery including liver resection for metastatic gastrointestinal stromal tumors or gastrointestinal leiomyosarcomas. *Jpn J Clin Oncol* 2005;35(6):338–41.

128. Xue A, Gao X, He Y, et al. Role of surgery in the management of liver metastases from gastrointestinal stromal tumors. *Front Oncol* 2022;12:903487.

129. Machairas N, Prodromidou A, Molmenti E, et al. Management of liver metastases from gastrointestinal stromal tumors: Where do we stand? *J Gastrointest Oncol* 2017;8(6):1100–8.

130. Du C-Y, Zhou Y, Song C, et al. Is there a role of surgery in patients with recurrent or metastatic gastro-intestinal stromal tumours responding to imatinib: A prospective randomised trial in China. *Eur J Cancer* 2014;50(10):1772–8.

131. Zalcberg JR, Verweij J, Casali PG, et al. Outcome of patients with advanced gastro-intestinal stromal tumours crossing over to a daily imatinib dose of 800 mg after progression on 400 mg. *Eur J Cancer* 2005;41(12):1751–7.

132. Casali PG, Zalcberg J, Le Cesne A, et al. Ten-year progression-free and overall survival in patients with unresectable or metastatic GI stromal tumors: Long-term analysis of the European Organisation for Research and Treatment of Cancer, Italian Sarcoma Group, and Australasian Gastrointestinal Trials Group Intergroup phase III randomized trial on imatinib at two dose levels. *J Clin Oncol* 2017;35(15):1713–20.

133. Demetri GD, von Mehren M, Blanke CD, et al. Efficacy and safety of imatinib mesylate in advanced gastrointestinal stromal tumors. *N Engl J Med* 2002;347:472–80.

134. Heinrich MC, Jones RL, von Mehren M, et al. Avapritinib in advanced PDGFRA D842V-mutant gastrointestinal stromal tumor (NAVIGATOR): A multicentre, open-label, phase 1 trial. *Lancet Oncol* 2020;21(7):935–46.

135. Drilon A, Laetsch TW, Kummar S, et al. Efficacy of Larotrectinib in TRK fusion-positive cancers in adults and children. *N Engl J Med* 2018;378:731–9.

136. Demetri GD, van Oosterom AT, Garrett CR, et al. Efficacy and safety of sunitinib in patients with advanced gastrointestinal stromal tumour after failure of imatinib: A randomised controlled trial. *Lancet* 2006;368:1329–38.

137. George S, Blay J-Y, Casali PG, et al. Clinical evaluation of continuous daily dosing of sunitinib malate in patients with advanced gastrointestinal stromal tumour after imatinib failure. *Eur J Cancer* 2009;45:1959–68.

138. Nishida T, Kanda T, Nishitani A, et al. Secondary mutations in the kinase domain of the KIT gene are predominant in imatinib-resistant gastrointestinal stromal tumor. *Cancer Sci* 2008;99(4):799–804.

139. Debiec-Rychter M, Cools J, Dumez H, et al. Mechanisms of resistance to imatinib mesylate in gastrointestinal stromal tumors and activity of the PKC412 inhibitor against imatinib-resistant mutants. *Gastroenterol* 2005;128(2):270–9.

140. Li J, Dang Y, Gao J, et al. PI3K/AKT/mTOR pathway is activated after imatinib secondary resistance in gastrointestinal stromal tumors (GISTs). *Med Oncol* 2015;32(4):111.

141. Bauer S, Jones RL, Blay J-Y, et al. Ripretinib versus sunitinib in patients with advanced gastrointestinal stromal tumor after treatment with imatinib (INTRIGUE): A randomized, open-label, phase III trial. *J Clin Oncol* 2022;40(34):3918–28.

142. Fudalej MM, Badowska-Kozakiewicz AM. Improved understanding of gastrointestinal stromal tumors biology as a step for developing new diagnostic and therapeutic schemes (Review). *Oncol Lett* 2021;21:417.

143. Falchook GS, Trent JC, Heinrich MC, et al. BRAF mutant gastrointestinal stromal tumor: First report of regression with BRAF inhibitor dabrafenib (GSK2118436) and whole exomic sequencing for analysis of acquired resistance. *Oncotarget* 2013;4(2):310–5.

144. Demetri G, Reichardt P, Kang Y-K, et al. Efficacy and safety of regorafenib for advanced gastrointestinal stromal tumours after failure of imatinib and sunitinib (GRID): An international, multicentre, randomised, placebo-controlled, phase 3 trial. *Lancet* 2013;381(9863):295–302.

145. Blay J-Y, Serrano C, Heinrich MC, et al. Ripretinib in patients with advanced gastrointestinal stromal tumours (INVICTUS): A double-blind, randomised, placebo-controlled, phase 3 trial. *Lancet Oncol* 2020;21(7):923–34.

146. Kang Y-K, Ryu M-H, Yoo C, et al. Resumption of imatinib to control metastatic or unresectable gastrointestinal stromal tumours after failure of imatinib and sunitinib (RIGHT): A randomised, placebo-controlled, phase 3 trial. *Lancet Oncol* 2013;14(12):1175–82.

147. Kang Y-K, George S, Jones RL, et al. Avapritinib versus regorafenib in locally advanced unresectable or metastatic GI stromal tumor: A randomized, open-label phase III study. *J Clin Oncol* 2021;39(28):3128–39.

148. Mir O, Cropet C, Toulmonde M, et al. Pazopanib plus best supportive care versus best supportive care alone in advanced gastrointestinal stromal tumours resistant to imatinib and sunitinib (PAZOGIST): A randomised, multicentre, open-label phase 2 trial. *Lancet Oncol* 2016;17(5):632–41.

149. Schoffski P, Mir O, Kasper B, et al. Activity and safety of the multi-target tyrosine kinase inhibitor cabozantinib in patients with metastatic gastrointestinal stromal tumour after treatment with imatinib and sunitinib: European Organisation for Research and Treatment of Cancer phase II trial 1317 'CaboGIST'. *Eur J Cancer* 2020;134:62–74.

150. Ricci R, Martini M, Ravegnini G, et al. Preferential MGMT methylation could predispose a subset of KIT/PDGFRA-WT GISTs, including SDH-deficient ones, to respond to alkylating agents. *Clin Epigenet* 2019;11:2.

9 Colorectal cancer

9.1 INTRODUCTION

9.1.1 EPIDEMIOLOGY

A GLOBOCAN database report estimated 1,148,515 new cases and 576,858 deaths from colorectal cancer (CRC) in 2020, with incidence age-adjusted standardized rates (ASRs) of colon and rectal cancer (RC) of 13.1 and 9.8/100,000 among males, 10.0 and 5.6 among females, whereas the mortality rates were 6.4/4.4 per 100,000 and 4.6/2.4 per 100,000, respectively [1]. The incidence ASR for CRC in Europe in 2022 was 79.7/100,000, with 356,154 new cases, and similar rates of mortality with ASR of 35.6/100,000 and 158,956 cancer deaths. The tumor was more prevalent among males with an incidence ASR of 92.7 vs. 58.2/100.000, and a mortality ASR of 42.8 vs. 24.6/100,000 [2].

A 9-fold variation in incidence rates by geographic areas has been reported, with the highest rates in Europe, Australia, and North America, except RCs which also had a peak in Eastern Asia [1].

The global reduction in the incidence of CRC is attributed to the change in lifestyle habits and screening. On the other hand, the reasons for the increased incidence of 1–4%/year in the <50-year-old population remain poorly understood [1]. More than 90% of CRC diagnoses occur at >50 [3, 4], but since 1994 in the US a progressive increase of CRCs in subjects <50 years old occurred, which were defined as early onset colorectal cancers (EO-CRCs), in contrast to general incidence reduction in the elderly, with a pronounced increase of RCs [5, 6]. Although the mutation rate in EO-CRC is lower than the average for CRC, in 30% there is a mutation typical of hereditary syndromes and in 20% (more common in <35 [7]) an increased familial risk, but no predisposing condition in the remaining 50% [8]. On the contrary, in the elderly, right-sided CRCs are more frequent [9–11], mostly in women.

Male sex is associated with a higher incidence of CRC [12] and precancerous lesions, maybe only be related to the higher prevalence of risk factors [13–15], but the lower incidence in females is a phenomenon that affects certain age groups, with women in childbearing age and on hormone replacement treatment having a lower risk of CRC [3, 16, 17].

9.1.2 STAGING OF METASTATIC DISEASE

Pancolonscopy+biopsy is the mainstay of diagnosis, and gives information about tumor location and other foci, clearing the colon of synchronous polyps. For these reasons, even if pancolonscopy was not performed before hemicolectomy, it should be done within 3–6 months.

Laboratory evaluation is necessary to exclude hemorrhage, to correct iron deficiency and to have an updated liver and kidney function, but also to provide prognostic factors (PFs), such as lactic dehydrogenase (LDH), alkaline phosphatase (ALP), albumin, and neutrophile-to-lymphocyte ratio (NLR). Serum carcinoembryonic antigen (CEA), although insufficient for diagnosis, should be evaluated at baseline and monitored [18–20].

Imaging should complete staging after diagnosis of CRC. The recommended investigations are chest-abdomen CT and pelvic MRI, in the case of intermediate and low RC. A more detailed liver evaluation could be necessary in the case of metastases, by hepato-specific contrast-enhanced MRI.

The reference staging system is TNM Classification (AJCC 8th edition 2017).

Based on the treatment plan of mCRC, other second-level investigations could be necessary, such as the biologic characterization of the mismatch repair (MMR) [21–23], the mutational status

DOI: 10.1201/9781032703350-9

of some genes (RAS and BRAF) [24–27], the analysis of di-hydro-pyrimidine-dehydrogenase (DPYD) pathogenetic polymorphisms for patients candidate to fluoropyrimidine-containing regimens [28]. In refractory disease, additional information will be useful about HER2 over-expression [29], NTRK fusion [30–33], and MAPK pathway, but due to the high level of molecular heterogeneity, the analysis of circulating tumor DNA (ctDNA) is the more appropriate tool for evaluating late metastatic disease.

9.1.3 PROGNOSIS OF METASTATIC DISEASE

Median overall survival (OS) of unresectable or metastatic colorectal cancer (mCRC) patients has increased from 7.7 months [34] to 36.2 months [35] from 1989 to 2023, with some studies reporting 5-year survival rates of 83.1% after radical resection of metastases [36].

However, the outcome of mCRC can be highly variable [37]. An analysis of 32 prospective NCCTG trials, from 1972 to 1995, documented that some mCRC patients (36/3407) had very long survival with a median OS of 10.6 years [38]. In this chapter the analyses will refer only to mCRC undergoing upfront treatment, reporting frequent disagreements in studies about PFs and their corresponding effect sizes (ES). Some studies and meta-analyses evaluated PFs of mCRC [39], but results of PFs analyses from prospective trials have been poorly reported.

9.2 ANALYSIS OF PROGNOSTIC VARIABLES IN EARLY METASTATIC DISEASE

A systematic review of phase III randomized clinical trials (RCTs) in patients with mCRC undergoing upfront therapy resulted in the selection of 112 studies, published from 1987 to 2022. In 42/112 an analysis of PFs was done, and in 39/112 a multivariate analysis was reported [34, 40–77]. With all the limitations related to the analysis of the PFs, whose choice for inclusion in individual studies was frequently arbitrary, this review analyzed their results (Table S1). It lists all PFs that have been reported in at least one study and the number of studies that found or did not a relationship between the PFs and OS.

In addition, the results of five pooled individual patient data analyses (IPDA) including patients enrolled in 12 RCTs are commented [78–82].

9.3 PATIENT-RELATED PROGNOSTIC FACTORS

9.3.1 PERFORMANCE STATUS

The ARCAD nomogram project analyzed performance status (PS), evaluating 12,123 patients with PS 0, 9,595 PS 1, and 956 PS 2 or greater. A significantly reduced OS was evident for both after the comparison, between patients with PS 1 vs. PS 0, and PS 2 vs. PS 0 [83]. Other three of five prospective data analyses supported the prognostic effect of PS [84–88], and a relationship with OS was evident also in three retrospective studies [89–91], but not among mCRC patients with resectable disease [92].

For frail patients or those with severe comorbidities, the interpretation of PS is challenging, due to cancer could be only a component of PS deterioration. An IPDA documented that patients with ECOG PS 2 had more chemotherapy toxicity, higher 60-day mortality, and reduced OS. On the other hand, the benefits of the experimental treatment arms were significantly greater than the control arm in every PS category [93], similarly to other studies and despite dose reductions [94]. Cohort studies document a 2.6-fold increased risk of death for frail patients [95, 96]. Only cohort studies suggest that comorbidity and frailty are indicators of OS and that a geriatric assessment (GA) may improve clinical oncology decisions [97], reducing the risk of overtreatment and severe toxicity [98].

TABLE S1

Prognostic factors analysed in selected clinical trials of patients with unresectable or metastatic colorectal cancer receiving upfront treatment

Variable	No. comparisons	Prognostic relationship	No prognostic relationship
Patient-related			
Performance status	29	24	5
Age	18	2	16
Sex	16	2	14
Anthropometric			
Physical activity	1	1	0
Geo & ethnic			
Geographic area	1	1	0
Institution	4	2	2
Ethnicity	1	0	1
Clinic			
Co-morbidity	1	0	1
Symptomatic	4	4	0
Weight loss	2	0	2
Lab			
Hemoglobin	4	2	2
Leukocyte-related	10	7	3
Platelet-related	3	1	2
Inflammation-related	2	2	0
Alkalyne phosphatase	12	11	1
Lactic dehydrogenase	8	5	3
Liver function	4	2	2
Tumor markers			
Carcinoembrionic antigen	12	6	6
Carbohydrate antigen 19-9	4	1	3
Tumor-related			
Tumor burden			
Tumor size	1	1	0
No. sites metatsases	14	13	1
No. liver metastases	1	1	0
Liver involvement %	4	4	0
Liver-limited disease	9	4	5
Lung-limited disease	2	0	2
Misurable disease	4	2	2
Location	19	4	15
Timing of metastasis			
Syn- vs. meta-chronous	6	1	5
Time diagnosis-to-CHT	6	0	6
Site of metastasis			
Liver metastases	7	4	3
Nodal metastases	2	1	1
Lung metastases	1	0	1
Pathology			
Grading	6	4	2
Dukes' stage	5	0	5
Previous treatments			
Primary tumor resection	9	3	6
Previous adjuvant therapy	8	0	8
Previous radiotherapy	4	1	3
Previous adjuvant CHT	6	0	6
Previous metastasectomy	2	1	1

9.3.1.1 Selected trials

Twenty-nine trials analyzed PS by different scales. Twenty-four studies had documented a significant prognostic relationship (Table 9.1). Considering the comparison of PS 1 or more vs. PS 0, a meta-analysis of 14 studies was performed. It confirmed a significant relationship between any PS deterioration and poor prognosis (HR 1.76, CI 1.56–1.98; Q = 29.91, p-value = 0.0049; I^2 = 56.5) (Figure 9.1).

All the five pooled analyses evaluated PS, but only in three it was an independent PF [78, 79, 81].

TABLE 9.1

Prognostic relationships of performance status in selected studies of patients with unresectable metastatic colorectal cancer receiving upfront treatment

Study [ref]	Phase	No. pts	Scale	Comparison	Prognostic relationship	Effect size
NCCTG 1989 [34]	III	419	WHO	2–3 vs. 0–1	Yes	NR
French CG 1992 [40]	III	163	WHO	1 vs. 0	Yes	NR
NCCTG 1994 [41]	III	362	ECOG	2–3 vs. 0–1	Yes	NR
EORTC 1996 [42]	III	297	WHO	1–2 vs. 0	Yes	RR 1.92
RMH 1997 [43]	III	198	ECOG	2 vs. 0–1	Yes	HR 2.63
EORTC-CCG1 2000 [44]	III	200	WHO	1–2 vs. 0	Yes	NR
FOLFOX 2000 [45]	III	420	WHO	continuous	Yes	HR 1.52
ISG 2000 [46]	III	679	ECOG	1–2 vs. 0	Yes	HR 1.79 (1.43–2.27)
V-303 2000 [47]	III	385	WHO	2–3 vs. 0–1	No	NR
ECOG 2290 2001 [48]	III	1047	ECOG	1 vs. 0	Yes	HR 1.36
		598		2 vs. 0		HR 2.57
MDACC 2001 [49]	III	605	KPS	70–80 vs. 100	Yes	HR 2.56
SO14796 2001 [50]	III	602	KPS	70–80 vs. 100	Yes	NR
FUMA 3008 2002 [51]	III	962	KPS	70–80 vs. 90–100	Yes	HR 1.69 (1.43–2.00)
HeCOG 2002 [52]	III	192	WHO	1 vs. 0	Yes	NR
ECOG 2200 2004 [53]	III	813	ECOG	1–2 vs. 0	Yes	HR 1.43 (1.28–1.54)
GERCOR C97.3 2004 [54]	III	220	WHO	1–2 vs. 0	Yes	NR
GOIM 9901 2005 [55]	III	349	ECOG	1 vs. 0	No	HR 1.09 (0.82–1.45)
		225		2 vs. 0		HR 1.65 (0.81–3.34)
EORTC-05963 2006 [56]	III	282	WHO	1–2 vs. 0	Yes	HR 1.72 (1.43–2.08)
FFCD-9601 2006 [58]	III	216	WHO	2 vs. 0–1	Yes	HR 2.00 (1.41–2.86)
OPTIMOX 1 2006 [59]	III	618	WHO	1–2 vs. 0	Yes	HR 1.61 (1.33–2.00)
AIO 22 2007 [60]	III	474	ECOG	1 vs. 0	Yes	NR
GONO 2007 [62]	III	244	ECOG	1–2 vs. 0	No	HR 1.43 (1.03–1.96)
HCOG 6A-05 2012 [68]	III	281	ECOG	1–2 vs. 0	Yes	HR 1.72 (1.16–2.50)
Nordic VII 2012 [69]	III	542	WHO	1 vs. 0	Yes	HR 1.64 (1.32–2.04)
		404		2 vs. 0		HR 3.45 (2.17–5.55)
FFCD 2001–02 2013 [70]	III	195	KPS	60–70 vs. 100	No	HR 1.39 (0.86–2.22)
		126		80–90 vs. 100		HR 1.12 (0.77–1.64)
FIRE 3 (*) 2014 [73]	III	400	ECOG	1–2 vs. 0	No	HR 1.15 (0.87–1.28)
TRIBE 2014 [74]	III	508	ECOG	1–2 vs. 0	Yes	HR 2.27 (1.61–3.23)
MARTHA 2017 [76]	III	198	ECOG	1 vs. 0	No	OR 1.05 (0.37–3.03)
TRIBE-2 [77]	III	520	ECOG	1–2 vs. 0	Yes	HR 2.17 (1.54–3.03)

Legend: ECOG, Eastern Cooperative Oncology Group. HR, hazard ratio. KPS, Karnofsky performance status. NR, not reported. OR, odds ratio. RR, risk ratio. WHO, World Health Organization. (*) RAS wild-type subgroup.

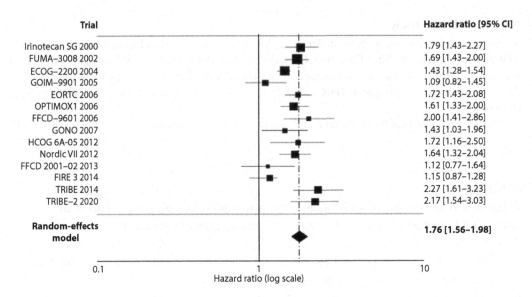

FIGURE 9.1   Forest plot of meta-analysis of performance status in prospective trials of patients with unresectable metastatic colorectal cancer

9.3.2   Demographic

9.3.2.1   Age

Although in clinical trials no age-related prognostic difference was found, both in the patients with EO-CRC and in the elderly [99], the prognosis of mCRC is poor.

EO-CRC presents peculiar characteristics and a late stage at onset [100, 101], with more synchronous metastases (SMs). A pooled analysis of 9 RCTs reported for patients <50 a poor PS, but similar OS and objective response rates (ORR), compared with the elderly [102], with a higher prevalence of poorly differentiated tumors [103] and delayed diagnosis [102, 103]. Conversely, better OS has been reported for <70-year-old patients from a large meta-analysis, with the authors explaining the results with the more aggressive treatments in the young patients [104].

Four population-based studies of patients with mCRC analyzed age at various cut-offs and concluded that it was associated with worse outcomes [105–108], whereas early death was more frequent in patients >50–58 [109, 110]. While the ARCAD database reported a reducing OS with increasing age [83], as two of five retrospective studies [90, 91, 111–113], another prospective study did not show different outcomes for patients >70 [87]. In resectable mCRC, two of three population-based [114–116] and one retrospective study [117] confirmed the poor prognosis of the elderly, while two prospective and four retrospective studies did not find differences [92, 118–122].

Other population-based studies described a further cancer-specific survival (CSS) reduction in patients aged 80 years or older [123, 124]. This subgroup of mCRC patients reported poor PS and nutritional status [125], with a possible detrimental effect from systemic inflammation response (SIR) and high CEA levels [125, 126], beyond the omitted or reduced treatments [127, 128]. For these patients treatment plans should be individualized taking into account the high complication rates of surgery [129], and the possible efficacy of sequential drug strategies [130, 131]. Despite the favorable studies [70, 132], GA is rarely performed in clinical practice, but a study reported that the timed up-and-go test was the only domain capable of predicting severe toxicities and treatment changes [133].

9.3.2.2   Sex

Metastases and mortality from mCRC are higher in males [134–137]. In females, the age group also plays a role in the prognosis as well as in the incidence. While young females have better OS than males, the opposite occurs among the elderly [138–140], with reduced 3-year survival rates and increased right-sided tumors [141].

Among patients with mCRC, two of four population-based studies documented longer OS for females [105–108], but no difference in early mortality [109, 110]. A better outcome for females with mCRC emerged from the CAIRO trial [85] and the ARCAD database [83], but not from prospective [87] or retrospective analyses [90, 91, 112]. In contrast, in the setting of resectable mCRC, OS was not associated with differences by sex [114–122].

Preclinical models support immune-associated differences in tumor response by sex [142], but the higher incidence of microsatellite instability-high (MSI-H) CRC in females could play a role.

Finally, some evidence suggests a possible predictive role of sex on the efficacy and toxicity of various antineoplastic drugs [143], due to different drug elimination mechanisms.

9.3.2.3 Other demographic variables

It can be stated that, despite differences in health care delivery, there is a geographic variation in CRC survival, but appropriate indicators to measure variations, regardless of the role of healthcare system-related variables, are unavailable.

According to some authors, rural patients may be viewed as a culture with their health determinants, that prefer individualized care in familial environments [144, 145]. Although this attitude could explain in part their reduced 5-year survival rates [146], moderate travel times to a specialized hospital have a prognostic role [147] and concur with the higher risk of dying from CRC reported by SEER [148].

Considering population studies on large geographical areas, different characteristics of the CRC can translate into prognostic differences [149]. This condition was reported for geographic differences of the MSI-H component, which ranges from <10% (South Korea and Taiwan) to 15% (US) [150–152], or of BRAF mutations, from 4–7% (Korea and China) to 13–15% (US) [150, 153, 154].

Ethnicity has been explored as a variable by the SEER database. For mCRC patients, such studies have documented poor OS among African-Americans vs. Whites [105–107]. These differences might reflect social disparities, but also epidemiological differences, because African-Americans appear more likely to have a diagnosis of an advanced and right-sided mCRC, low-grade tumors in the cecum, early age of onset, and higher KRAS mutation rates [155]. Still, the MSI-H component was more relevant in the White vs. Black patients (16.9% vs. 11.3%) [153].

Some analyses of the SEER database report poor outcomes of mCRC patients among the unmarried [105, 115], while it is unclear whether cancer-related early death increases [109, 110].

9.3.2.4 Selected trials

Eighteen studies evaluated age, but only two found a prognostic relationship, with longer OS in younger patients [41, 60] (Table 9.2). Three of the pooled analyses assessed age, which in none was an independent variable.

Sixteen studies investigated the effect of sex, and only two documented a better survival of females (Table 9.3). Of the three pooled analyses that assessed sex, only one reported a prognostic role [82].

One study demonstrated different outcomes by geographic origin (Western Europe+Canada+Australia vs. rest of the world) [64], while the ethnic variable did not affect prognosis [46].

9.3.3 Anthropometric

Among the studies that have reported the results of body mass index (BMI) on OS in mCRC, retrospective evaluations were negative [90, 117], but the prospective data of the ARCAD database documented a prognostic relationship with an L-shaped pattern [156]. The risk of progression/death was increased for low BMI (<28 kg/m^2), then the risk decreased and plateaued, with the relationship of

TABLE 9.2

Prognostic relationships of age in selected studies of patients with unresectable metastatic colorectal cancer receiving upfront treatment

Study [ref]	Phase	No. pts	Comparison	Prognostic relationship	Effect size
NCCTG 1989 [34]	III	419	<50 vs. 50–70 vs. >70	No	NR
NCCTG 1994 [41]	III	362	<50 vs. 50–70 vs. >70	Yes	NR
EORTC 1996 [42]	III	297	< vs. >58	No	RR 0.98 (0.77–1.23)
EORTC-CCG1 2000 [44]	III	200	continuous	No	NR
FOLFOX 2000 [45]	III	420	continuous	No	NR
ISG 2000 [46]	III	679	< vs. >65	No	HR 1.22 (0.98–1.54)
V-303 2000 [47]	III	385	< vs. >58	No	HR 0.78 (0.61–1.01)
GOIM 9901 2005 [55]	III	349	continuous	No	HR 1.01 (0.99–1.02)
EORTC-CCG2 2006 [56]	III	282	< vs. >50	No	HR 1.05 (0.83–1.35)
FFCD-9601 2006 [58]	III	216	< vs. >65	No	HR 0.91 (0.68–1.22)
AIO 22 2007 [60]	III	474	< vs. >70	Yes	NR (°)
GONO 2007 [62]	III	244	continuous	No	HR 1.00 (0.99–1.02)
PRIME 2010 [64]	III	475	< vs. ≥65	No	OR 1.69 (0.98–2.91)
HCOG 6A-05 2012 [68]	III	281	< vs. >60	No	NR
FFCD 2001–02 2013 [70]	III	195	< vs. >80	No	HR 0.98 (0.77–1.26)
SOFT 2013 [72]	III	511	< vs. >70	No	HR 0.94 (0.73–1.22)
FIRE 3 2014 [73] (*)	III	400	continuous	No	HR 1.01 (0.99–1.03)
MARTHA 2017 [76]	III	200	continuous	No	OR 1.00 (0.94–1.04)

Legend: HR, hazard ratio. NR, not reported. OR, odds ratio. RR, risk ratio. (°) p-value <0.05. (*) RAS wild-type subgroup.

low BMI with OS more pronounced among males. The authors hypothesized that cancer-associated cachexia syndrome (CACS) was the explanation for the poor prognosis in low BMI patients since CACS affects 50% of mCRCs and is associated with 20% mortality [157], but other possible mechanisms can not be excluded [156].

On the other hand, a negative interaction between obesity and mCRC prognosis has been suggested for some subgroups, such as those with high serum LDH or IL-8 [158], SIR activation [159] or transcriptomic-dependent mechanisms [160]. Metabolic reasons could explain the relationship of physical activity with the outcome.

9.3.3.1   Selected trials

One study assessed physical activity and showed a trend of better OS for patients with >18 metabolic equivalent task (MET) hours per week than those with <3 MET hours (HR 0.85, CI 0.71–1.02) [75], with better tolerance to treatments for more than 9 MET hours per week [161].

A pooled analysis of the TRIBE and TRIBE-2 evaluated 1,160 patients and did not find any effect of BMI on OS [162].

9.3.4   Clinic

9.3.4.1   Comorbidities

In mCRC patients, symptoms seem more to identify the tumor burden (TB) than a symptom-related prognostic difference.

A meta-analysis documented that comorbidities increased mortality risk and CRC-specific mortality, in particular in frail patients [163]. CO.17 investigated the Charlson Comorbidity Index (CCI),

TABLE 9.3

Prognostic relationships of sex in selected studies of patients with unresectable metastatic colorectal cancer receiving upfront treatment

Study [ref]	Phase	No. pts	Comparison	Prognostic relationship	Effect size
NCCTG 1989 [34]	III	419	M vs. F	No	NR
EORTC 1996 [42]	III	297	M vs. F	No	HR 1.05 (0.83–1.33)
EORTC-CCG1 2000 [44]	III	200	M vs. F	No	NR
FOLFOX 2000 [45]	III	420	M vs. F	No	NR
ISG 2000 [46]	III	679	M vs. F	No	NR
V-303 2000 [47]	III	385	M vs. F	No	NR
GERCOR C97.3 2004 [54]	III	220	M vs. F	Yes	NR
GOIM 9901 2005 [55]	III	349	M vs. F	No	HR 0.95 (0.72–1.24)
EORTC-CCG2 2006 [56]	III	282	M vs. F	No	HR 1.15 (0.88–1.51)
FFCD-9601 2006 [58]	III	216	M vs. F	No	HR 0.90 (0.66–1.23)
GONO 2007 [62]	III	244	M vs. F	No	HR 1.25 (0.98–1.59)
FFCD 2001–02 2013 [70]	III	195	M vs. F	No	HR 0.93 (0.73–1.20)
SOFT 2013 [72]	III	511	M vs. F	No	HR 0.89 (0.71–1.12)
FIRE 3 2014 [73] (*)	III	400	M vs. F	No	HR 1.05 (0.78–1.42)
MARTHA 2017 [76]	III	198	M vs. F	No	OR 1.89 (0.76–4.70)
TRIBE-2 2020 [77]	III	520	M vs. F	Yes	HR 1.43 (1.11–1.85)

Legend: F, females. HR, hazard ratio. M, males. NR, not reported. OR, odds ratio. (*) RAS wild-type subgroup.

which was predicted by increasing age, but was not prognostic [164]. Conversely, in a retrospective analysis, the number of CIRS-G comorbidities predicted OS, while TRS correlated with OS only for the subgroup of RCs [165].

Among co-morbid conditions, metabolic syndrome induces a chronic inflammatory state and is associated with increased CRC risk, but also the risk of all-cause and CRC-specific mortality increased, proportionally to the number of metabolic risk factors [166]. A cohort of 378 diabetic patients with mCRC, enrolled in the CALGB-80405 trial, reported a significant OS reduction despite good tolerance to oncological therapies [167].

9.3.4.2 Predisposing conditions

Other clinical conditions increase the risk of CRC but their prognostic role is unclear.

Although the prognosis of patients with hereditary nonpolyposis colorectal cancer (HNPCC) follows that of the MSI-H subgroup, little is known about the prognosis of patients with microsatellite stable (MSS) mCRC arising in the context of familial predisposition, but no data on mCRC are known [168].

Inflammatory bowel diseases are associated with a 2–8-fold increased risk of CRC, but there is insufficient data about their effect on OS [169, 170].

Some cohorts reported poor prognosis of mCRC patients receiving upfront chemotherapy in the presence of a vitamin-D deficit [171, 172], and high-dose vitamin-D improved post-chemotherapy PFS [173].

9.3.4.3 Selected trials

All studies evaluating the prognostic role of CRC-related symptoms showed a significant relationship with survival (Table 9.4).

TABLE 9.4

Prognostic relationships of baseline symptoms occurrence in selected studies of patients with unresectable metastatic colorectal cancer receiving upfront treatment

Study [ref]	Phase	No. pts	Comparison	Prognostic relationship	Effect size
NCCTG 1989 [34]	III	419	Yes vs. not	Yes	NR
NCCTG 1994 [41]	III	362	Yes vs. not	Yes	NR
ECOG 2290 2001 [48]	III	1098	Yes vs. not	Yes	HR 1.28
FUMA 3008 2002 [51]	III	962	Yes vs. not	Yes	HR 0.64 (0.54–0.75)

Legend: HR, hazard ratio. NR, not reported.

No effect of 5% and 10% weight loss was found in RCTs [42, 47], and any effect of comorbidity in the elderly population according to the CCI was not evident in the FFCD trial [70, 174].

9.3.5 LABORATORY

9.3.5.1 Hematology

In mCRC, anemia was independently associated with poor OS [83, 84, 89]. Leukocytosis proved to be a negative PF, with variable cut-offs between 8,000–10,000/mcL [83, 74, 175, 176], but not at an 11,000/mcL cut-off [91]. Similar results have been suggested for neutrophil count [83], and polymorphonuclear count in resectable mCRC [92]. Two prospective and two retrospective studies, with cut-offs ranging from 2.68 to 5, documented a relationship of NLR with prognosis [86, 88, 90, 91], while the relationship was not significant in the setting of resectable disease with lung metastases [118] and in a retrospective analysis of two RCTs [177].

Platelet count was independently associated with a poor prognosis in RCTs [83, 84] and in a retrospective study [90]. Interestingly, platelet count >400/nL predicted poor outcomes after intermittent chemotherapy compared with continuous chemotherapy, suggesting avoiding stop-and-go strategies in these patients [178].

9.3.5.2 Chemistry

Serum albumin (SA) was inversely related to OS in mCRCs [83, 111], and similarly various inflammation-related indexes [90, 118, 179, 180].

High serum levels of liver enzymes, as well as ALP and LDH, have been associated with poor prognosis of mCRC [39, 78, 181]. Baseline serum ALP >300 U/L was associated with poor outcome in one study [84], but not in others [87, 175].

Even though early mortality was not increased by high levels of LDH, this enzyme was associated with reduced OS in three studies [85, 87, 91], a relationship that was not confirmed in resectable mCRC [92]. An analysis of the AMORIS study evaluated serum LDH in samples taken three years before cancer diagnosis. The study reported 450 mCRC deaths, with a resulting increased death risk for subjects with high LDH and a more pronounced relationship as LDH was measured near the diagnosis of CRC [182]. A meta-analysis of seven studies, enrolling 1,219 patients, comparing chemotherapy+bevacizumab vs. chemotherapy, documented that an LDH increase was associated with lower PFS and OS in the chemotherapy+bevacizumab arm [183].

9.3.5.3 Tumor markers

CEA is a glycoprotein that is upregulated in >75% of mCRCs [184, 185]. It was often associated with a poor prognosis, although according to some studies only in SMs [105], and its increase is less pronounced in the case of EHD [186]. CEA also acts as a negative predictor of the efficacy of chemotherapy [187, 188] and combination of chemotherapy+bevacizumab [73, 189]. Population-based studies have documented poor prognosis in mCRC patients with increased CEA [105–107, 109], as well as two prospective analyses [175, 176]. Despite the various cut-offs, retrospective studies also agree on the negative prognostic role of elevated CEA [89, 90, 111]. In resectable mCRC, two population-based studies documented a worse prognosis for patients with increased CEA [114, 115], but not at cut-offs of 100–200 ng/mL [92, 116]. Retrospective studies in resectable mCRC did not yield concordant results on baseline CEA [119, 121] but reported worse outcomes for a postoperative value >10 ng/mL [121] or when increased after neoadjuvant chemotherapy [122].

Elevated serum carbohydrate antigen 19-9 (CA 19-9) concentrations correlated with TB and are a useful marker for <10% of mCRC patients who have normal CEA [190]. The prognostic value of CA 19-9 is independent of CEA [89, 191], with a study reporting that high CA 19-9 levels predicted poor OS in mCRC patients with normal CEA, with a more pronounced effect in patients with lung metastases [192].

9.3.5.4 Selected trials

Four studies evaluated hemoglobin, with two documenting a negative prognostic effect for anemia [62, 76]. Six studies evaluated leukocyte count, and four reported a correlation between the increased count with poor OS (Table 9.5). NLR was shown to be closely associated with OS in the two RCTs that analyzed it [65, 71]. No effect on OS from platelet count was found [73, 76], while a PLR >169 correlated with poor OS [71]. Pooled analyses assessed leukocyte count [78, 79] and lymphocyte count [79], but no effect on OS was found in any case.

Twelve studies evaluated the relationship of baseline ALP with OS, as resumed in Table 9.6. Eleven of the 12 studies documented a relationship with poor survival for high ALP. A meta-analysis allowed us to calculate an overall ES (HR 1.80, CI 1.27–2.56; Q = 27.66, p-value<0.0001; I^2 = 81.9%) (Figure 9.2). One of the pooled analyses evaluated ALP, without detecting a prognostic role [78], whereas another combined analysis of two prospective trials confirmed a poor outcome of patients with baseline ALP >2ULN [193].

LDH was evaluated by eight studies (Table 9.6). Five studies found a significant association between increased LDH and poor OS. Therefore, a meta-analysis, which included the four studies

---

TABLE 9.5

Prognostic relationships of hematologic parameters in selected studies of patients with unresectable metastatic colorectal cancer receiving upfront treatment

Study [ref]	No. pts	Cut-off	Comparison	Prognostic relationship	Effect size
Hemoglobin (g/dL)					
ISG 2000 [46]	665	11	<11 vs. ≥11	No	NR
GONO 2007 [62]	122	10	<10 vs. ≥10	Yes	HR 0.59 (0.40–0.87)
FIRE 3 2014 [73] (*)	392	11	≤11 vs. >11	No	HR 0.95 (0.89–1.02)
MARTHA 2017 [76]	198	-	high vs. low	Yes	OR 0.77 (0.60–0.99)
Leukocyte count (x10³/mL)					
ISG 2000 [46]	665	8	<8 vs. ≥8	Yes	HR 0.65 (0.52–0.82)
AIO 22 2007 [60]	482	8	<8 vs. ≥8	Yes	NR
GONO 2007 [62]	122	8	<8 vs. ≥8	No	NR
FFCD 2001–02 2013 [70]	123	11	≤11 vs. >11	Yes	HR 0.63 (0.46–0.87)
FIRE 3 2014 [73] (*)	392	10	≤10 vs. >10	Yes	HR 1.09 (1.02–1.16)
MARTHA 2017 [76]	198	-	low vs. high	No	OR 1.12 (0.97–1.29)

Legend: HR, hazard ratio. NR, not reported. OR, odds ratio. (*) RAS wild-type subgroup.

TABLE 9.6

Prognostic relationships of serum chemistry variables in selected studies of patients with unresectable metastatic colorectal cancer receiving upfront treatment

Study [ref]	Phase	No. pts	Comparison	Prognostic relationship	Effect size
Alkaline phosphatase (U/L)					
FOLFOX 2000 [45]	III	415	≤ULN vs. >ULN	Yes	RR 1.59
MDACC 2001 [49]	III	605	≤ULN vs. >ULN	Yes	NR
SO14796 2001 [50]	III	602	low vs. high	Yes	NR
GERCOR C97.3 2004 [54]	III	202	<ULN vs. ≥ULN	Yes	NR
FFCD-9601 2006 [58]	III	216	≤300 vs. >300	Yes	HR 1.73 (1.23–2.42)
OPTIMOX 1 2006 [59]	III	613	≤ULN vs. >ULN	Yes	HR 1.28 (1.02–1.61)
AIO 22 2007 [60]	III	474	≤300 vs. >300	Yes	NR
GONO 2007 [62]	III	244	≤300 vs. >300	Yes	HR 1.75 (1.28–2.44)
Nordic VII 2012 [69]	III	586	≤ULN vs. >ULN	Yes	HR 1.91 (1.57–2.34)
FFCD 2001–02 2013 [70]	III	123	≤2 vs. >2 ULN	Yes	HR 3.33 (2.50–4.54)
FIRE 3 2014 [73] (*)	III	388	≤300 vs. >300	Yes	HR 1.42 (1.05–1.91)
MARTHA 2017 [76]	III	198	≤ULN vs. >ULN	No	OR 1.59 (0.24–5.56)
Lactate dehydrogenase (U/L)					
FOLFOX 2000 [45]	III	359	≤ULN vs. >ULN	Yes	RR 1.94
ISG 2000 [46]	III	606	≤ULN vs. >ULN	Yes	HR 2.13 (1.67–2.78)
GERCOR C97.3 2004 [54]	III	220	<ULN vs. ≥ULN	Yes	NR
OPTIMOX 1 2006 [59]	III	307	≤ULN vs. >ULN	Yes	HR 1.82 (1.45–2.27)
GONO 2007 [62]	III	57	<ULN vs. ≥ULN	No	NR
ITACa 2013 [71]	III	344	<ULN vs. ≥ULN	Yes	HR 1.55 (1.18–2.04)
FIRE 3 2014 [73] (*)	III	244	≤250 vs. >250	No	HR 1.18 (0.87–1.59)
MARTHA 2017 [76]	III	198	≤ULN vs. >ULN	No	OR 1.20 (0.56–2.63)

Legend: HR, hazard ratio. NR, not reported. OR, odds ratio. RR, risk ratio. ULN, upper limit normal. (*) RAS wild-type subgroup.

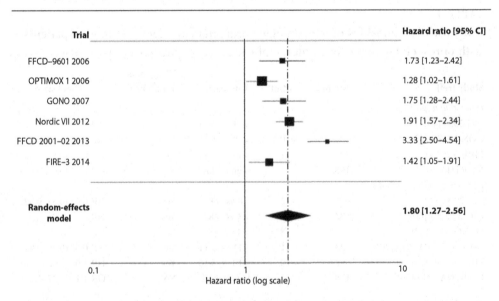

FIGURE 9.2   Forest plot of meta-analysis of alkaline phosphatase in prospective trials of patients with unresectable metastatic colorectal cancer

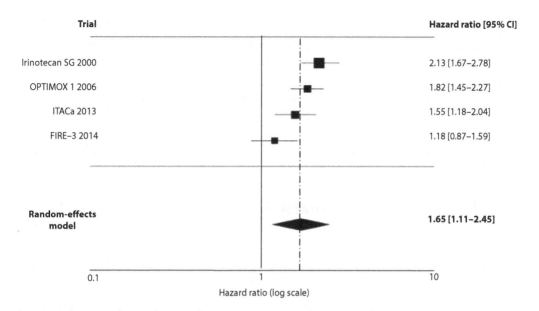

FIGURE 9.3   Forest plot of meta-analysis of lactic dehydrogenase in prospective trials of patients with unresectable metastatic colorectal cancer

TABLE 9.7

Prognostic relationships of serum carcinoembryonic antigen in selected studies of patients with unresectable metastatic colorectal cancer receiving upfront treatment

Study [ref]	Phase	No. pts	Comparison	Prognostic relationship	Effect size
EORTC 2000 [44]	III	192	≤ vs. > 10	No	NR
FOLFOX 2000 [45]	III	404	<5 vs. 5–50 vs. >50	Yes	RR 1.48
ISG 2000 [46]	III	656	< vs. ≥ 100	No	NR
GERCOR C97.3 2004 [54]	III	207	< vs. ≥ 10	Yes	NR
EORTC-CCG2 2006 [56]	III	513	≤ vs. > 10	Yes	NR
FFCD-9002 2006 [57]	III	171	≤ vs. >5	Yes	OR 0.65 (0.42–1.00)
FFCD-9601 2006 [58]	III	216	≤ vs. >30	No	HR 1.04 (0.75–1.46)
OPTIMOX-1 2006 [59]	III	589	≤ vs. >10	Yes	HR 0.57 (0.45–0.73)
GONO 2007 [62]	III	94	< vs. ≥100	No	NR
FFCD 2001–02 2013 [70]	III	123	≤ vs. >2UNL	Yes	HR 0.52 (0.39–0.69)
FIRE-3 2014 [73] (*)	III	356	≤ vs. > 6.4	No	HR 0.96 (0.88–1.05)
MARTHA 2017 [76]	III	200	continuous	No	OR 1.00 (0.99–1.00)

Legend: HR, hazard ratio. NR, not reported. OR, odds ratio. RR, risk ratio. ULN, upper limit normal. (*) RAS wild-type subgroup.

reporting HR, confirmed the significant overall ES (HR 1.65, CI 1.11–2.45; Q = 9.43, p-value = 0.0241; I^2 = 68.2%) (Figure 9.3). Two pooled analyses evaluated LDH and in both cases, a significant relationship with OS was highlighted [78, 79].

Each one among bilirubin [46], AST/ALT [45], and C-reactive protein (CRP) [71], reported a significant relationship with OS in single studies.

Twelve studies evaluated CEA, with cut-offs ranging from 5 to 100 ng/mL. Only six studies documented a prognostic relationship (Table 9.7). The meta-analysis of four studies reporting HR

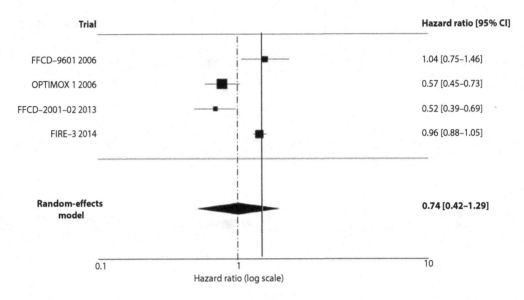

FIGURE 9.4 Forest plot of meta-analysis of carcinoembryonic antigen in prospective trials of patients with unresectable metastatic colorectal cancer

resulted in a not-significant relationship (HR 0.74, CI 0.42–1.29; Q = 30.11, p-value <0.0001; I^2 = 90.0%) (Figure 9.4). The conclusions of the pooled analyses are conflicting, with one reporting no relationship between CEA and OS [78] and the other correlating CEA >200 ng/mL with OS [82].

In the four studies evaluating CA 19-9, the cut-off was variable, and only in one case patients with elevated CA 19-9 had poor prognosis [70].

9.4 TUMOR-RELATED PROGNOSTIC FACTORS

9.4.1 TUMOR BURDEN

TB is inversely related to OS, but it remains difficult to measure. Primary tumor size is not a reliable criterion, given the inconsistent measurability, but some population-based studies reported a relationship [106, 107, 110], as for T4-stage [106], but not retrospective studies [112, 194]. In resectable mCRC, population-based studies documented a worse outcome for T4 [114] but not for tumor size [114, 115], similar to a prospective study [92]. In five retrospective studies, N-stage [117, 121] but not T-stage and tumor size [117, 119–122] correlated with poor OS.

A TB definition based on the area of liver metastases (LMs) >10 cm² was used in an RCT, but it needed to stratify the sample by the presence of LMs [195]. In patients with resectable LMs, an increasing number of resected LMs [117, 119] and maximum size >10 cm [117] were associated with poor prognosis.

Another issue with the TB measurement is the composition of the metastasis. The Immunoscore (IS) was inversely related to the number of metastases, but also to their size, due to the global immune densities change with the metastasis size. IS tends to be low in small metastases and affects more time to progression than metastasis size, as suggested by a study reporting that patients with high IS had longer OS despite having larger metastasis size, while mean immune cell density was higher in patients with more metastases [196].

Other not imaging-related variables have been used as a surrogate for TB, such as the mean number of metastatic sites, which increases from 1.4 at baseline to 2.6 at the time of the third mCRC progression [197]. Data from population-based registries [108, 198] and prospective studies confirmed the unfavorable prognosis with the increasing number of organs affected by the disease [83–85, 87], except for two studies [86, 88]. Similar conclusions came from 3/5 retrospective studies [89–91, 112,

113]. Even in resectable mCRC, the involvement of more than one organ has been associated with reduced OS [114], although not always significant [86, 121].

9.4.1.1 Selected trials

RCTs evaluated many TB-related PFs, such as number of metastasis sites (14 studies), liver-limited disease (LLD, 9 studies), presence of measurable disease (4 studies), percentage of liver involvement (LI, 4 studies), and lung-limited disease (2 studies) [72, 73], while the number of LMs [40], the number of metastases [52] were each evaluated in a single study.

The original Dukes stage did not affect the prognosis of patients with mCRC [43, 44, 56, 73].

In 13/14 studies that evaluated the number of sites of metastasis, the higher number of organs involved was significantly associated with OS (Table 9.8). Single vs. multiple site comparisons were available for 9 RCTs, and the meta-analysis concluded for a significant overall ES (HR 1.47, CI 1.31–1.65; $Q = 9.23$, p-value = 0.3232; $I^2 = 13.3\%$) (Figure 9.5). Among the five pooled analyses, three assessed the number of metastasis sites, and in all cases, this variable demonstrated a relationship with OS [78, 79, 82].

Nine studies reported the presence of LLD vs. LMs+EHD, of which five documented a worse prognosis for the second subgroup (Table 9.9), and a significant global ES (HR 0.77, CI 0.68–0.88; $Q = 2.63$, p-value = 0.6221; $I^2 = 0\%$) (Figure 9.6).

The presence of lung-limited disease was analyzed in two studies, and it did not correlate with OS [72, 73]. Conversely, divergent results reported the trials that investigated nodal-limited disease vs. other sites of metastasis [48, 72].

LI by mCRC was defined at a cut-off of 25% [44, 56, 62] or 30% [40], and in all RCTs, the relationship with poor prognosis was significant for patients with >25–30% LI.

The number of LMs was also associated with poor prognosis [40].

Four studies compared the prognosis of patients with measurable versus nonmeasurable disease, reporting two positive relationships with poor [34, 48] and two not [41, 72].

TABLE 9.8

Prognostic relationships of the number of sites of metastasis in selected studies of patients with unresectable metastatic colorectal cancer receiving upfront treatment

Study [ref]	Phase	No. pts	Comparison	Prognostic relationship	Effect size
EORTC 2000 [44]	III	200	≥3 vs. 2 vs. 1	Yes	NR
FOLFOX 2000 [45]	III	420	≥2 vs. 1	Yes	RR 1.34
ISG 2000 [46]	III	679	≥2 vs. 1	Yes	HR 1.49 (1.20–1.85)
V-303 2000 [47]	III	385	≥3 vs. 1–2	Yes	HR 1.56 (1.09–2.23)
MDACC 2001 [49]	III	605	≥2 vs. 1	Yes	NR
SO14796 2001 [50]	III	602	≥2 vs. 1	Yes	NR
GOIM 9901 2005 [55]	III	360	≥2 vs. 1	Yes	HR 1.35 (1.02–1.77)
EORTC-CC G2 2006 [56]	III	564	≥2 vs. 1	Yes	HR 1.67 (1.37–2.00)
FFCD-9002 2006 [57]	III	171	≥3 vs. 1–2	Yes	OR 1.97 (1.11–3.51)
FFCD-9601 2006 [58]	III	216	≥2 vs. 1	Yes	HR 1.49 (1.10–2.00)
OPTIMOX 1 2006 [59]	III	619	≥2 vs. 1	Yes	HR 1.28 (1.04–1.56)
HCOG 2012 [68]	III	251	2 vs. 1	Yes	HR 1.58 (1.05–2.37)
		202	≥3 vs. 1	Yes	HR 2.60 (1.50–4.50)
FFCD 2001–02 2013 [70]	III	217	≥2 vs. 1	Yes	HR 1.85 (1.33–2.56)
		182	>2 vs. 2	Yes	HR 1.64 (1.16–2.27)
SOFT 2013 [72]	III	511	≥2 vs. 1	No	HR 1.04 (0.72–1.54)

Legend: HR, hazard ratio. NR, not reported. OR, odds ratio. RR, risk ratio.

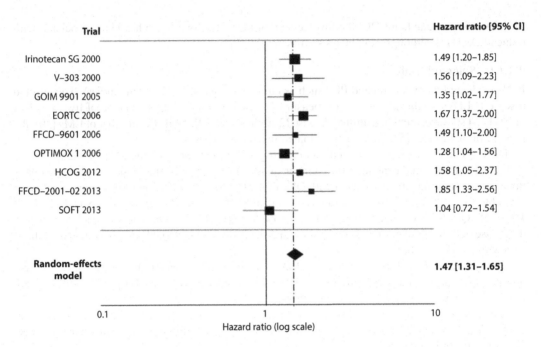

FIGURE 9.5   Forest plot of meta-analysis of the number of sites of metastasis in prospective trials of patients with unresectable metastatic colorectal cancer

9.4.2   Primary tumor location

The classification of tumor location along the colon has shifted from a categorization in colon vs. rectum to right- vs. left-sided tumors, separated by splenic flexure. Most of the evidence argues for a worse prognosis of right-sided CRC, and this would be valid regardless of gender and age, except for the oldest. However, the large bowel should be considered as a continuum rather than as two or three subsections in terms of molecular and clinical-pathologic features [154], and only cecal tumors, very rich in RAS mutations, could be considered a different subgroup [199].

Various population-based studies reported a poor prognosis of right-sided tumors [106, 107, 109, 110, 200], and only one article a reduced OS of colic vs. rectal cancers [105]. Among prospective analyses, one documented longer OS for RCs [84], while others did not find differences between colic and rectal sites [85, 175], or between right and left-sided [88]. According to the AIO-KRK-0104 trial, the favorable prognosis of left-sided mCRC could be limited to wild-type KRAS tumors [201]. One of two retrospective studies found worse outcomes for right-sided [90, 113], but the outcome of colic and rectal mCRCs was superimposable [91, 112]. Even in resectable mCRC, the right-sided tumors expressed shorter median OS [115, 117], while similar outcomes were found between colon vs. rectum [92, 116, 119–121].

The pattern of metastases differed too, since left-sided mCRCs were predominantly associated with liver and lung metastases, while right-sided with peritoneal and other sites [201]. Mucinous carcinoma was more frequent among right-sided [150, 192, 202], as well as MSI-H. Despite minimal differences between the colon and rectum [203], clinical and molecular characteristics between the various CRC locations were significant, as Consensus Molecular Subgroups 1 (CMS1) prevails in the right colon and CMS2 in the left [202].

Primary tumor location is also a predictive variable, as palliative primary tumor resection (PTR) improved survival of left-sided CRC patients but not right-sided [205], and anti-EGFR antibodies are more active in left-sided tumors [35].

TABLE 9.9
Prognostic relationships of liver-limited disease in selected studies of patients with unresectable metastatic colorectal cancer receiving upfront treatment

Study [ref]	Phase	No. pts	Comparison	Prognostic relationship	Effect size
EORTC-CCG1 2000 [44]	III	200	LLD vs. liver-plus	No	NR
V-303 2000 [47]	III	338	LLD vs. other sites	No	NR
FUMA-3008 2002 [51]	III	981	LLD vs. other	Yes	HR 0.83 (0.70–0.97)
GERCOR C97.3 2004 [54]	III	220	LLD vs. other	Yes	NR (°)
GONO 2007 [62]	III	122	LLD vs. not	No	HR 0.75 (0.49–1.15)
PRIME 2010 [64]	III	475	LLD vs. liver plus	No	OR 0.28 (0.04–2.26)
			LLD vs. other only	Yes	OR 0.11 (0.01–0.85)
FIRE-3 2014 [73] (*)	III	400	LLD vs. non-LLD	Yes	HR 0.67 (0.49–0.91)
TRIBE 2014 [74]	III	508	LLD vs. not	Yes	HR 0.66 (0.49–0.90)
TRIBE-2 2020 [77]	III	520	LLD vs. not	No	HR 0.79 (0.60–1.03)

Legend: HR, hazard ratio. LLD, liver-limited disease. NR, not reported. OR, odds ratio. (°), p-value <0.05. (*) RAS wild-type subgroup.

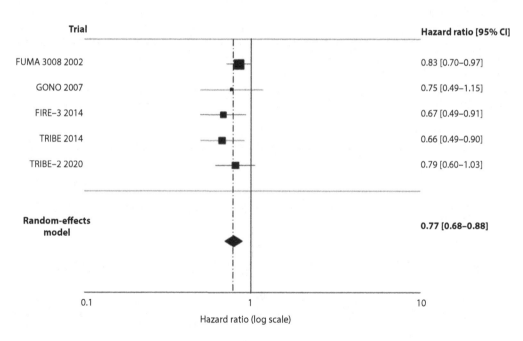

FIGURE 9.6   Forest plot of meta-analysis of liver-limited disease in prospective trials of patients with unresectable metastatic colorectal cancer

9.4.2.1   Selected trials

Nineteen trials evaluated the location of the primary tumor (Table 9.10). Due to the different comparisons, two separate analyses were done, colon vs. rectum and right-sided vs. left-sided. The first meta-analysis resulted in reduced OS for patients with colon cancer, with a significant overall ES (HR 1.16, CI 1.01–1.32; Q = 1.25, p-value = 0.7408; I^2 = 0%), while the other resulted in a poor prognosis of proximal malignancies (HR 1.31, CI 1.04–1.65; Q = 3.11, p-value = 0.3754; I^2 = 3.5%) (Figure 9.7).

TABLE 9.10

Prognostic relationships of the primary tumor location in selected studies of patients with unresectable metastatic colorectal cancer receiving upfront treatment

Study [ref]	Phase	No. pts	Comparison	Prognostic relationship	Effect size
EORTC 1996 [42]	III	276	Colon vs. Rectosigm	No	RR 0.84 (0.65–1.10)
RMH 1997 [43]	III	195	Colon vs. Rectum	No	NR
EORTC 2000 [44]	III	200	Colon vs. Rectum	No	NR
FOLFOX 2000 [45]	III	416	Colon vs. Rectum	No	NR
ISG 2000 [46]	III	671	Colon vs. Rectum	No	NR
V-303 2000 [47]	III	385	Colon vs. Rectum	No	NR
ECOG 2290 2001 [48]	III	1120	Right vs. Left	Yes	HR 1.50
EORTC-CCG2 2006 [56]	III	813	Colon vs. Rectum	No	NR
FFCD-9002 2006 [57]	III	171	Desc vs. Rect+asc	No	OR 1.52 (0.98–2.36)
FFCD-9601 2006 [58]	III	172	Proximal vs. Distal	Yes	HR 1.52 (1.08–2.13)
		105	Proximal vs. Rectum		HR 1.67 (1.08–2.50)
GONO 2007 [62]	III	244	Colon vs. Rectum	No	HR 1.16 (0.88–1.56)
FIRE 1 2011 [67]	III	423	Midgut vs. Hindgut	Yes	HR 1.54
HCOG 2012 [68]	III	262	Colon vs. Rectum	No	NR
Nordic VII 2012 [69]	III	457	Colon vs. Rectum	No	HR 1.20 (0.99–1.47)
SOFT 2013 [72]	III	342	Colon vs. Rectosigm	No	HR 1.19 (0.87–1.64)
		423	Colon vs. Rectum	No	HR 1.03 (0.80–1.33)
FIRE 3 2014 [73] (*)	III	566	Colon vs. Rectum	No	HR 1.27 (0.92–1.76)
TRIBE 2014 [74]	III	508	Right vs. Left	Yes	HR 1.47 (1.15–1.89)
MARTHA 2017 [76]	III	201	Right vs. Left	No	OR 1.51 (0.57–4.04)
TRIBE-2 2020 [77]	III	520	Right vs. Left	No	HR 1.14 (0.88–1.45)

Legend: HR, hazard ratio. NR, not reported. OR, odds ratio. RR, risk ratio. (*) RAS wild-type subgroup.

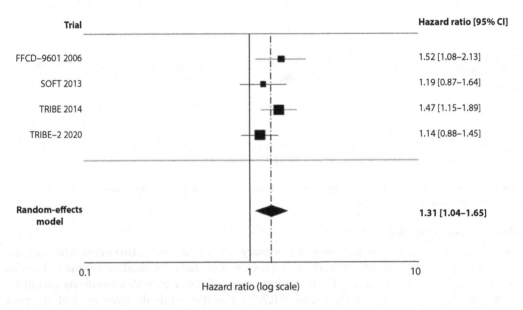

FIGURE 9.7 Forest plot of meta-analysis of primary tumor location in prospective trials of patients with unresectable metastatic colorectal cancer

Of the five pooled analyses, three evaluated primary tumor location, but only one reported a prognostic effect [82]. Furthermore, another pooled analysis of six trials of RAS wild-type mCRC receiving chemotherapy+EGFRi, showed a poor outcome of right-sided, with left-sidedness predicting the efficacy of EGFRi [206].

9.4.3 TIMING OF METASTASIS

To date, there is no clear definition of SMs in mCRC [207, 208], with a meta-analysis identifying 17 different definitions and an increasing percentage of SMs in clinical trials [208]. Approximately 15–25% of patients with CRC are diagnosed with SMs and another 10–20% develop metachronous metastases (MMs) [108, 209, 210]. Generally, data relating to MMs derive from studies of hospital units, but a population-based cohort from a French registry revealed a progressive MMs reduction from 18.6% in 1976–1980 to 10% in 2006–2011, contrary to SMs which remained at 17% [211]. Conversely, a Dutch population study reported an increasing percentage of SMs over time, mainly lung metastases [209].

As expected from the mortality data, the incidence of SMs is higher in males [135–137, 211], with more pronounced differences in the elderly in a Chinese study [212] but not in a Taiwanese exploring resectable mCRC [120].

Various population-based studies have reported a poor prognosis for SMs vs. MMs [108, 136, 209, 211, 214, 215], despite similar trends of improving 5-year survival [216]. The progressive OS improvement of mCRC patients with MMs [211] seems controversial for "late MMs", occurring after at least 12 months after CRC diagnosis [136, 213]. In most cases, the analyses of the single studies concluded that no prognostic role was played by the timing of metastases [45, 46, 54, 55, 212, 217] or for better outcomes of MMs [218–221]. Two of four retrospective studies suggested longer OS for patients with MMs [113, 117, 120, 122]. On the contrary, in studies of resectable mCRCs, no survival difference by timing of metastasis was evident [92, 118].

Despite reporting conflicting outcomes, clinical trials confirm the more aggressive characteristics of SMs [85, 222] as tumor registries [223] but did not suggest distinctive biological features of SMs [222]. In general, the differences that could explain the poor prognosis, or at least the different biology, of SM vs. MM, have been poorly studied [120, 224]. R0 resection appeared more likely in patients with MMs, and the OS improvement could be limited to the subgroup not receiving chemotherapy [108].

The explanations proposed by the various authors regarding the poor prognosis of SMs are not univocal. According to some authors, a significant moderating effect on the relationship is played by the primary tumor, because only in the presence of a primary tumor SMs were associated with poor prognosis [85, 225–227]. This finding was confirmed by a meta-analysis [228], and an IPDA [229]. On the other hand, PTR is not a significant PF in other studies with unresectable SMs [230, 231], even though after PTR other authors confirm an improvement in the prognosis of SMs mCRC patients [85, 222, 227, 232, 233]. A study of patients with LMs demonstrated that in the presence of the primary tumor, the liver adjacent to the metastasis replicated a proangiogenic environment [234].

Other characteristics might influence differently the SM and MM outcome, such as CEA expression [235–237], sidedness [238], size, number, and distribution of LMs [120]. For MM, the lymph node status of the resected primary tumor [235, 237], T-stage [120, 226, 227], symptoms and a lead time bias [239] could also affect outcomes.

While KRAS does not interfere with SM vs. MM [240], MSI-H correlates with a reduced risk of SMs [241], that was limited to LMs. However, MSI-H mCRC patients with SMs had similar outcomes of MSS [241].

9.4.3.1 Selected trials

Six studies evaluated the timing of metastasis (Table 9.11). Only one study found a significant OS reduction for patients with SMs [74]. Three of the five pooled analyses assessed timing, without detecting a relationship with OS [79, 81, 82].

TABLE 9.11

Prognostic relationships of the timing of metastasis in selected studies of patients with unresectable metastatic colorectal cancer receiving upfront treatment

Study [ref]	Phase	No. Pts	Comparison	Prognostic relationship	Effect size
EORTC-CCG1 2000 [44]	III	200	Metachr vs. Synchr	No	NR
FOLFOX 2000 [45]	III	414	Metachr vs. Synchr	No	NR
GOIM 9901 2005 [55]	III	360	Metachr vs. Synchr	No	HR 1.05 (0.76–1.46)
FIRE-3 2014 [73] (*)	III	400	Metachr vs. Synchr	No	HR 0.97 (0.64–1.45)
TRIBE 2014 [74]	III	508	Metachr vs. Synchr	Yes	HR 0.61 (0.36–1.06)
TRIBE-2 2020 [77]	III	520	Metachr vs. Synchr	No	HR 1.10 (0.75–1.61)

Legend: HR, hazard ratio. Metachr, metachronous. NR, not reported. Synchr, synchronous. (*) RAS wild-type subgroup.

9.4.4 SITE OF METASTASIS

Generally, LMs represent the most frequent site of metastasis, followed by lung, lymph node, and peritoneum, while other sites are rare [197], but primary tumor location and timing of metastases influence the pattern. In general, peritoneal, brain, and bone metastases were reported to have a poor prognosis [242], while lung metastases seem to be associated with better OS than LMs [243–245].

Extra-hepatic metastases are predominantly localized in the peritoneum and lung, and are more frequent among females, with different metastatic patterns according to age. Female genital tract localizations prevail in young women, while lymph node and bone metastases are more frequent among males [141].

The TNM classification distinguishes three categories of M1, and a series of 814 mCRC patients confirmed the prognostic validity of the M1 categories, with 2-year survival rates of 52%, 39% and 22%, respectively [246].

Molecular characteristics of mCRC differ by site of metastasis too. Besides CEA expression, higher in the primary tumor and in LMs and lower in lung metastases [247], among KRAS-mutated mCRC, the lung was more frequent as the first site of metastasis than liver and lymph nodes [242, 248], with increasing KRAS mutation discordance between primary tumor and lung metastases compared to that between primary tumor and metastases in other sites (32% vs. 12%) [248]. On the other hand, BRAF mutation was strongly related to peritoneal metastases and rarely present in lung and liver metastases, while LMs were less frequent among MSI-H mCRC patients [242].

9.4.4.1 Liver metastases

A large NCDB analysis concluded that in mCRC patients LMs predicted a shorter OS than lung metastases [249]. Other population-based analyses confirmed the poor OS of mCRC with LMs [83, 106, 109, 110]. The prognostic role was confirmed by others [84, 111], but not by every study [86, 90, 112]. Among patients with resectable mCRC, only one of three retrospective studies reported a poor OS for patients with bilateral LMs [119, 120, 122], whereas the occurrence of LMs conferred the same prognosis as other sites of metastases in other experiences [118, 121].

Up to 70% of R0-resected mCRC patients with LMs have a recurrence [250]. After radical resection of LMs, a study documented how progression is predominantly hepatic, but is more related to systemic dissemination than to failure of local therapy [251].

The possibility of a cure after liver metastasectomy has led to the development of a series of composite indicators to predict the prognosis of patients with LMs from CRC [252–254]. Nevertheless, all prognostic scores are not predictive of OS in patients undergoing multimodal treatments [255].

High NLR and dNLR resulted in unfavorable PFs in a series of 302 patients with resectable LMs [256]. KRAS and MSI-H were associated with poor OS in the case of LLD whether the primary tumor was left-sided or rectal [249]. In resectable mCRC, a meta-analysis concluded that the occurrence of RAS or BRAF mutation was negative PF [257–259].

9.4.4.2 Lung metastases

Lung metastases did not show a clear prognostic effect in mCRC. Population-based studies suggest a poor prognosis [106] with increased rates of early death [109, 110], as does a retrospective study [111]. Conversely, other authors report favorable outcomes [84, 113]. In resectable disease, the presence of lung metastases in patients with LMs does not seem to reduce OS [117]. Pulmonary metastasectomy was associated with a 5-year survival rate of 50% [260].

The single lesion was the most important favorable PF, while there was an inverse correlation between the number of metastases, hilar/mediastinal nodal involvement, CEA levels and OS [261]. Other studies investigated different variables, suggesting a favorable prognostic effect for low serum CEA levels [262], and left-sided primary tumors [242, 249], but rectal origin [242, 249] and inflammatory parameters [118] were controversial.

The lung microenvironment suppresses CEA expression and promotes the nuclear localization of beta-catenin by favoring the WNT pathway [247], but the relationship between RAS mutations and lung metastases is unclear. However, mCRC patients with RAS mutation in codon-12 reported longer survival after lung resection [263].

9.4.4.3 Peritoneal metastases

Up to 15% of mCRC patients are diagnosed with peritoneal metastases, and a general global improvement in their prognosis has been registered [264].

The occurrence of peritoneal metastases was independently associated with poor prognosis [83]. Similar conclusions were reached by prospective [84] and retrospective studies [90, 111, 112], also in resectable mCRC [121]. The extent of peritoneal involvement [265] and the presence of of extra-peritoneal disease [266, 267] furtherly reduced OS. After peritoneal surgery and hyperthermic intraperitoneal chemotherapy, a meta-analysis documented only three PFs (primary tumor obstruction/perforation, peritoneal extension, completeness of cytoreduction) [268].

Among the patients with peritoneal-limited disease, the female gender prevailed, but also colic vs. rectal origin and poor PS [269], as well as right-sided tumors [242]. Other studies suggested a prognostic effect also for N-stage, PS and histotype [267], rectal origin [270].

Tumor cells in peritoneal metastases display peculiar characteristics: they can survive as floating single cells, adhere and invade, create an angiogenesis-driven microenvironment, and evade immunosurveillance. In the context of CMS, peritoneal metastases are predominantly CMS4 (75%) [271], furtherly classified into three molecular subgroups (PM.A or RAS-mutated; PM.B or mucinous; PM.C or inflammation-related) [272]. RAS-mutated mCRC with peritoneal dissemination has a poor prognosis [273], but BRAF mutations are more represented among patients with peritoneal dissemination [269].

9.4.4.4 Ovarian metastases

Ovarian metastases are rare in mCRC (3.4%) [274], are present at diagnosis in 0.6–1.1% [275], and are associated with high lethality [274]. The risk appears to be higher in young and premenopausal patients. A cohort of young patients (<55 years) evaluated in six Dutch hospitals documented a risk of ovarian metastases from CRC of 5% (10/200 patients), with a 5-year survival of 40% [276]. The role of prophylactic salpingo-oophorectomy in postmenopausal patients with CRC is unclear [277].

9.4.4.5 Bone metastases

Bone involvement is rare, interesting 5% or less of mCRC patients [278, 279], and is usually associated with high TB. However, its incidence is increasing [280], and population-based studies suggest poor prognosis [106], higher early death rates [109, 110], with similar findings from retrospective analyses [111], and median OS of 17 months, that is reduced when synchronous [279].

Bone metastases occur often in left-sided and rectal tumors [242]. They are multiple in 73% and associated with extra-osseous disease in 87% [279], with their increasing number having a negative impact on OS [281].

9.4.4.6 Brain metastases

Brain metastases affect 2% of mCRC patients [282], up to 14.6% in late mCRC, but a brain-limited disease at the onset of mCRC is rare [283]. In 70% they originate from a left-sided CRC, prevail in males and at a median age of 60 [282].

Population-based studies documented poor prognosis [106, 109, 110]. Some unfavorable PFs have been reported, such as the high number of metastases, advanced age, poor PS, left-sided tumors [282, 284, 285], pre-existing lung metastases [282], high CEA levels [286], extra-cerebral metastases and lack of regional treatments [287].

Brain metastases from CRC are localized in the posterior regions or cerebellum [288]. From a molecular point of view, they seem to express clones independent from those of the primary tumor [289]. The primary tumors more often present RAS mutations and RAS mutations increase even more in brain metastasis, while the lymphocytic infiltration of CD3 and CD8 decreases [290].

9.4.4.7 Selected trials

Seven studies investigated the prognostic role of LMs, as resumed in Table 9.12. Five studies evaluated LMs, even in the presence of other sites, comparing cases with LI vs. not [45, 46, 48, 52, 72], reporting in two studies a significant poor OS for LI [48, 52], while two evaluated the "liver predominant" disease, which in both correlated with poor prognosis [49, 50].

An analysis of the TRIBE and TRIBE-2 trials showed the occurrence of bone metastases in 41/1187 patients (3.5%), with a significant OS reduction, even more pronounced when bone metastasis was the first site of relapse [291].

9.4.5 PATHOLOGY

Most data reported in mCRC studies refer to pathological variables found in the previously resected primary tumor or to limited biopsy examination. However, other histopathological characteristics of the metastases have been more studied.

TABLE 9.12

Prognostic relationships of the liver involvement in selected studies of patients with unresectable metastatic colorectal cancer receiving upfront treatment

Study [ref]	Phase	No. pts	Comparison	Prognostic relationship	Effect size
FOLFOX 2000 [45]	III	420	Liver involvement vs. not	No	NR
ISG 2000 [46]	III	683	Liver involvement vs. not	No	NR
ECOG 2001 [48]	III	1098	Liver metastasis vs. not	Yes	NR
MDACC 2001 [49]	III	605	Liver predominant vs. not	Yes	NR
SO14796 2001 [50]	III	602	Liver predominant vs. not	Yes	NR
HeCOG 2002 [52]	III	191	Liver metastasis vs. not	Yes	NR
SOFT 2013 [72]	III	311	Liver metastasis vs. not	No	HR 1.27 (0.90–1.78)

Legend: HR, hazard ratio. NR, not reported.

9.4.5.1 Histology

Adenocarcinoma is the prevalent histotype. In three population-based studies, non-adenocarcinomas were associated with reduced OS [106] and increased early death rates [110], but prognostic differences did not occur in other studies [85, 112]. In resectable mCRC, reports on the outcome of mucinous neoplasms and signet ring cell carcinoma are discordant [114, 115].

The mucinous variant of adenocarcinoma is the most frequent (10–15%) [292], prevailing in females and early stages [293]. It has been related to a poor prognosis [107, 294], similar for both sexes, with less difference in the elderly, which in part can be explained by the primary tumor location [150, 192, 202].

Physiologically, the production of mucin is higher in the right colon, and consequently, the mucinous variants are more frequent among right-sided CRC [293, 294], with increased MSI-H tumors up to 33% [153]. Increased chemoresistance is typical of the mucinous phenotype, as it shows differential expression of metabolism and drug resistance genes. Genes related to fluorouracil metabolism (TYMS, TYMP, DYPD) and other genes were more expressed, while oxaliplatin-related genes (ATP7B, SRPK1) were reduced [295].

9.4.5.2 Tumor grade

Tumor grading is a variable that includes tumor differentiation, degree of anaplasia, nature of the tumor margin, and small vessel invasion. Although related, tumor grading and tumor differentiation are not super-imposable. In addition to the changing definition over time, tumor grading is consistently dependent on the judgment of the pathologist.

Various studies have reported an independent prognostic effect of tumor grading in CRC [296–299], but there are few evaluations in mCRC. Six population-based analyses found a poor prognosis of patients with G3 or G3–G4 tumors [105–107, 198], and an increasing early death rate [109, 110]. Except the CAIRO trial [85], other retrospective experiences support the negative prognostic role of G3 [90, 111]. Even among resectable mCRC patients a G3 or G3–G4 predicted poor outcomes in almost all the analyses [114, 115, 120, 121, 300].

9.4.5.3 Other pathological variables

Some patient-related variables, mostly linked to the composition of the tumor microenvironment (TME), have been studied in mCRC.

IS is a score based on the quantization of cytotoxic and memory T-cells in the core of the primary tumor and its invasive margin [301]. This score has also been evaluated in mCRC and has been associated with fewer metastases, suggesting that immunity within metastases was not lost [196]. IS predicts OS after curative resection of the metastases [302]. In some molecular subgroups of mCRC, this influence on prognosis was so important that IS outperformed other variables, such as MSI-H, in predicting OS [303]. However, it is difficult to conclude about the utility of IS in treatment-refractory mCRC, considering the complexity of the immune landscape. IS is heterogeneous among metastases from the same patient, but the density of CD8 and CD20 is rather homogeneous within the same metastasis, high-density CD8 and low-density CD20 being associated with longer OS, but higher is the CD8 spatial heterogeneity poorer is the prognosis [196]. In addition to the relationship with the number and size of metastases [302], a higher IS in the most recent metastases correlated with a lower number of metastases. In turn, the composition of the infiltrative margin of the metastases was affected by the previous exeresis of primary tumor and metastases. Although IS does not predict the efficacy of systemic treatment, in RAS wild-type mCRC the lymphocyte composition and activated genes change depending on the upfront regimen (EGFRi- or bevacizumab-based), with higher IS after EGFRi [196].

Differently than lymphovascular invasion in localized disease [304], the distribution of lymphocyte populations within metastases was poorly studied, but changes of specific immune densities within the tumor are common [305]. The favorable prognostic role of tumor-infiltrating lymphocytes (TILs) is related to their presence and density in the primary tumor and metastases [112, 303,

306, 307]. Similarly, the presence of tertiary lymphoid structures (TLS) in the TME was associated with longer OS, with TLS at the metastasis margin of LMs associated with PFS, in particular CD3+ T-cells [308]. Besides different TLS compositions by site of metastasis, the spatial location of TLS was important [309–311], suggesting that the antigen-presenting cells must be close to T-cell activation sites and that this mechanism could drive response to treatments [307, 312, 313].

Finally, the histopathological growth pattern (HGP) of LMs is a morphological classification of how tumor cells interact with surrounding normal liver tissue. Three morphological features have been distinguished, as desmoplastic, pushing, and replacement [314, 315]. Various studies have reported an effect of HGPs on mCRC prognosis [316], with the pushing pattern associated with shorter OS [317], while other authors identified the replacement pattern as predictive and PF [318, 319], and various authors describing HGP-specific immune responses [320, 321].

9.4.5.4 Molecular biology

Any deficit of the MMR system produces the typical DNA phenotype of MSI-H, which is associated with different cancerogenesis and tumor prognosis. MSI-H was reported in 3.1% of mCRC patients [322], with higher rates in the elderly [212]. Despite its rarity, MSI-H has been independently associated with OS and predicted response to immunotherapy [323]. Within MSI-H mCRC patients, two subgroups have been suggested, that have common clinicopathologic features, but differ by age, multifocality, stage, and BRAF mutations [324].

Various alterations at the MAPK pathway are relevant, both for prognostic and predictive roles. Beyond their role in mCRC diagnosis, the MAPK pathway by ctDNA is increasingly evaluated in the management of late mCRC. RAS mutation is present in 40–50% of mCRC. Mutation rates vary by primary tumor location and by geographical area [322]. Data from prospective studies agree on the poor prognosis of patients with RAS mutated [83, 87], but it is more relevant as a predictive variable of non-response to EGFRi. BRAF gene has a mutation in 10% of mCRC. The mutational state of BRAF-V600E is a well-characterized predictive and PF, because V600E mutation results in aggressive tumors reporting less chemotherapy activity [83, 113], whereas mCRCs with a BRAF non-V600E mutation have different characteristics [325]. Genetic profiles suggested two different molecular subgroups among BRAF-V600E-mutated mCRC [326], and a less pronounced prognostic effect in patients with a concomitant MSI-H [327]. In the upfront setting, BRAF mutation status predicts resistance to anti-EGFR antibodies too, and, after the introduction of encorafenib in the treatment of refractory mCRC in 2019, it defines the therapeutic strategy.

The CMS system is a transcriptome-based classifier of CRC. These genetic profiles were defined on a sample of localized CRCs [328], but in mCRC CMSs reported different impacts and profiles [204, 329]. In particular, in mCRC, except peritoneal metastases, the transcriptome analysis of primary tumors and metastases showed that the metastases are depleted of CMS1 and CMS3 and rich in CMS4 [330] so some authors have also proposed a colorectal adenocarcinoma metastasis-specific gene-expression signature [331], while others suggest introducing subtype-specific prognostic biomarkers [332]. LMs are predominantly CMS2 (>60%) or CMS4 and analysis of transcriptomic profiles revealed differences with the primary tumor and similarities with normal liver tissue [333]. A retrospective analysis of the FIRE-3 trial evaluated CMS confirming the prognostic role of the classification, and detecting predictive effects, as CMS4 and CMS3 were associated with more activity of EGFRi vs. bevacizumab [204]. Other posthoc analyses of RCTs revealed that EGFRi is active in association with irinotecan in left tumors with CMS2/3 and CMS4 and in right-sided with CMS4, while the association of EGFRi with oxaliplatin was active in the right-sided tumors with a CMS2/3 [334]. Other evidence about the predictive effect of CMS concerns various drugs, such as irinotecan for CMS4 [329, 335, 336], bevacizumab [337] or pembrolizumab [323] for CMS1, EGFRi for CMS2, bevacizumab for CMS2 and CMS3 [338].

Although CIMP is defined by a phenotype of global genome hypermethylation in CpG islands, the complex network of silencing of multiple genes has made its interpretation considerably complicated [339]. A recent systematic review of large studies reported that 18.3% of mCRC were

CIMP-H, and had a significantly poor OS in patients with a stage III-IV MSS CRC [340], with fluorouracil resistance.

9.4.5.5 Selected trials

Six RCTs evaluated tumor grade (Table 9.13). Four studies found a relationship between grade and OS.

Of the selected studies, four evaluated RAS mutational status, which correlated with prognosis in three [61, 69, 74, 75], as in a pooled analysis of five AIO trials [341].

Among the selected trials, the BRAF mutation was always associated with a significantly poor outcome in all the five studies and the pooled analysis that evaluated it [61, 64, 69, 71, 75, 341].

A retrospective analysis of the FIRE-3 study evaluated CMS, which was a significant PF for all outcome measures [204]. The prognostic role of CMS appears independent of that of other variables such as RAS and BRAF, as reported by an analysis of the TRIBE study [77].

9.4.6 PREVIOUS TREATMENTS

9.4.6.1 Primary tumor resection

With the expansion of therapeutic options for mCRC, a SEER-based analysis documented a reduction over time of PTR, but a better OS/CSS [342]. The reduction of PTR has been progressive [343], and practice changes could have reduced and made the benefit of PTR hardly noticeable.

Recently, two RCTs did not report any benefit from PTR in asymptomatic mCRC with unresectable metastases [344, 345]. On the contrary, various small non-randomized studies and a meta-analysis documented a prognostic benefit from PTR [346], that appeared particularly accentuated with low LI and in females, especially if they received more intense chemotherapy regimens [347]. Still, three population-based analyses support the favorable effect of PTR on OS [105, 106, 110], and other studies on PFS after chemotherapy, without OS improvement [347, 348], as well as posthoc analyses of RCTs [233, 349] and some retrospective studies [350–352] while other did not [353–356].

Several authors have documented a positive predictive effect of PTR on bevacizumab-based regimen activity [351, 357–363], but other studies did not [354, 355, 364]. In addition, PTR was associated with more pronounced chemosensitivity of the RAS-mutated mCRCs [350–352, 355, 356].

Primary tumors can favor SIR, which in turn promotes drug resistance, as inferred by high values of inflammatory indices [365, 366], or by NLR reduction in 55% of mCRC patients undergoing PTR [367]. Other authors suggest evaluating the possible role of other variables in the selection of PTR candidates, such as CEA [111, 368], LDH [233, 368], site of metastases, albumin, and histological features.

TABLE 9.13

Prognostic relationships of the tumor grading in selected studies of patients with unresectable metastatic colorectal cancer receiving upfront treatment

Study [ref]	Phase	No. pts	Scale	Comparison	Prognostic relationship	Effect size
NCCTG 1989 [34]	III	419	Broder	G1/G2 vs. G3/G4	Yes	NR (°)
NCCTG 1994 [41]	III	362	Broder	G1/G2 vs. G3/G4	Yes	NR (°)
RMH 1997 [43]	III	187	Differ	G1 vs. G2 vs. G3	No	NR
ECOG-2290 2001 [48]	III	1120	Differ	G1 vs. G2 vs. G3	Yes	NR (°)
SOFT 2013 [72]	III	293	Differ	G1/G2 vs. G3	Yes	HR 2.72 (1.67–4.44)
MARTHA 2017 [76]	III	200	Differ	G1/G2 vs. G3	No	OR 1.84 (0.89–3.80)

Legend: Differ, differentiation grade. G, grade. HR, hazard ratio. NR, not reported. OR, odds ratio. (°). P-value <0.05.

9.4.6.2   Previous adjuvant therapies

The prognostic effect on patients with mCRC of prior adjuvant chemotherapy is unclear, with a favorable effect on OS from population-based [106, 107] but not in prospective studies [87, 175], that rather report detrimental effects from previous adjuvant chemotherapy [83].

Timing from adjuvant chemotherapy to relapse appears crucial in affecting mCRC prognosis, particularly in stage III younger patients receiving fewer cycles of oxaliplatin-based adjuvant chemotherapy [369], even though early relapse was more important than oxaliplatin dose [370]. Similarly, in the pre-oxaliplatin era, the ACCENT data set also documented that progression within 6 months was associated with poor OS [371]. However, a possible relationship of OS with the overall regimen intensities can not be excluded [370, 372, 373].

Prior adjuvant radiotherapy has been evaluated in population-based studies as being associated with better outcomes of mCRC [105, 106, 110], while it did not change the prognosis of patients enrolled in the MACRO trial [135].

9.4.6.3   Previous treatments of metastatic disease

In population-based studies, previous resection of metastases had an unfavorable impact on prognosis if incomplete [108, 198]. However, mCRC patients who had previously received intervention for metastatic disease often had better outcomes [89, 105, 113] and reduced risk of early death [109].

In resectable disease, the benefit of neo-adjuvant chemotherapy emerged in some studies [115] but not in others [92, 117, 118, 122], and some emphasize the absence of progression as PF [117]. Similarly, positive [116, 117] and negative results are reported for postoperative adjuvant chemotherapy [92, 116–118, 121, 122].

9.4.6.4   Selected trials

Nine studies evaluated PTR, and only three documented a significant favorable prognostic effect (Table 9.14). A pooled analysis of the four trials that calculated an ES, resulted in a not statistically significant relationship (HR 0.67, CI 0.39–1.16; Q = 11.41, p-value = 0.0097; I^2 = 73.7%) (Figure 9.8). Two of the selected five pooled analyses evaluated PTR among the PFs, and in one it was significantly associated with longer OS [81]. Trials investigating a previous R0-surgery of the metastases were discordant, with no relationship in one [44] and a better outcome after R0-resection in the other [73].

None of the eight RCTs assessing previous adjuvant chemotherapy documented a relationship to OS (Table 9.14). Similarly, only one [73] of the four studies that evaluated previous adjuvant radiotherapy found a prognostic effect [42, 44, 45]. Nine studies analyzed the variable "previous adjuvant therapy" and did not find a prognostic effect [47, 55, 56, 62, 66, 73, 74, 77], except one [51].

Finally, from the studies that constructed a "DFI" variable between the diagnosis of mCRC and the start of chemotherapy [47, 76] or between diagnosis and recurrence [46, 47, 62], no significant relationship emerged with OS.

9.5   PROGNOSTIC FACTORS IN DECISION-MAKING

The mCRC is not always a lethal disease, but when a cure is possible this happens through local control of metastases, usually by surgery. Consequently, the goals of treatment of mCRC change depending on resectability, with different roles for PFs (Table 9.15).

9.5.1   RESECTABLE DISEASE

Current recommendations consist of surgery eventually associated with perioperative chemotherapy.

Although perioperative chemotherapy according to the FOLFOX regimen achieved the endpoint of improving DFS, it did not prolong OS [374], and the benefit was higher in patients with high TB

TABLE 9.14

Prognostic relationships of previous treatments in selected studies of patients with unresectable metastatic colorectal cancer receiving upfront treatment

Study [ref]	Phase	No. pts	Comparison	Prognostic relationship	Effect size
Primary tumor resection					
EORTC 1996 [42]	III	159	Not vs. Yes	Yes	RR 0.60
EORTC-CCG1 2000 [44]	III	200	Not vs. Yes	No	NR
V-303 2000 [47]	III	338	Not vs. Yes	No	NR
EORTC-CCG2 2006 [56]	III	560	Not vs. Yes	No	NR
FFCD-9601 2006 [58]	III	216	Not vs. Yes	Yes	HR 0.42 (0.30–0.60)
FIRE-3 2014 [73] (*)	III	396	Not vs. Yes	No	HR 0.98 (0.67–1.43)
TRIBE 2014 [74]	III	508	Not vs. Yes	Yes	HR 0.67 (0.55–0.82)
MARTHA 2017 [76]	III	200	Not vs. Yes	No	OR 1.58 (0.66–3.80)
TRIBE-2 2020 [77]	III	679	Not vs. Yes	No	HR 0.75 (0.56–1.01)
Adjuvant chemotherapy					
EORTC-CCG1 2000 [44]	III	200	Not vs. Yes	No	NR
FOLFOX 2000 [45]	III	420	Not vs. Yes	No	NR
Irinotecan SG 2000 [46]	III	683	Not vs. Yes	No	NR
HeCOG 2002 [52]	III	191	Not vs. Yes	No	NR
HeCOG 2012 [68]	III	285	Not vs. Yes	No	NR
SOFT 2013 [72]	III	511	Not vs. Yes	No	HR 1.20 (0.87–1.69)
MARTHA 2017 [76]	III	200	Not vs. Yes	No	OR 0.49 (0.16–1.49)
TRIBE-2 2020 [77]	III	679	Not vs. Yes	No	HR 0.67 (0.26–1.69)

Legend: HR, hazard ratio. NR, not reported. OR, odds ratio. RR, risk ratio. (*) RAS wild-type subgroup.

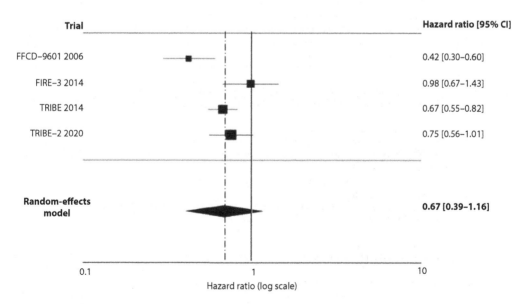

FIGURE 9.8 Forest plot of meta-analysis of primary tumor resection in prospective trials of patients with unresectable metastatic colorectal cancer

TABLE 9.15

Prognostic and predictive variables in clinical decision-making of microsatellite-stable unresectable metastatic colorectal cancer

Patients with potential conversion

1   Primary tumor status
- Resected (left-sided, RAS wt): EGFRi+CHT favored (EGFRi+CHT is better than CHT +/- BEV)
- Resected (liver-limited): triplet+BEV favored (triplet+BEV is better than doublet+BEV)

2   Primary tumor sidedness
- Right-sided: triplet+BEV favored (triplet+BEV is better than doublet+BEV)
- Right-sided (RAS wt, BRAF wt): consider EGFRi-based doublet as an option
- Left-sided: triplet+BEV favored (triplet+BEV is better than doublet+BEV)
- Left-sided (RAS wt): EGFRi+CHT favored (EGFRi+CHT is better than CHT +/- BEV)

3   Site of metastasis
- Liver-limited (RAS wt): EGFRi+CHT favored (EGFRi+CHT is better than CHT)
- Liver-limited: SIRT+CHT favored (SIRT+CHT is better than CHT)

4   Low tumor burden
- Consider pre-operative regional approaches (HAI, RFA)

Patients without potential conversion

A. Upfront systemic treatment

1   Local symptoms
- Occlusion / hemorrhage (high risk): consider primary tumor resection

2   Primary tumor sidedness
- Right-sided: triplet+BEV favored (triplet+BEV is better than doublet+BEV)
- Left-sided (RAS wt): EGFRi+CHT favored (EGFRi+CHT is better than CHT +/- BEV)
- Left-sided (RAS mt): triplet+BEV favored (triplet+BEV is better than doublet+BEV)

3   Site of metastasis
- Liver-limited (RAS wt): EGFRi+CHT favored (EGFRi+CHT is better than CHT)
- Liver-limited: SIRT+CHT favored (SIRT+CHT is better than CHT)

4   Uneligibility for doublets
- FUP+BEV favored (FUP+BEV is better than FUP)

B. Treatment of refractory disease

1   BRAF
- Mutated (V600E): encorafenib+cetuximab favored (encorafenib+cetuximab is better than FOLFIRI+cetuximab)

2   Previous upfront regimen
- BEV-based (PFS >9 months): doublet+BEV favored (doublet+BEV is better than doublet)
- Not BEV-based: doublet+aflibercept favored (doublet+aflibercept is better than doublet)
- Not EGFRi-based (RAS wt): EGFRi+irinotecan-based favored (EGFRi+irinotecan-based regimens are better than irinotecan-based)

3   Site of metastasis
- Liver-limited: consider TARE (TheraSphere) or SIRT (right-sided tumors)

4   Sex
- Male: doublet+BEV favored (doublet+BEV is better than doublet)
- Female: FOLFIRI+ramucirumab favored (FOLFIRI+ramucirumab is better than FOLFIRI)

C. Third-line treatment

1   Biologic characterization (liquid biopsy)
- HER2 over-expression: consider HER2-directed therapy
- RAS wt: consider EGFRi-based regimen rechallenge

2   Site of metastasis
- Liver-limited: DEBIRI favored (DEBIRI is better than CHT)

3   Previous upfront regimen
- No progression after upfront regimen: consider upfront regimen rechallenge
- Long TFI from EGFRi: consider EGFRi-based regimen rechallenge

4   Age
- Younger (<65): REG or FRU favored (REG/FRU are better than placebo)
- Elderly (>65): TAS-102 favored (TAS-102 is better than placebo)

Legend: BEV, bevacizumab. CHT, chemotherapy. DEBIRI, irinotecan-loaded drug-eluting beads. EGFRi, epidermal growth factor receptor inhibitor. FRU, fruquitinib. FUP, fluoropyrimidine. HAI, hepatic artery infusion. mt, mutated. PFS, progression-free survival. REG, regorafenib. RFA, radiofrequency ablation. SIRT, selective internal radiation therapy. TARE, trans-arterial radio-embolization. TAS-102, trifluridine/tipiracil. TFI, treatment-failure interval. wt, wild type.

(CEA >5; metastasis diameter >3 cm) and excellent PS [375]. In contrast, in wild-type RAS adding cetuximab to the doublet significantly reduced OS [376].

There is less evidence for lung metastases, with some retrospective data supporting regional ablative therapy, in particular for patients who are not candidates for surgery, males, those with lung-limited disease, and age >69 [377].

Similarly, systemic therapy after R0-surgery achieved DFS but no OS improvement, with 12 FOLFOX cycles improving DFS in young, males, left-sided, SMs, low TB (<4 metastases, size < 5 cm) and chemo-naive tumors [36].

9.5.2 Unresectable disease

In this clinical setting, it is necessary to define the reasons for non-resectability to understand whether cytoreduction may convert the disease to resectable. Outside contraindications related to patient characteristics, never-resectable cases are difficult to define at baseline, so conversion therapy is often proposed.

9.5.2.1 Potentially resectable disease

Conversion chemotherapy with response assessment every 2 months, possibly followed by surgery/locoregional treatment, is recommended. Chemotherapy may convert mCRC to resectable or at least amenable to a regional control with other treatment options [378].

The most appropriate conversion drug regimen varies depending on the characteristics of the patient and tumor, such as tumor sidedness and RAS status.

Although EGFRi+doublet was effective only in wild-type RAS mCRC, higher ORRs and early tumor shrinkage (ETS) occurred in left-sided tumors [379], and in CMS3/CMS4 [204]. However, conversion rates increase regardless of the biologic drug associated with chemotherapy [380], while the subgroup of right-sided mCRCs that benefit from doublet+EGFRi is undefined [381].

In unselected and RAS-mutated mCRC the triplet is superior to the doublet, especially for LMs [62, 382]. Bevacizumab-based combinations improved conversion rates [383, 384], and triplet+bevacizumab vs. doublet+bevacizumab improved ORR/ETS and OS, particularly in right-sided [385]. Among mCRC with unresectable LLD, OS correlated with R0/R1-resection of metastases but also with PTR and good PS [386]. Still, the combination of radiofrequency ablation with chemotherapy can improve outcomes in the presence of up to 9 LMs [387], and more and more studies are available for stereotactic ablative radiotherapy [388, 389]. Responses [379] and ablation margins [390] differ by metastasis sites.

9.5.2.2 Never resectable disease

Therapeutic plans in MSS mCRC without potential conversion, generally consist of a sequential strategy.

The occurrence of local symptoms supports the appropriateness of including PTR. In asymptomatic patients, PTR is usually not recommended, particularly in patients with ECOG PS 1/more and right-sided tumors [344, 391], and may increase 60-day mortality in the presence of increased AST/ALT, LDH and neutrophil count >8,300/mcL [392].

Although certain variables such as frailty and patient preference shall influence treatment strategies, tumor and patient characteristics help guide on the optimal sequence.

In the context of mCRC amenable only to medical therapy, a 2009 meta-analysis concluded that sequential rather than concomitant use of the available drugs did not reduce OS [93]. Consequently, many treatment studies in this setting used PFS and not OS as endpoints, and only recently have triplet+bevacizumab combinations as an upfront regimen shown increased OS [393].

9.5.2.2.1 Upfront treatment

Although 20% of MSI-H mCRC patients report poor early PFS with pembrolizumab compared to chemotherapy [394], it is impossible to identify these patients, so pembrolizumab should be considered the standard of care for every MSI-H mCRC patient, with OS benefit particularly pronounced in young males with ECOG PS 0 [395]. In contrast, in the PFS analysis, there was no benefit from pembrolizumab over chemotherapy in elderly patients with ECOG PS 1 and RAS-mutated, while data on patients with left-sided mCRC are limited [323].

In MSS mCRC patients, a wild-type RAS predicts a benefit from adding EGFRi to an upfront doublet, both vs. chemotherapy+bevacizumab [35, 396] or chemotherapy alone [396]. The improvement was limited to left-sided mCRC patients [35, 206, 396]. In particular, better OS/PFS was reported vs. chemotherapy alone in LLD [26, 397, 398], but not vs. chemotherapy+bevacizumab [143]. Other isolated subgroup analyses should be confirmed, as they suggest that an EGFRi-based regimen would also be preferable in CMS2 [329], PTR [35], in combination with FOLFOX more than FOLFIRI [399], in patients with normal leukocyte counts [398], low TB [397, 398], high CEA [400]. On the other hand, triplet+EGFRi was not superior to doublet+EGFRi, but the limited number of right-sided and female patients do not allow conclusions on these subgroups [401].

For right-sided mCRCs with a wild-type RAS bevacizumab-based regimens are recommended, except when an ORR is required [402], due to the unfavorable results of EGFRi [399]. This indication could also be supported by the different kinetics of response between EGFRi-based and bevacizumab-based regimens, with superior ETS and deepness of response with EGFRi in the subgroup of patients with right-sided tumors, but among right-sided mCRC patients who will have a response to the EGFRi-based regimen remains unpredictable [403].

In RAS unknown or mutated mCRC patients, adding bevacizumab to chemotherapy is a well-established approach. Bevacizumab improved OS in patients with non-over-expressed TP53 [404] and in those with CMS2 and CMS3 [338]. Large trials underreported results of RAS-mutated subgroups, and when reported suggest that bevacizumab improved outcomes regardless of KRAS [405, 406]. However, the superiority of bevacizumab-based vs. EGFRi-based regimens is not always clear even in patients with KRAS-mutated mCRC, as revealed by the FIRE-3 trial for males, with low leucocyte count and SMs [143]. Still, doublet+bevacizumab combination did not improve the results of fluoropyrimidine+bevacizumab in left-sided mCRC patients, but only in right-sided and RAS wild-type [407], while triplet+bevacizumab vs. doublet+bevacizumab improved OS only in RAS-mutated mCRC regardless of sidedness [408], suggesting that the chemorefractoriness of RAS-mutated might be confined to midgut tumors.

Several studies compared the best chemotherapy regimen to combine with bevacizumab. A recent IPDA documented that FOLFOXIRI was superior to doublet, with benefits distributed evenly among subgroups [81], with RCTs not reporting consistent predictors [74, 408, 409]. Even among patients with BRAF-mutated mCRC, the prognosis did not improve after bevacizumab-based triplet vs. doublet [408]. Whenever patients are not amenable to FOLFOXIRI+bevacizumab, the reference regimen is not unique [410] and its activity could differ according to CMS [329], although some studies are more favorable to irinotecan-based regimens [406], especially in the presence of a single site of metastasis [411].

For patients who are not eligible to doublets, the combination of capecitabine+bevacizumab has been shown to be superior to capecitabine alone in the elderly (age >70), particularly in left-sided malignancies without previous PTR [412]. In addition, the trifluridine/tipiracil (TAS-102)+bevacizumab combination is better tolerated than capecitabine+bevacizumab, with similar results and feasibility even in the presence of DPYD deficits [413], with a more pronounced effect in females, left-sided tumours without a previous PTR.

The combination of selective internal radiation therapy (SIRT) on LMs did not improve the results of upfront systemic therapy. However, analysis of three RCTs documented some OS differences favoring right-sided mCRCs and females, especially in the presence of limited LI, age <65 and prior PTR [414]. Other authors suggested higher activity of SIRT in combination with bevacizumab and in MMs without EHD [415].

9.5.2.2.2   Maintenance treatment

When conversion failed, the upfront regimen, especially if oxaliplatin-based, should be depotentiated.

This strategy proved to be slightly superior to complete discontinuation of chemotherapy, although the subgroups of patients for whom discontinuation is a valid option differed in the European and Asian studies [416–418].

The role of bevacizumab in maintenance regimens remains questioned. Bevacizumab maintenance was inferior to the upfront regimen continuation [419] and similar to observation only [420, 421], in particular among ECOG PS 1–2, females, age <70, single-site metastases, wild-type RAS and after ORR [420], and was inferior to the fluoropyrimidine+bevacizumab maintenance [420].

After induction with EGFRi-based regimen, data on optimal maintenance treatment are more limited, but generally with inferior outcomes for EGFRi alone vs. induction regimen [69, 422–425], and support the continuation of the induction regimen in aggressive mCRCs (e.g., MAPK pathway mutations) [424], but also in elderly, right-sided, non-LLD, MM with prior PTR and adjuvant chemotherapy [425]. On the contrary, a maintenance with panitumumab+fluorouracil vs. fluorouracil improved PFS in males, <65 years, with multiple metastatic sites, in stable disease after induction, especially if no panitumumab dose reductions were required [426, 427].

9.5.2.2.3   Treatment of refractory disease

9.5.2.2.3.1   Second-line regimens   MSI-H mCRCs progressing to pembrolizumab should be enrolled in immunotherapy trials or receive upfront regimens of MSS disease.

For MSS mCRCs refractory to upfront therapy, the second-line regimen depends on the previously reported variables and the drugs received upfront. Patients with BRAF-mutated tumors may benefit from the encorafenib+cetuximab regimen, whose activity remains doubtful for MSI-H mCRC, and reduced PS 0 and increased CRP [428].

In patients with RAS-unknown/mutated mCRC or wild-type progressing to EGFRi-based regimen, the regimen of choice should include an antiangiogenic antibody-based regimen with a doublet including a drug not received upfront. While bevacizumab appeared more effective in patients who had received a bevacizumab-based upfront regimen with PFS >9 months, PS 0 and males [429], aflibercept was effective in all subgroups particularly when bevacizumab was not received upfront [430]. Ramucirumab in combination with FOLFIRI reported better results among females and patients with multiple sites of metastasis [431]. Finally, transarterial radioembolisation has been shown to improve PFS in patients with disease refractory to upfront treatment [432].

9.5.2.2.3.2   Further lines regimens   RAS wild-type mCRCs should receive a reevaluation of RAS and HER2 status, possibly by liquid biopsy [433, 434]. A RAS wild-type status or a previous EGFRi-based regimen response [435] supports an EGFRi rechallenge [433, 435], with/without irinotecan [436, 437] or TAS-102 [438], while in case of HER2 overexpression, a HER2-directed therapy should be proposed [439–442].

Registration studies of EGFRi in the third-line setting, have documented a more pronounced benefit in good PS, left-sided mCRC patients [443]. Furthermore, the time to progression and the reasons for discontinuation of upfront therapy might suggest the usefulness of a rechallenge of the upfront chemotherapy.

Patients with MSS mCRC could benefit from further treatment with anti-angiogenics (regorafenib and fruquitinib) or TAS-102+/-bevacizumab. Anti-angiogenics proved to be more effective in young patients, but other characteristics varied between studies [444–447]. Although regorafenib is also well tolerated, in the elderly an alternative low-dose regimen has been developed [448]. TAS-102 was more effective in patients with time since diagnosis >18 months [449, 450], while the

TABLE 9.16

Prognostic factors evaluated in prospective trials of upfront treatment in patients with unresectable metastatic colorectal cancer

Suggested	Not suggested	Needing study
Performance status	Age	Frailty assessment
Symptoms		Nutritional assessment
Alkaline phosphatase		Sex
Lactic dehydrogenase		Inflammation indexes
		Carcinoembrionary antigen
Number of sites of metastasis	Site of metastasis	Sum of tumor diameters
Liver limited disease		Timing of metastasis
Liver involvement >25%		Primary tumor resection
Location (right vs. left-sided)		
Timing + Primary tumor resection		
Immunoscore		

combination TAS-102+bevacizumab was more active in left-sided RAS-mutated mCRCs with at least three sites of metastasis [451].

In patients eligible to regional treatments, SIRT protocols (DEBIRI) were effective in combination with systemic therapy, also in terms of distant control and not only on LMs [452, 453], although the optimal therapeutic role remains unclear.

9.6   CONCLUSION

From a more articulated combination of the various PFs examined, and summarized in Table 9.16, prognostic and predictive subgroups could be defined, but mostly it could improve our understanding of the course of disease after upfront treatments, especially resectable disease. Molecular and TME analysis of metastases after resection is a unique condition, to infer new information on TME, molecular features, and kinetics of response to treatments. For example, the controversial prognostic role of RAS mutation might have an explanation if evaluated according to the site of metastasis. Liver-limited vs. lung-limited metastasis site, in addition to primary tumor location, might better predict the efficacy of MAPK-directed therapy.

In patients at risk of progression, the CMS2/CMS4 ratio in metastases has still been poorly investigated and could contribute to better defining the upfront drug regimen in the individual patient, as well as prognosis, especially in certain subgroups such as early onset mCRC or patients with R0 resection.

Finally, though IS is prognostic for mCRC, resectable and unresectable, it has been poorly reported in RCTs. Furthermore, the relationship with other PFs (MSI, CMS, number of metastatic sites, PTR+timing, inflammatory and nutritional indices), and especially with response to treatments, has been little studied. In addition to improving the prediction of outcome, a greater understanding of IS in early mCRC could allow for guidance on the intensity of treatments to be offered.

REFERENCES

1. Sung H, Ferlay J, Siegel RL, et al. Global cancer statistics 2020: GLOBOCAN estimates of incidence and mortality worldwide for 36 cancers in 185 countries. *CA Cancer J Clin* 2021;71:209–49.
2. ECIS – European Cancer Information System, available at: https://ecis.jrc.ec.europa.eu, accessed October 27, 2023.
3. Barzi A, Lenz AM, Labonte MJ, Lenz H-J. Molecular pathways: Estrogen pathway in colorectal cancer. *Clin Cancer Res* 2013;19:5842–8.

4. Maingi JW, Tang S, Liu S, et al. Targeting estrogen receptors in colorectal cancer. *Sci Rep* 2020;47:4087–91.
5. Siegel RL, Miller KD, Fuchs HE, et al. Cancer statistics, 2022. *CA Cancer J Clin* 2022; 72(1):7–33.
6. Patil PS, Saklani A, Gambhire P, et al. Colorectal cancer in India: An audit from a tertiary center in a low prevalence area. *Indian J Surg Oncol* 2017;8(4):484–90.
7. Cercek A, Chatila WK, Yaeger R, et al. A comprehensive comparison of early-onset and average-onset colorectal cancers. *J Natl Cancer Inst* 2021;113(12):1683–92.
8. Mauri G, Sartore-Bianchi A, Russo AG, et al. Early-onset colorectal cancer in young individuals. *Mol Oncol* 2019;13(2):109–31.
9. Nawa T, Kato J, Kawamoto H, et al. Differences between right- and left-sided colon cancer in patient characteristics, cancer morphology and histology. *J Gastroenterol Hepatol* 2008;23:418–23.
10. Cheng L, Eng C, Nieman LZ, et al. Trends in colorectal cancer incidence by anatomic site and disease stage in the United States from 1976 to 2005. *Am J Clin Oncol* 2011;34:573–80.
11. Li Y, Feng Y, Dai W, et al. Prognostic effect of tumor sidedness in colorectal cancer: A SEER-based analysis. *Clin Colorectal Cancer* 2019;18:e104–16.
12. Nguyen SP, Bent S, Chen Y-H, et al. Gender as a risk factor for advanced neoplasia and colorectal cancer: A systematic review and meta-analysis. *Clin Gastroenterol Hepatol* 2009;7:676–81.
13. White A, Ironmonger L, Steele RJC, et al. A review of sex-related differences in colorectal cancer incidence, screening uptake, routes to diagnosis, cancer stage and survival in the UK. *BMC Cancer* 2018;18:906.
14. Brenner H, Kloor M, Pox CP. Colorectal cancer. *Lancet* 2014;383(9927):1490–502.
15. Waldmann E, Heinze G, Ferlitsch A, et al. Risk factors cannot explain the higher prevalence rates of precancerous colorectal lesions in men. *Br J Cancer* 2016;115(11):1421–9.
16. Matarrese P, Mattia G, Pagano MT, et al. The sex-related interplay between TME and cancer: On the critical role of estrogen, microRNA and autophagy. *Cancers* 2021;13(13):3287.
17. Williams C, DiLeo A, Niv Y, et al. Estrogen receptor beta as target for colorectal cancer prevention. *Cancer Lett* 2016;372(1):48–56.
18. Konishi T, Shimada Y, Hsu M, et al. Association of preoperative and postoperative serum carcinoembryonic antigen and colon cancer outcome. *JAMA Oncol* 2018;4:309–15.
19. Duffy MJ, van Dalen A, Haglund C, et al. Clinical utility of biochemical markers in colorectal cancer: European Group on Tumour Markers (EGTM) guidelines. *Eur J Cancer* 2003;39(6):718–27.
20. Locker GY, Hamilton S, Harris J, et al. ASCO 2006 update of recommendations for the use of tumor markers in gastrointestinal cancer. *J Clin Oncol* 2006;24(33):5313–27.
21. Le DT, Uram JN, Wang H, et al. PD-1 blockade in tumors with mismatch-repair deficiency. *N Engl J Med* 2015;372(26):2509–20.
22. Andrè T, Shiu K-K, Kim TW, et al. Pembrolizumab in microsatellite-instability-high advanced colorectal cancer. *N Engl J Med* 2020;383(23):2207–18.
23. Stjepanovic N, Moreira L, Carneiro F, et al. Hereditary gastrointestinal cancers: ESMO clinical practice guidelines for diagnosis, treatment and follow-up. *Ann Oncol* 2019;30(10):1558–71.
24. Amado RG, Wolf M, Peeters M, et al. Wild-type KRAS is required for panitumumab efficacy in patients with metastatic colorectal cancer. *J Clin Oncol* 2008;26(10):1626–34.
25. Karapetis CS, Khambata-Ford S, Jonker DJ, et al. K-ras mutations and benefit from cetuximab in advanced colorectal cancer. *N Engl J Med* 2008;359(17):1757–65.
26. Douillard J-Y, Siena S, Cassidy J, et al. Randomized, phase III trial of panitumumab with infusional fluorouracil, leucovorin, and oxaliplatin (FOLFOX4) versus FOLFOX4 alone as first-line treatment in patients with previously untreated metastatic colorectal cancer: The PRIME study. *J Clin Oncol* 2010;28(31):4697–705.
27. Normanno N, Esposito Abate R, Lambiase M, et al. RAS testing of liquid biopsy correlates with the outcome of metastatic colorectal cancer patients treated with first-line FOLFIRI plus cetuximab in the CAPRI-GOIM trial. *Ann Oncol* 2018;29(1):112–8.
28. Henricks LM, Lunenburg CATC, de Man FM, et al. DPYD genotype-guided dose individualisation of fluoropyrimidine therapy in patients with cancer: A prospective safety analysis. *Lancet Oncol* 2018;19:1459–67.
29. Sartore-Bianchi A, Trusolino L, Martino C, et al. Dual-targeted therapy with trastuzumab and lapatinib in treatment-refractory, KRAS codon 12/13 wild-type, HER2-positive metastatic colorectal cancer (HERACLES): A proof-of-concept, multicentre, open-label, phase 2 trial. *Lancet Oncol* 2016;17(6):738–46.
30. Pietrantonio F, Di Nicolantonio F, Schrock AB, et al. ALK, ROS1, and NTRK rearrangements in metastatic colorectal cancer. *J Natl Cancer Inst* 2017;109(12):djx089.

31. Marchiò C, Scaltriti M, Ladanyi M, et al. ESMO recommendations on the standard methods to detect NTKR fusions in daily practice and clinical research. *Ann Oncol* 2019;30(9):1417–27.
32. Hong DS, DuBois SG, Kummar S, et al. Larotrectinib in patients with TRK fusion-positive solid tumours: A pooled analysis of three phase 1/2 clinical trials. *Lancet Oncol* 2020;21(4):531–40.
33. Doebele RC, Drilon A, Paz-Ares L, et al. Entrectinib in patients with advanced or metastatic NTRK fusion-positive solid tumours: Integrated analysis of three phase 1–2 trials. *Lancet Oncol* 2020;21(2):271–82.
34. Poon MA, O'Connell MJ, Moertel CG, et al. Biochemical modulation of fluorouracil: Evidence of significant improvement of survival and quality of life in patients with advanced colorectal carcinoma. *J Clin Oncol* 1989;7:1407–17.
35. Watanabe J, Muro K, Shitara K, et al. Panitumumab vs bevacizumab added to standard first-line chemotherapy and overall survival among patients with RAS wild-type, left-sided metastatic colorectal cancer. A randomized clinical trial. *JAMA* 2023;329(15):1271–82.
36. Kanemitsu Y, Shimizu Y, Mizusawa J, et al. Hepatectomy followed by mFOLFOX6 versus hepatectomy alone for liver-only metastatic colorectal cancer (JCOG0603): A phase II or III randomized controlled trial. *J Clin Oncol* 2021;39:3789–99.
37. Poston GJ, Figueras J, Giuliante F, et al. Urgent need for a new staging system in advanced colorectal cancer. *J Clin Oncol* 2008;26:4828–33.
38. Dy GK, Hobday TJ, Nelson G, et al. Long-term survivors of metastatic colorectal cancer treated with systemic chemotherapy alone: A North Central Cancer Treatment Group review of 3811 patients, N0144. *Clin Colorectal Cancer* 2009;8(2):88–93.
39. Stillwell AP, Ho Y-H, Veitch C. Systematic review of prognostic factors related to overall survival in patients with stage IV colorectal cancer and unresectable metastases. *World J Surg* 2011;35:684–92.
40. Rougier P, Laplanche A, Huguier M, et al. Hepatic arterial infusion of floxuridine in patients with liver metastases from colorectal carcinoma: Long-term results of a prospective randomized trial. *J Clin Oncol* 1992;10:1112–8.
41. Buroker TR, O'Connell MJ, Wieand HS, et al. Randomized comparison of two schedules of fluorouracil and leucovorin in the treatment of advanced colorectal cancer. *J Clin Oncol* 1994;12:14–20.
42. Blijham G, Wagener T, Wils J, et al. Modulation of high-dose infusional fluorouracil by low-dose methotrexate in patients with advanced or metastatic colorectal cancer: Final results of a randomized European Organization for Research and Treatment of Cancer study. *J Clin Oncol* 1996;14:2266–73.
43. Ross P, Norman A, Cunningham D, et al. A prospective randomised trial of protracted venous infusion 5-fluorouracil with or without mitomycin C in advanced colorectal cancer. *Ann Oncol* 1997;8:995–1001.
44. Giacchetti S, Perpoint B, Zidani R, et al. Phase III multicenter randomized trial of oxaliplatin added to chronomodulated fluorouracil-leucovorin as first-line treatment of metastatic colorectal cancer. *J Clin Oncol* 2000;18:136–47.
45. de Gramont A, Figer A, Seymour M, et al. Leucovorin and fluorouracil with or without oxaliplatin as first-line treatment in advanced colorectal cancer. *J Clin Oncol* 2000;18:2938–47.
46. Saltz LB, Cox JV, Blanke C, et al. Irinotecan plus fluorouracil and leucovorin for metastatic colorectal cancer. *N Engl J Med* 2000;343:905–14.
47. Douillard JY, Cunningham D, Roth AD, et al. Irinotecan combined with fluorouracil compared with fluorouracil alone as first-line treatment for metastatic colorectal cancer: A multicentre randomised trial. *Lancet* 2000;355:1041–7.
48. O'Dwyer PJ, Manola J, Valone FH, et al. Fluorouracil modulation in colorectal cancer: Lack of improvement with N-phosphonoacetyl-l-aspartic acid or oral leucovorin or interferon, but enhanced therapeutic index with weekly 24-hour infusion schedule – An Eastern Cooperative Oncology Group / Cancer and Leukemia Group B study. *J Clin Oncol* 2001;19:2413–21.
49. Hoff PM, Ansari R, Batist G, et al. Comparison of oral capecitabine versus intravenous fluorouracil plus leucovorin as first-line treatment in 605 patients with metastatic colorectal cancer: Results of a randomized phase III study. *J Clin Oncol* 2001;19:2282–92.
50. Van Cutsem E, Twelves C, Cassidy J, et al. Oral capecitabine compared with intravenous fluorouracil plus leucovorin in patients with metastatic colorectal cancer: Results of a large phase III study. *J Clin Oncol* 2001;19:4097–106.
51. Schilsky RL, Levin J, West WH, et al. Randomized, open-label, phase III study of a 28-day oral regimen of eniluracil plus fluorouracil versus intravenous fluorouracil plus leucovorin as first-line therapy in patients with metastatic/advanced colorectal cancer. *J Clin Oncol* 2002;20:1519–26.

52. Kalofonos HP, Nicolaides C, Samantas E, et al. A phase III study of 5-fluorouracil versus 5-fluorouracil plus interferon alpha 2 b versus 5-fluorouracil plus leucovorin in patients with advanced colorectal cancer. *An J Clin Oncol* 2002;25(1):23–30.

53. Hurwitz H, Fehrenbacher L, Novotny W, et al. Bevacizumab plus irinotecan, fluorouracil, and leucovorin for metastatic colorectal cancer. *N Engl J Med* 2004;350:2335–42.

54. Tournigand C, André T, Achille E, et al. FOLFIRI followed by FOLFOX6 or the reverse sequence in advanced colorectal cancer: A randomized GERCOR study. *J Clin Oncol* 2004;22:229–37.

55. Colucci G, Gebbia V, Paoletti G, et al. Phase III randomized trial of FOLFIRI versus FOLFOX4 in the treatment of advanced colorectal cancer: A multicenter study of the Gruppo Oncologico dell'Italia Meridionale. *J Clin Oncol* 2005;23:4866–75.

56. Giacchetti S, Bjarnason G, Garufi C, et al. Phase III trial comparing 4-day chronomodulated therapy versus 2-day conventional delivery of fluorouracil, leucovorin, and oxaliplatin as first-line chemotherapy of metastatic colorectal cancer: The European Organisation for Research and Treatment of Cancer chronotherapy group. *J Clin Oncol* 2006;24:3562–9.

57. Portier G, Elias D, Bouche O, et al. Multicenter randomized trial of adjuvant fluorouracil and folinic acid compared with surgery alone after resection of colorectal liver metastases: FFCD ACHBTH AURC 9002 trial. *J Clin Oncol* 2006;24:4976–82.

58. Ferrand F, Malka D, Bourredjem A, et al. Impact of primary tumor resection on survival of patients with colorectal cancer and synchronous metastases treated by chemotherapy: Results from the multicenter, randomised trial Federation Francophone de Cancerologie Digestive 9601. *Eur J Cancer* 2013;49:90–7.

59. Tournigand C, Cervantes A, Figer A, et al. OPTIMOX1: A randomized study of FOLFOX4 or FOLFOX7 with oxaliplatin in a stop-and-go fashion in advanced colorectal cancer – A GERCOR study. *J Clin Oncol* 2006;24:394–400.

60. Porschen R, Arkenau H-T, Kubicka S, et al. Phase III study of capecitabine plus oxaliplatin compared with fluorouracil and leucovorin plus oxaliplatin in metastatic colorectal cancer: A final report of the AIO colorectal study group. *J Clin Oncol* 2007;25:4217–23.

61. Richman SD, Seymour MT, Chambers P, et al. KRAS and BRAF mutations in advanced colorectal cancer are associated with poor prognosis but do not preclude benefit from oxaliplatin or irinotecan: Results from the MRC FOCUS trial. *J Clin Oncol* 2009;27(35):5931–7.

62. Masi G, Vasile E, Loupakis F, et al. Randomized trial of two induction chemotherapy regimens in metastatic colorectal cancer: An updated analysis. *J Natl Cancer Inst* 2011;103:21–30.

63. Glimelius B, Sorbye H, Balteskard L, et al. A randomized phase III multicenter trial comparing irinotecan in combination with the Nordic bolus 5-FU and folinic acid schedule or the bolus/infused de Gramont schedule (Lv5FU2) in patients with metastatic colorectal cancer. *Ann Oncol* 2008;19:909–14.

64. Peeters M, Price T, Taieb J, et al. Relationships between tumour response and primary tumour location, and predictors of long term survival, in patients with RAS wild-type metastatic colorectal cancer receiving first-line panitumumab therapy: Retrospective analyses of the PRIME and PEAK clinical trials. *Br J Cancer* 2018;118:303–12.

65. Grenader T, Nash S, Adams R, et al. Derived neutrophil lymphocyte ratio is predictive of survival from intermittent therapy in advanced colorectal cancer: A post hoc analysis of the MRC COIN study. *Br J Cancer* 2016;114:612–5.

66. Penichoux J, Michiels S, Bouché O, et al. Taking into account successive treatment lines in the analysis of a colorectal cancer randomised trial. *Eur J Cancer* 2013;49(8):1882–8.

67. Fischer von Weikersthal L, Schalhorn A, Stauch M, et al. Phase III trial of irinotecan plus infusional 5-fluorouracil/folinic acid versus irinotecan plus oxaliplatin as first-line treatment of advanced colorectal cancer. *Eur J Cancer* 2011;47:206–14.

68. Pectasides L, Papaxoinis G, Kalogeras KT, et al. XELIRI-bevacizumab versus FOLFIRI-bevacizumab as first-line treatment in patients with metastatic colorectal cancer: A Hellenic Cooperative Oncology Group phase III trial collateral biomarker analysis. *BMC Cancer* 2012;12:271.

69. Tveit KM, Guren T, Glimelius B, et al. Phase III trial of cetuximab with continuous or intermittent fluorouracil, leucovorin, and oxaliplatin (Nordic FLOX) versus FLOX alone in first-line treatment of metastatic colorectal cancer: The NORDIC-VII study. *J Clin Oncol* 2012;30:1755–62.

70. Aparicio T, Jouve J-L, Teillet L, et al. Geriatric factors predict chemotherapy feasibility: Ancillary results of FFCD 2001–02 phase III study in first-line chemotherapy for metastatic colorectal cancer in elderly patients. *J Clin Oncol* 2013;31:1464–70.

71. Passardi A, Scarpi E, Tamberi S, et al. Impact of pre-treatment lactate dehydrogenase levels on prognosis and bevacizumab efficacy in patients with metastatic colorectal cancer. *PLoS ONE* 2015;10(8):e0134732.

72. Yamada Y, Muro K, Takahashi K, et al. Impact of sex and histology on the therapeutic effects of fluo-ropyrimidines and oxaliplatin plus bevacizumab for patients with metastatic colorectal cancer in the SOFT trial. *Global Health Med* 2020;2(4):240–6.

73. Holch JW, Ricard I, Stintzing S, et al. Relevance of liver-limited disease in metastatic colorectal cancer: Subgroup findings of the FIRE-3/AIO KRK0306 trial. *Int J Cancer* 2018;142:1047–55.

74. Loupakis F, Cremolini C, Masi G, et al. Initial therapy with FOLFOXIRI and bevacizumab for meta-static colorectal cancer. *N Engl J Med* 2014;371:1609–18.

75. Guercio BJ, Zhang S, Ou F-S, et al. Associations of physical activity with survival and progression in metastatic colorectal cancer: Results from Cancer and Leukemia Group B (Alliance)/SWOG 80405. *J Clin Oncol* 2019;37:2620–31.

76. Formica V, Ionta MT, Massidda B, et al. Predictive factors for 6 vs 12 cycles of FOLFIRI-bevacizumab in metastatic colorectal cancer. *Oncotarget* 2018;9(2):2876–86.

77. Borelli B, Fontana E, Giordano M, et al. Prognostic and predictive impact of consensus molecular sub-types and CRCAssigner classifications in metastatic colorectal cancer: A translational analysis of the TRIBE2 study. *ESMO Open* 2021;6(2):100073.

78. Chibaudel B, Bonnetain F, Tournigand C, et al. Simplified prognostic model in patients with oxaliplatin-based or irinotecan-based first-line chemotherapy for metastatic colorectal cancer: A GERCOR study. *Oncologist* 2011;16:1228–38.

79. Claret L, Gupta M, Han K, et al. Evaluation of tumor-size response metrics to predict overall sur-vival in Western and Chinese patients with first-line metastatic colorectal cancer. *J Clin Oncol* 2013;31(17):2110–14.

80. Jary M, Lecomte T, Bouché O, et al. Prognostic value of baseline seric Syndecan-1 in ini-tially unresectable metastatic colorectal cancer patients: A simple biological score. *Int J Cancer* 2016;139(10):2325–35.

81. Cremolini C, Casagrande M, Loupakis F, et al. Efficacy of FOLFOXIRI plus bevacizumab in liver-limited metastatic colorectal cancer: A pooled analysis of clinical studies by Gruppo Oncologico del Nord Ovest. *Eur J Cancer* 2017;73:74–84.

82. Sunakawa Y, Ichikawa W, Tsuji A, et al. Prognostic impact of primary tumor location on clinical out-comes of metastatic colorectal cancer treated with cetuximab plus oxaliplatin-based chemotherapy: A subgroup analysis of the JACCRO CC-05/06 trials. *Clin Colorectal Cancer* 2017;16(3):e171–80.

83. Sjoquist KM, Renfro LA, Simes RJ, et al. Personalizing survival predictions in advanced colorectal cancer: The ARCAD nomogram project. *J Natl Cancer Inst* 2018;110(6):638–48.

84. Kohne C-H, Cunningham D, Di Costanzo F, et al. Clinical determinants of survival in patients with 5-fluorouracil-based treatment for metastatic colorectal cancer: Results of a multivariate analysis of 3825 patients. *Ann Oncol* 2002;13:308–17.

85. Mekenkamp LJM, Koopman M, Teerenstra S, et al. Clinicopathological features and outcome in advanced colorectal cancer patients with synchronous vs metachronous metastases. *Br J Cancer* 2010;103:159–64.

86. Clarke SJ, Burge M, Feeney K, et al. The prognostic role of inflammatory markers in patients with metastatic colorectal cancer treated with bevacizumab: A translational study [ASCENT]. *PLoS ONE* 2020;15(3):e0229900.

87. Diaz-Rubio E, Gomez-Espana A, Massuti B, et al. Role of Kras status in patients with metastatic colorectal cancer receiving first-line chemotherapy plus bevacizumab: A TTD Group Cooperative study. *PLoS ONE* 2012;7(10):e47345.

88. Sunakawa Y, Yang D, Cao S, et al. Immune-related genes to dominate neutrophil-lymphocyte ratio (NLR)associated with survival of cetuximab treatment in metastatic colorectal cancer. *Clin Colorectal Cancer* 2018;17(4):e741–9.

89. Tampellini M, Ottone A, Alabiso I, et al. The prognostic role of baseline CEA and CA 19–9 values and their time-dependent variations in advanced colorectal cancer patients submitted to first-line therapy. *Tumor Biol* 2015;39:1519–27.

90. Shimura T, Toiyama Y, Saigusa S, et al. Inflammation-based prognostic scores as indicators to select candidates for primary site resection followed by multimodal therapy among colorectal cancer patients with multiple metastases. *Int J Clin Oncol* 2017;22:758–66.

91. Chen Z-Y, Raghav K, Lieu CH, et al. Cytokine profile and prognostic significance of high neutrophil-lymphocyte ratio in colorectal cancer. *Br J Cancer* 2015;112:1088–97.

92. Makhloufi S, Turpin A, el Amrani M, et al. Fong's score in the era of modern perioperative chemo-therapy for metastatic colorectal cancer: A post hoc analysis of the GERCOR-MIROX phase III trial. *Ann Surg Oncol* 2020;27:877–85.

93. Sargent D, Kohne CH, Sanoff HK, et al. Pooled safety and efficacy analysis examining the effect of performance status on outcomes in nine first-line treatment trials using individual data from patients with metastatic colorectal cancer. *J Clin Oncol* 2009;27:1948–55.

94. Teixeira MC, Marques DF, Ferrari AC, et al. The effects of palliative chemotherapy in metastatic colorectal cancer patients with an ECOG performance status of 3 and 4. *Clin Colorectal Cancer* 2015;14(1):52–7.

95. Boakye D, Rillmann B, Walter V, et al. Impact of comorbidity and frailty on prognosis in colorectal cancer patients: A systematic review and meta-analysis. *Cancer Treat Rev* 2018;64:30–9.

96. Van Cutsem E, Nayer RJ, Laurent S, et al. The subgroups of the phase III RECOURSE trial of trifluridine/tipiracil (TAS-102) versus placebo with best supportive care in patients with metastatic colorectal cancer. *Eur J Cancer* 2018;90:63–72.

97. Dotan E, Browner I, Hurria A, Denlinger C. Challenges in the management of older patients with colon cancer. *J Natl Compr Canc Netw* 2012;10(2):213–24.

98. Feliu J, Espinosa E, Basterretxea L, et al. Undertreatment and overtreatment in older patients treated with chemotherapy. *J Geriatr Oncol* 2020;12(3):381–7.

99. Sorbye H, Cvancarova M, Qvortrup C, et al. Age-dependent improvement in median and long-term survival in unselected population-based Nordic registries of patients with synchronous metastatic colorectal cancer. *Ann Oncol* 2013;24(9):2354–60.

100. Davidson KW, Barry MJ, Mangione CM, et al. Screening for colorectal cancer: US Preventive Services Task Force recommendation statement. *J Am Med Assoc* 2021;325:1965–77.

101. Boardman LA, Vilar E, You YN, et al. AGA clinical practice update on young adult-onset colorectal cancer diagnosis and management: Expert review. *Clin Gastroenterol Hepatol* 2020;18(11):2415–24.

102. Blanke CD, Bot BM, Thomas DM, et al. Impact of young age on treatment efficacy and safety in advanced colorectal cancer: A pooled analysis of patients from nine first-line phase III chemotherapy trials. *J Clin Oncol* 2011;29:2781–6.

103. Kim TJ, Kim ER, Hong SN, et al. Long-term outcome and prognostic factors of sporadic colorectal cancer in young patients. *Medicine* 2016;95(19):e3641.

104. Dagher M, Sabidò M, Zollner Y. Effect of age on the effectiveness of the first-line standard of care treatment in patients with metastatic colorectal cancer: Systematic review of observational studies. *J Cancer Res Clin Oncol* 2019;145:2105–14.

105. Dawood S, Sirohi B, Shrikhande SV, et al. Potential prognostic impact of baseline CEA level and surgery of primary tumor among patients with synchronous stage IV colorectal cancer: A large population based study. *Indian J Surg Oncol* 2015;6(3):198–206.

106. Han L, Dai W, Mo S, et al. Nomogram of conditional survival probability of long-term survival for metastatic colorectal cancer: A real-world data retrospective cohort study from SEER database. *Int J Surg* 2021;92:106013.

107. Zhang Q, Li B, Zhang S, et al. Prognostic impact of tumor size on patients with metastatic colorectal cancer: A large SEER-based retrospective cohort study. *Updated Surg* 2023;75:1135–47.

108. Ghiringhelli F, Hennequin A, Drouillard A, et al. Epidemilogy and prognosis of synchronous and metachronous colon cancer metastases: A French population-based study. *Dig Liver Dis* 2014;46:854–8.

109. Wang X, Mao M, Xu G, et al. The incidence, associated factors, and predictive nomogram for early death in stage IV colorectal cancer. *Int J Colorectal Dis* 2019;34:1189–201.

110. Zhang Y, Zhang Z, Wei L, Wei S. Construction and validation of nomograms combined with novel machine learning algorithms to predict early death of patients with metastatic colorectal cancer. *Front Public Health* 2022;10:1008137.

111. Dorajoo SR, Tan WJH, Koo SX, et al. A scoring model for predictiong survival following primary tumour resection in stage IV colorectal cancer patients with unresectable metastasis. *Int J Colorectal Dis* 2016;31:235–45.

112. Shibutani M, Maeda K, Nagahara H, et al. Tumor-infiltrating lymphocytes predict the chemotherapeutic outcomes in patients with stage IV colorectal cancer. *In Vivo* 2018;32:151–8.

113. Rumpold H, Niedersub-Beke D, Heiler C, et al. Prediction of mortality in metastatic colorectal cancer in a real-life population: A multicenter explorative analysis. *BMC Cancer* 2020;20:1149.

114. Zhang J, Gong Z, Gong Y, et al. Development and validation of nomograms for prediction of overall survival and cancer-specific survival of patients with stage IV colorectal cancer. *Jpn J Clin Oncol* 2019;49(5):438–46.

115. Jin X, Wu Y, Feng Y, et al. A population-based predictive model identifying optimal candidates for primary and metastasis resection in patients with colorectal cancer with liver metastatic. *Front Oncol* 2022;12:899659.

116. Beppu T, Kobayashi S, Itabashi M, et al. Validation study of the JSHBPS nomogram for patients with colorectal liver metastases who underwent hepatic resection in the recent era – A nationwide survey in Japan. *J Hepatobiliary Pancreat Sci* 2023;30:591–601.

117. Dasari BVM, Raptis D, Syn N, et al. Development and validation of a novel risk score to predict overall survival following surgical clearance of bilobar colorectal liver metastases. *BJS Open* 2023;7(5):zrad085.

118. Ghanim B, Schweiger T, Jedamzik J, et al. Elevated inflammatory parameters and inflammation scores are associated with poor prognosis in patients undergoing pulmonary metastasectomy for colorectal cancer. *Interact Cardiovasc Thor Surg* 2015;21:616–23.

119. Tocchi A, Mazzoni G, Brozzetti S, et al. Hepatic resection in stage IV colorectal cancer: Prognostic predictors of outcome. *Int J Colorectal Dis* 2004;19:580–5.

120. Tsai M-S, Su Y-H, Ho M-C, et al. Clinicopathological features and prognosis in resectable synchronous and metachronous colorectal liver metastasis. *Ann Surg Oncol* 2007;14:786–94.

121. Kawai K, Ishihara S, Yamaguchi H, et al. Nomograms for predicting the prognosis of stage IV colorectal cancer after curative resection: A multicenter retrospective study. *Eur J Surg Oncol* 2015;41(4):457–65.

122. Neofytou K, Giakoustidis A, Costa Neves M, et al. Increased carcinoembryonic antigen (CEA) following neoadjuvant chemotherapy predicts poor prognosis in patients that undergo hepatectomy for liver-only colorectal metastases. *Langenbecks Arch Surg* 2017;402(4):599–605.

123. Liu W, Zhang M, Wu J, et al. Oncologic outcome and efficacy of chemotherapy in colorectal cancer patients aged 80 years or older. *Front Med* 2020;7:525421.

124. Kumar R, Jain K, Beeke C, et al. A population-based study of metastatic colorectal cancer in individuals aged ≥80 years. *Cancer* 2013;119:722–8.

125. Hisada H, Takahashi Y, Kubota M, et al. Clinical and therapeutic features and prognostic factors of metastatic colorectal cancer over age 80: A retrospective study. *BMC Gastroenterol* 2021;21:199.

126. Numata K, Ono Y, Toda S, et al. Modified Glasgow prognostic score and carcinoembryonic antigen predict poor prognosis in elderly patients with colorectal cancer. *Oncol Res Treat* 2020;43:125–32.

127. Jung YH, Kim JY, Jang YN, et al. Clinical characteristics and treatment propensity in elderly patients aged over 80 years with colorectal cancer. *Korean J Intern Med* 2018;33:1182–93.

128. Parakh S, Wong H-L, Rai R, et al. Patterns of care and outcomes for elderly patients with metastatic colorectal cancer in Australia. *J Geriatr Oncol* 2015;6(5):387–94.

129. de Angelis N, Baldini C, Brustia R, et al. Surgical and regional treatments for colorectal cancer metastases in older patients: A systematic review and meta-analysis. *PLoS ONE* 2020;15(4):e0230914.

130. Landre T, Uzzan B, Nicolas P, et al. Doublet chemotherapy vs. single-agent therapy with 5FU in elderly patients with metastatic colorectal cancer: A meta-analysis. *Int J Colorectal Dis* 2015;30(10):1305–10.

131. Seymour MT, Thompson LC, Wasan HS, et al. Chemotherapy options in elderly and frail patients with metastatic colorectal cancer (MRC FOCUS2): An open-label, randomised factorial trial. *Lancet* 2011;377(9779):1749–59.

132. Aparicio T, Gargot D, Teillet L, et al. Geriatric factors analyses from FFCD 2001–02 phase III study of first-line chemotherapy for elderly metastatic colorectal cancer patients. *Eur J Cancer* 2017;74:98–108.

133. van der Vlies E, Kurk SA, Roodhart JML, et al. The relevance of geriatric assessment for older patients receiving palliative chemotherapy. *J Geriatr Oncol* 2020;11:482–7.

134. Ferlay J, Soerjomataran I, Dikshit R, et al. Cancer incidence and mortality worldwide: Sources, methods and major patterns in GLOBOCAN 2012. *Int J Cancer* 2015;136(5):E359–86.

135. Engstrand J, Nilsson H, Stromberg C, Jonas E, Freedman J. Colorectal cancer liver metastases – A population-based study on incidence, management and survival. *BMC Cancer* 2018;18(1):78.

136. Varyrynen V, Wirta E-V, Seppala T, et al. Incidence and management of patients with colorectal cancer and synchronous and metachronous colorectal metastases: A population-based study. *BJS Open* 2020;4(4):685–92.

137. Meyer Y, Olthof PB, Grunhagen DJ, et al. Treatment of metachronous colorectal cancer metastases in the Netherlands: A population-based study. *Eur J Surg Oncol* 2022;48(5):1104–9.

138. Hendifar A, Yang D, Lenz F, et al. Gender disparities in metastatic colorectal cancer survival. *Clin Cancer Res* 2009;15(20):6391–7.

139. Koo JH, Jalaludin B, Wong SKC, et al. Improved survival in young women with colorectal cancer. *Am J Gastroenterol* 2008;103(6):1488–95.

140. Majek O, Gondos A, Jansen L, et al. Sex differences in colorectal cancer survival: Population-based analysis of 164,996 colorectal cancer patients in Germany. *PLoS ONE* 2013;8(7):e68077.

141. Perotti V, Fabiano S, Contiero P, et al. Influence of sex and age on site of onset, morphology, and site of metastasis in colorectal cancer: A population-based study on data from four Italian cancer registries. *Cancers* 2023;15:803.

142. Ray AL, Nofchissey RA, Khan MA, et al. The role of sex in the innate and adaptive immune environment of metastatic colorectal cancer. *Br J Cancer* 2020;123:624–32.

143. Heinemann V, Fischer von Weikersthal L, Decker T, et al. FOLFIRI plus cetuximab versus FOLFIRI plus bevacizumab as first-line treatment for patients with metastatic colorectal cancer (FIRE-3): A randomised, open-label, phase 3 trial. *Lancet Oncol* 2014;15(10):1065–75.

144. Hartley D. Rural health disparities, population health, and rural culture. *Am J Public Health* 2004;94(10):1675–8.

145. Humber N, Dickinson P. Rural patients' experiences accessing surgery in British Columbia. *Can J Surg* 2010;53(6):373–8.

146. Crawford-Williams F, March S, Goodwin BC, et al. Geographic variations in stage at diagnosis and survival for colorectal cancer in Australia: A systematic review. *Eur J Cancer Care* 2019;28(3):e13072.

147. Murchie P, Falborg AZ, Turner M, et al. Geographic variation in diagnostic and treatment interval, cancer stage and mortality among colorectal patients – An international comparison between Denmark and Scotland using data-linked cohorts. *Cancer Epidemiol* 2021;74:102004.

148. Panchal JM, Lairson DR, Chan W, Du XL. Geographic variation in oxaliplatin chemotherapy and survival in patients with colon cancer. *Am J Ther* 2016;23(3):e720–9.

149. Jiang Y, Yuan H, Li Z, et al. Global pattern and trends of colorectal cancer survival: A systematic review of population-based registration data. *Cancer Biol Med* 2021;19(2):175–86.

150. Lochhead P, Kuchiba A, Imamura Y, et al. Microsatellite instability and BRAF mutation testing in colorectal cancer prognostication. *J Natl Cancer Inst* 2013;105(15):1151–6.

151. Lynch HT, de la Chapelle A. Hereditary colorectal cancer. *N Engl J Med* 2003;348(10):919–32.

152. Fujita S, Moriya Y, Sugihara K, et al. Prognosis of hereditary nonpolyposis colorectal cancer (HNPCC) and the role of Japanese criteria for HNPCC. *Jpn J Clin Oncol* 1996;26(5):351–5.

153. Gutierrez C, Ogino S, Meyerhardt JA, Iorgulescu JB. The prevalence and prognosis of microsatellite instability-high/mismatch repair-deficient colorectal adenocarcinomas in the United States. *JCO Precis Oncol* 2023;7:e2200179.

154. Bae JM, Kim JH, Cho N-Y, et al. Prognostic implication of the CpG island methylator phenotype in colorectal cancers depends on tumour location. *Br J Cancer* 2013;109(4):1004–12.

155. Lee GH, Malietzis G, Askari A, et al. Is right-sided colon cancer different to left-sided colorectal cancer? – A systematic review. *Eur J Surg Oncol* 2015;41(3):300–8.

156. Renfro LA, Loupakis F, Adams RA, et al. Body mass index is prognostic in metastatic colorectal cancer: Pooled analysis of patients from first-line clinical trials in the ARCAD database. *J Clin Oncol* 2016;34:144–50.

157. Argiles JM, Busquets S, Stemmler B, Lopez-Soriano FJ. Cancer cachexia: Understanding the molecular basis. *Nat Rev Cancer* 2014;14(11):754–62.

158. Shah MS, Fogelman DR, Raghav KPS, et al. Joint prognostic effect of obesity and chronic systemic inflammation in patients with metastatic colorectal cancer. *Cancer* 2015;121(17):2968–7.

159. Davis JS, Chavez JC, Kok M, et al. Association of prediagnosis obesity and postdiagnosis aspirin with survival from stage IV colorectal cancer. *JAMA Netw Open* 2022;5(10):e2236357.

160. Greene MW, Abraham PT, Kuhlers PC, et al. Consensus molecular subtype differences linking colon adenocarcinoma and obesity revealed by a cohort transcriptomic analysis. *PLoS ONE* 2022;17:e0268436.

161. Guercio BJ, Zhang S, Ou F-S, et al. Associations of physical activity with survival and progression in metastatic colorectal cancer: Results from cancer and leukemia group B (Alliance)/SWOG 80405. *J Clin Oncol* 2021;37(29):2620–31.

162. Dell'Aquila E, Rossini D, Galletti A, et al. Prognostic and predictive role of body mass index (BMI) in metastatic colorectal cancer (mCRC): A pooled analysis of Tribe and Tribe-2 studies by GONO. *Clin Colorectal Cancer* 2022;21(3):220–8.

163. Boakye D, Rillmann B, Walter V, et al. Impact of comorbidity and frailty on prognosis in colorectal cancer patients: A systematic review and meta-analysis. *Cancer Treat Rev* 2018;64:30–9.

164. Asmis TR, Powell E, Karapetis CS, et al. Comorbidity, age and overall survival in cetuximab-treated patients with advanced colorectal cancer (ACRC)--Results from NCIC CTG CO.17: A phase III trial of cetuximab versus best supportive care. *Ann Oncol* 2011;22(1):118–26.

165. Kim KH, Lee JJ, Kim J, et al. Association of multidimensional comorbidities with survival, toxicity, and unplanned hospitalizations in older adults with metastatic colorectal cancer treated with chemotherapy. *J Geriatr Oncol* 2019;10(5):733–41.

166. Lu B, Qian J-M, Li J-N. The metabolic syndrome and its components as prognostic factors in colorectal cancer: A meta-analysis and systematic review. *J Gastroenterol Hepatol* 2023;38(2):187–96.

167. Brown JC, Zhang S, Ou F-S, et al. Diabetes and clinical outcome in patients with metastatic colorectal cancer: CALGB 80405 (Alliance). *JNCI Cancer Spectr* 2019;4(1):pkz078.

168. Choi Y-H, Lakhal-Chaieb L, Krol A, et al. Risk of colorectal cancer and cancer-related mortality in familial colorectal cancer type X and Lynch syndrome families. *J Natl Cancer Inst* 2019;111(7):djy159.

169. Olen O, Erichsen R, Sachs MC, et al. Colorectal cancer in ulcerative colitis: A Scandinavian population-based cohort study. *Lancet* 2020;395(10218):123–31.

170. Han YD, Al Bandar MH, Dulskas A, et al. Prognosis of ulcerative colitis colorectal cancer vs. sporadic colorectal cancer: Propensity score matching analysis. *BMC Surg* 2017;17:28.

171. Ng K, Sargent DJ, Goldberg RM, et al. Vitamin D status in patients with stage IV colorectal cancer: Findings from Intergroup trial N9741. *J Clin Oncol* 2011;29(12):1599–606.

172. Yuan C, Sato K, Hollis BW, et al. Plasma 25-hydroxyvitamin D levels and survival in patients with advanced or metastatic colorectal cancer: Findings from CALGB/SWOG 80405 (Alliance). *Clin Cancer Res* 2019;25(24):7497–505.

173. Ng K, Nimeiri HS, McCleary NJ, et al. Effect of high-dose vs standard-dose vitamin D3 supplementation on progression-free survival among patients with advanced or metastatic colorectal cancer. The SUNSHINE randomized clinical trial. *JAMA* 2019;321(14):1370–9.

174. Aparicio T, Lavau-Denes S, Phelip JM, et al. Randomized phase III trial in elderly patients comparing LV5FU2 with or without irinotecan for first-line treatment of metastatic colorectal cancer (FFCD 2001–02). *Ann Oncol* 2016;27:121–7.

175. Giessen C, Graeven U, Laubender RP, et al. Prognostic factors for 60-day mortality in first-line treatment of metastatic colorectal cancer (mCRC): Individual patient analysis of four randomised, controlled trials by the AIO colorectal cancer study group. *Ann Oncol* 2013;24(12):3051–5.

176. Aparicio T, Bennouna J, Le Malicot K, et al. Predictive factors for early progression during induction chemotherapy and chemotherapy-free interval: Analysis from PRODIGE 9 trial. *Br J Cancer* 2020;122:957–62.

177. Fucà G, Guarini V, Antonioyyi C, et al. The Pan-Immune-Inflammation Value is a new prognostic biomarker in metastatic colorectal cancer: Results from a pooled-analysis of the Valentino and TRIBE first-line trials. *Br J Cancer* 2020;123:403–9.

178. Adams RA, Meade AM, Seymour MT, et al. Intermittent versus continuous oxaliplatin and fluoropyrimidine combination chemotherapy for first-line treatment of advanced colorectal cancer: Results of the randomised phase 3 MRC COIN trial. *Lancet Oncol* 2011;12(7):642–53.

179. Takamizawa Y, Shida D, Boku N, et al. Nutritional and inflammatory measures predict survival of patients with stage IV colorectal cancer. *BMC Cancer* 2020;20(1):1092.

180. Mitani S, Taniguchi H, Sugiyama K, et al. The impact of the Glasgow Prognostic Score on survival in second-line chemotherapy for metastatic colorectal cancer patients with BRAF V600E mutation. *Ther Adv Med Oncol* 2019;11:1–11.

181. Giessen C, Stintzing S, Laubender RP, et al. Analysis for prognostic factors of 60-day mortality: Evaluation of an irinotecan-based phase III trial performed in the first-line treatment of metastatic colorectal cancer. *Clin Colorectal Cancer* 2011;10(4):317–24.

182. Wulaningsih W, Holmberg L, Garmo H, et al. Serum lactate dehydrogenase and survival following cancer diagnosis. *Br J Cancer* 2015;113(9):1389–96.

183. Feng W, Wang Y, Zhu X. Baseline serum lactate dehydrogenase level predicts survival benefit in patients with metastatic colorectal cancer receiving bevacizumab as first-line chemotherapy: A systematic review and meta-analysis of 7 studies and 1,219 patients. *Ann Transl Med* 2019;7(7):133.

184. Iwanicki-Caron I, Di Fiore F, Roque I, et al. Usefulness of the serum carcinoembryonic antigen kinetic for chemotherapy monitoring in patients with unresectable metastasis of colorectal cancer. *J Clin Oncol* 2008;26(22):3681–6.

185. Duffy MJ. Carcinoembryonic antigen as a marker for colorectal cancer: Is it clinically useful? *Clin Chem* 2001;47(4):624–30.

186. Pakdel A, Malekzadeh M, Naghibalhossaini F. The association between preoperative serum CEA concentrations and synchronous liver metastasis in colorectal cancer patients. *Cancer Biomarkers* 2016;16:245–52.

187. Lin JZ, Zeng ZF, Wu XJ, et al. Phase II study of pre-operative radiotherapy with capecitabine and oxaliplatin for rectal cancer and carcinoembryonic antigen as a predictor of pathological tumour response. *J Int Med Res* 2010;38(2):645–54.

188. Li M, Li J-Y, Zhao A-L, et al. Comparison of carcinoembryonic antigen prognostic value in serum and tumour tissue of patients with colorectal cancer. *Colorectal Dis* 2009;11(3):276–81.

189. Eftekar E, Naghibalhossaini F. Carcinoembryonic antigen expression level as a predictive factor for response to 5-fluorouracil in colorectal cancer. *Mol Biol Rep* 2014;41(1):459–66.

190. Stiksma J, Grootendorst DC, van der Linden PWG. CA 19–9 as a marker in addition to CEA to monitor colorectal cancer. *Clin Cororectal Cance* 2014;13(4):239–44.

191. Selcukbiricik F, Bilici A, Tural D, et al. Are high initial CEA and CA 19–9 levels associated with the presence of K-ras mutation in patients with metastatic colorectal cancer? *Tumor Biol* 2013;34:2233–9.

192. Lin C-C, Lai Y-L, Lin T-C, et al. Clinicopathologic features and prognostic analysis of MSI-high colon cancer. *Int J Colorectal Dis* 2012;27(3):277–86.

193. Mitry E, Douillard J-Y, Van Cutsem E, et al. Predictive factors of survival in patients with advanced colorectal cancer: An individual data analysis of 602 patients included in irinotecan phase III trials. *Ann Oncol* 2004;15:1013–7.

194. Shimura T, Toiyama Y, Saigusa S, et al. Inflammation-based prognostic scores as indicators to select candidates for ptimary site resection followed by multimodal therapy among colorectal cancer patients with multiple metastases. *Int J Clin Oncol* 2017;22(4):758–66.

195. Colucci G, Maiello E, Gebbia V, et al. 5-fluorouracil and levofolinic acid with or without recombinant interferon-2b in patients with advanced colorectal carcinoma: A randomized multicenter study with stratification for tumor burden and liver involvement by the Southern Italy Oncology Group. *Cancer* 1999;85(3):535–45.

196. van den Eynde M, Mlecnik B, Bindea G, et al. The link between the multiverse of immune microenvironments in metastases and the survival of colorectal cancer patients. *Cancer Cell* 2018;34:1012–26.

197. Holch JW, Demmer M, Lamersdorf C, et al. Pattern and dynamics of distant metastases in metastatic colorectal cancer. *Visc Med* 2017;33(1):70–5.

198. Marschner N, Frank M, Vach W, et al. Development and validation of a novel prognostic score to predict survival in patients with metastatic colorectal cancer: The metastatic colorectal cancer score (mCCS). *Colorectal Dis* 2019;21(7):816–26.

199. Yamauchi M, Morikawa T, Kuchiba A, et al. Assessment of colorectal cancer molecular features along bowel subsites challenges the conception of distinct dichotomy of proximal versus distal colorectum. *Gut* 2012;61:847–54.

200. Price TJ, Beeke C, Ullah S, et al. Does the primary site of colorectal cancer impact outcomes for patients with metastatic disease? *Cancer* 2015;121:830–5.

201. Hugen N, Nagtegaal ID. Distinct metastatic patterns in colorectal cancer patients based on primary tumor location. *Eur J Cancer* 2017;75:3–4.

202. Hanna MC, Go C, Roden C, et al. Colorectal cancers from distinct ancestral populations show variations in BRAF mutation frequency. *PLoS ONE* 2013;8(9):e74950.

203. Sanz-Pamplona R, Cordero D, Berenguer A, et al. Gene expression differences between colon and rectum tumors. *Clin Cancer Res* 2011;17(23):7303–12.

204. Stintzing S, Wirapati P, Lenz H-J, et al. Consensus molecular subgroups (CMS) of colorectal cancer (CRC) and first-line efficacy of FOLFIRI plus cetuximab or bevacizumab in the FIRE3 (AIO KRK-0306) trial. *Ann Oncol* 2019;30:1796–803.

205. Zhang R-X, Ma W-J, Gu Y-T, et al. Primary tumor location as a predictor of the benefit of palliative resection for colorectal cancer with unresectable metastasis. *World J Surg Oncol* 2017;15:138.

206. Arnold D, Lueza B, Douillard J-Y, et al. Prognostic and predictive value of primary tumor side in patients with RAS wild-type metastatic colorectal cancer treated with chemotherapy and EGFR directed antibodies in six randomized trials. *Ann Oncol* 2017;28:1713–29.

207. Martin R, Paty P, Fong Y, et al. Simultaneous liver and colorectal resections are safe for synchronous colorectal liver metastasis. *J Am Coll Surg* 2003;197(2):233–41.

208. Goey KKH, 't Lam-Boer J, de Wilt JHW, et al. Significant increase of synchronous disease in first-line metastatic colorectal cancer trials: Results of a systematic review. *Eur J Cancer* 2016;69:166–77.

209. van der Geest LGM, 't Lam-Boer J, Koopman M, et al. Nationwide trends in incidence, treatment and survival of colorectal cancer patients with synchronous metastases. *Clin Exp Metastasis* 2015;32(5):457–65.

210. Elferink MA, de Jong KP, Klaase JM, et al. Metachronous metastases from colorectal cancer: A population-based study in North-East Netherlands. *Int J Colorectal Dis* 2014;30(2):205–12.

211. Reboux N, Jooste V, Goungounga J, et al. Incidence and survival in synchronous and metachronous liver metastases from colorectal cancer. *JAMA Netw Open* 2022;5(10):e2236666.

212. Chen H, Yin S, Xiong Z, et al. Clinicopathologic characteristics and prognosis of synchronous colorectal cancer: A retrospective study. *BMC Gastroenterol* 2022;22(1):120.

213. Engstrand J, Stromberg C, Nilsson H, et al. Synchronous and metachronous liver metastases in patients with colorectal cancer – Towards a clinically relevant definition. *World J Surg Oncol* 2019;17(1):228.

214. Kumar R, Price TJ, Beeke C, et al. Colorectal cancer survival: An analysis of patients with metastatic disease synchronous and metachronous with the primary tumor. *Clin Colorectal Cancer* 2014;13(2):87–93.

215. Mitry E, Guiu B, Cosconea S, et al. Epidemiology, management and prognosis of colorectal cancer with lung metastases: A 30-year population-based study. *Gut* 2010;59(10):1383–8.

216. Wisneski AD, Jin C, Huang C-Y, et al. Synchronous versus metachronous colorectal liver metastasis yields similar survival in modern era. *J Surg Res* 2020;256:476–85.

217. Kemeny N, Niedzwiecki D, Shurgot B, Oderman P. Prognostic variables in patients with hepatic metastases from colorectal cancer. Importance of medical assessment of liver involvement. *Cancer* 1989;63(4):742–7.

218. Nordic Gastrointestinal Tumor Adjuvant Therapy Group. Expectancy or primary chemotherapy in patients with advanced asymptomatic colorectal cancer: A randomized trial. *J Clin Oncol* 1992;10(6):904–11.

219. Graf W, Bergstrom R, Pahlman L, Glimelius B. Appraisal of a model for prediction of prognosis in advanced colorectal cancer. *Eur J Cancer* 1994;30A(4):453–7.

220. Freyer G, Rougier P, Bugat R, et al. Prognostic factors for tumour response, progression-free survival and toxicity in metastatic colorectal cancer patients given irinotecan (CPT-11) as second-line chemotherapy after 5FU failure. CPT-11 F205, F220, F221 and V222 study groups. *Br J Cancer* 2000;83(4):431–7.

221. Etienne-Grimaldi M-C, Formento J-L, Francoual M, et al. K-Ras mutations and treatment outcome in colorectal cancer patients receiving exclusive fluoropyrimidine therapy. *Clin Cancer Res* 2008;14(15):4830–5.

222. Slesser AAP, Georgiou P, Brown G, Mudan S, et al. The tumour biology of synchronous and metachronous colorectal liver metastases: A systematic review. *Clin Exp Metastasis* 2013;30(4):457–70.

223. Zhu Y-J, Chen Y, Hu H-Y, et al. Predictive risk factors and online nomograms for synchronous colon cancer with liver metastasis. *Front Oncol* 2020;10:1681.

224. Bokhorn M, Frilling A, Fruhauf NR, et al. Survival of patients with synchronous and metachronous colorectal liver metastases – Is there a difference? *J Gastrointest Surg* 2008;12(8):1399–405.

225. Koopman M, Antonini NF, Vreugdenhil G, et al. Resection of the primary tumor as an independent prognostic factor for survival in patients with advanced colorectal cancer, CAIRO study of the Dutch Colorectal Cancer Group (DCCG). *Eur J Cancer Suppl* 5:250 (abstract Po3047).

226. Ng WWC, Cheung YS, Wong J, et al. A preliminary analysis of combined liver resection with new chemotherapy for synchronous and metachronous colorectal liver metastases. *Asian J Surg* 2009;32(4):189–97.

227. van der Pool AEM, Lalmahomed ZS, Ozbay Y, et al. 'Staged' liver resection in synchronous and metachronous colorectal hepatic metastases: Differences in clinicopathological features and outcome. *Colorectal Dis* 2010;12(10):229–35.

228. Stillwell AP, Buettner PG, Ho YH. Meta-analysis of survival of patients with stage IV colorectal cancer managed with surgical resection versus chemotherapy alone. *World J Surg* 2010;34(4):797–807.

229. van Rooijen KL, Shi Q, Goey KKH, et al. Prognostic value of primary tumor resection in synchronous metastatic colorectal cancer: Individual patient data analysis of first-line randomised trials from the ARCAD database. *Eur J Cancer* 2018;91:99–106.

230. Alawadi Z, Phatak UR, Hu C-Y, et al. Comparative effectiveness of primary tumor resection in patients with stage IV colon cancer. *Cancer* 2017;123(7):1124–33.

231. Wong SF, Wong HL, Field KM, et al. Primary tumor resection and overall survival in patients with metastatic colorectal cancer treated with palliative intent. *Clin Colorectal Cancer* 2016;15(3):e125–32.

232. Simkens LHJ, van Tinteren H, May A, et al. Maintenance treatment with capecitabine and bevacizumab in metastatic colorectal cancer (CAIRO3): A phase 3 randomised controlled trial of the Dutch Colorectal Cancer Group. *Lancet* 2015;385:1843–52.

233. Venderbosch S, de Wilt JH, Teerenstra S, et al. Prognostic value of resection of primary tumor in patients with stage IV colorectal cancer: Retrospective analysis of two randomized studies and a review of the literature. *Ann Surg Oncol* 2011;18(12):3252–60.

234. van der Wal GE, Gouw A, Kamps JAAM, et al. Angiogenesis in synchronous and metachronous colorectal liver metastases. The liver as a permissive soil. *Ann Surg* 2012;255:86–94.

235. Chuang S-C, Su Y-C, Lu C-Y, et al. Risk factors for the development of metachronous liver metastasis in colorectal cancer patients after curative resection. *World J Surg* 2011;35:424–9.

236. Iizasa T, Suzuki M, Yoshida S, et al. Prediction of prognosis and surgical indications for pulmonary metastasectomy from colorectal cancer. *Ann Thorac Surg* 2006;82(1):254–60.

237. Hoshino Y, Terashima S, Teranishi Y, et al. Ornithine decarboxylase activity as a prognostic marker for colorectal cancer. *Fukushima J Med Sci* 2007;53(1):1–9.

238. Yahagi M, Okabayashi K, Hasegawa H, et al. The worse prognosis of right-sided compared with left-sided colon cancers: A systematic review and meta-analysis. *J Gastrointest Surg* 2016;20(3):648–55.

239. Pantaleo MA, Astolfi A, Nannini M, et al. Gene expression profiling of liver metastases from colorectal cancer as potential basis for treatment choice. *Br J Cancer* 2008;99(10):1729–34.

240. Rose JS, Serna DS, Martin LK, et al. Influence of KRAS mutation status in metachronous and synchronous metastatic colorectal adenocarcinoma. *Cancer* 2012;118:6243–52.

241. Nordholm-Carstensen A, Krarup P-M, Morton D, Harling H. Mismatch repair status and synchronous metastases in colorectal cancer: A nationwide cohort study. *Int J Cancer* 2018;137(9):2139–48.

242. Prasanna T, Karapetis CS, Roder D, et al. The survival outcome of patients with metastatic colorectal cancer based on the site of metastases and the impact of molecular markers and site of primary cancer on metastatic pattern. *Acta Oncol* 2018;57(11):1438–44.

243. Kwon MJ, Lee SE, Kang SY, Choi Y-L. Frequency of KRAS, BRAF, and PIK3CA mutations in advanced colorectal cancers: Comparison of peptide nucleic acid-mediated PCR clamping and direct sequencing in formalin-fixed, paraffin-embedded tissue. *Pathol Res Pract* 2011;207(12):762–8.

244. Li L, Ma BB. Colorectal cancer in Chinese patients: Current and emerging treatment options. *Onco Targets Ther* 2014;7:1817–28.

245. Sawayama H, Miyamoto Y, Hiyoshi Y, et al. Overall survival after recurrence in stage I–III colorectal cancer patients in accordance with the recurrence organ site and pattern. *Ann Gastroenterol Surg* 2021;5(6):813–22.

246. Merkel S, Weber K, Croner RS, et al. Distant metastases in colorectal carcinoma: A proposal for a new M1 subclassification. *Eur J Surg Oncol* 2016;42(9):1337–42.

247. Rao US, Hoerster NS, Thirumala S, Rao PS. The influence of metastatic site on the expression of CEA and cellular localization of β-catenin in colorectal cancer. *J Gastroenterol Hepatol* 2013;28(3):505–12.

248. Kim M-J, Lee HS, Kim JH, et al. Different metastatic pattern according to the KRAS mutational status and site-specific discordance of KRAS status in patients with colorectal cancer. *BMC Cancer* 2012;12:347.

249. Cavallaro P, Bordeianou L, Stafford C, et al. Impact of single-organ metastasis to the liver or lung and genetic mutation status on prognosis in stage IV colorectal cancer. *Clin Colorectal Cancer* 2020;19(1):e8–17.

250. de Jong MC, Pulitano C, Ribero D, et al. Rates and patterns of recurrence following curative intent surgery for colorectal liver metastasis: An international multi-institutional analysis of 1669 patients. *Ann Surg* 2009;250(3):440–8.

251. Pugh SA, Bowers M, Ball A, et al. Patterns of progression, treatment of progressive disease and post-progression survival in the New EPOC study. *Br J Cancer* 2016;115(4):420–4.

252. Spelt L, Andersson B, Nilsson J, Andersson R. Prognostic models for outcome following liver resection for colorectal cancer metastases: A systematic review. *Eur J Surg Oncol* 2012;38(1):16–24.

253. Matias M, Casa-Nova M, Faria M, et al. Prognostic factors after liver resection for colorectal liver metastasis. *Acta Med Port* 2015;28(3):357–69.

254. Buisman FE, Giardiello D, Kemeny NE, et al. Predicting 10-year survival after resection of colorectal liver metastases; an international study including biomarkers and perioperative treatment. *Eur J Cancer* 2022;168:25–33.

255. Schreckenbach T, Malkomes P, Bechstein WO, et al. The clinical relevance of the Fong and the Nordlinger scores in the era of effective neoadjuvant chemotherapy for colorectal liver metastasis. *Surg Today* 2015;45(12):1527–34.

256. Neal CP, Cairns V, Jones MJ, et al. Prognostic performance of inflammation-based prognostic indices in patients with resectable colorectal liver metastases. *Med Oncol* 2015;32(5):590.

257. Tosi F, Magni E, Amatu A, et al. Effect of KRAS and BRAF mutations on survival of metastatic colorectal cancer after liver resection: A systematic review and meta-analysis. *Clin Colorectal Cancer* 2017;16(3):e153–63.

258. Vauthey J-N, Zimmitti G, Kopetz SE, et al. RAS mutation status predicts survival and patterns of recurrence in patients undergoing hepatectomy for colorectal liver metastases. *Ann Surg* 2013;258(4):619–26.

259. Kemeny NE, Chou JF, Capanu M, et al. KRAS mutation influences recurrence patterns in patients undergoing hepatic resection of colorectal metastases. *Cancer* 2014;120(24):3965–71.

260. Pfannschmidt J, Dienemann H, Hoffmann H. Surgical resection of pulmonary metastases from colorectal cancer: A systematic review of published series. *Ann Thorac Surg* 2007;84(1):324–38.

261. Tsitsias T, Toufektzian L, Routledge T, Pilling J. Are there recognized prognostic factors for patients undergoing pulmonary metastasectomy for colorectal carcinoma? *Inter Cardiovasc Thorac Surg* 2016;23:962–9.
262. Osoegawa A, Kometani T, Fukuyama S, et al. Prognostic factors for survival after resection of pulmonary metastases from colorectal carcinoma. *Ann Thorac Cardiovasc Surg* 2016;22:6–11.
263. Renaud S, Guerrera F, Seitlinger J, et al. KRAS exon 2 codon 13 mutation is associated with a better prognosis than codon 12 mutation following lung metastasectomy in colorectal cancer. *Oncotarget* 2017;8(2):2514–24.
264. Foster JM, Zhang C, Rehman S, et al. The contemporary management of peritoneal metastasis: A journey from the cold past of treatment futility to a warm present and a bright future. *CA Cancer J Clin* 2023;73(1):49–71.
265. Mulsow J, Merkel S, Agaimy A, Hohenberger W. Outcomes following surgery for colorectal cancer with synchronous peritoneal metastases. *Br J Surg* 2011;98(12):1785–91.
266. Lemmens VE, Klaver YL, Verwaal VJ, et al. Predictors and survival of synchronous peritoneal carcinomatosis of colorectal origin: A population-based study. *Int J Cancer* 2011;128(11):2717–25.
267. Kwakman R, Schrama AM, van Olmen JP, et al. Clinicopathological parameters in patient selection for cytoreductive surgery and hyperthermic intraperitoneal chemotherapy for colorectal cancer metastases: A meta-analysis. *Ann Surg* 2016;263(6):1102–11.
268. Hallam S, Tyler R, Price M, et al. Meta-analysis of prognostic factors for patients with colorectal peritoneal metastasis undergoing cytoreductive surgery and heated intraperitoneal chemotherapy. *BJS Open* 2019;3:585–94.
269. Franko J, Shi Q, Meyers JP, et al. Prognosis of patients with peritoneal metastatic colorectal cancer given systemic therapy: An analysis of individual patient data from prospective randomised trials from the Analysis and Research in Cancers of the Digestive System (ARCAD) database. *Lancet Oncol* 2016;17(12):1709–19.
270. Chen H, Zhou S, Bi J, et al. Does the primary tumour location affect the prognosis of patients with colorectal cancer peritoneal metastases treated with cytoreductive surgery and hyperthermic intraperitoneal chemotherapy? *World J Surg Oncol* 2021;19(1):253.
271. Ubink I, van Eden WJ, Snaebjornsson P, et al. Histopathological and molecular classification of colorectal cancer and corresponding peritoneal metastases. *Br J Surg* 2018;105(2):e204–11.
272. Lenos KJ, Bach S, Ferreira Moreno L, et al. Molecular characterization of colorectal cancer related peritoneal metastatic disease. *Nat Commun* 2022;13:4443.
273. Arjona-Sanchez A, Rodriguez-Ortiz L, Baratti D, et al. RAS mutation decreases overall survival after optimal cytoreductive surgery and hyperthermic intraperitoneal chemotherapy of colorectal peritoneal metastasis: A modification proposal of the peritoneal surface disease severity score. *Ann Surg Oncol* 2019;26(8):2595–604.
274. Pitt J, Dawson PM. Oophorectomy in women with colorectal cancer. *Eur J Surg Oncol* 1999;25(4):432–8.
275. Segelman J, Floter-Radestad A, Hellborg H, et al. Epidemiology and prognosis of ovarian metastases in colorectal cancer. *Br J Surg* 2010;97:1704–9.
276. van der Meer R, Bakkers C, Wegdam JA, et al. Ovarian metastases in young women with colorectal cancer: A retrospective multicenter cohort study. *Int J Colorectal Dis* 2022;37(8):1865–73.
277. Van der Meer R, de Hingh IHJT, Bloemen JG, et al. Role of Ovarian Metastases in Colorectal Cancer (ROMIC): A Dutch study protocol to evaluate the effect of prophylactic salpingo-oophorectomy in postmenopausal women. *BMC Women Health* 2022;22(1):441.
278. Rihimaki M, Hemminki A, Sundquist J, Hemminki K. Patterns of metastasis in colon and rectal cancer. *Sci Rep* 2016;6:29765.
279. Baek S-J, Hur H, Min B-S, et al. The characteristics of bone metastasis in patients with colorectal cancer: A long-term report from a single institution. *World J Surg* 2016;404(4):982–6.
280. Santini D, Tampellini M, Vincenzi B, et al. Natural history of bone metastasis in colorectal cancer: Final results of a large Italian bone metastases study. *Ann Oncol* 2012;23(8):2072–7.
281. Kanthan R, Loewy J, Kanthan SC. Skeletal metastases in colorectal carcinomas: A Saskatchewan profile. *Dis Colon Rectum* 1999;42(12):1592–7.
282. Muller S, Kohler F, Hendricks A, et al. Brain metastases from colorectal cancer: A systematic review of the literature and meta-analysis to establish a guideline for daily treatment. *Cancers* 2021;13(4):900.
283. Shindorf ML, Jafferji MS, Goff SL. Incidence of asymptomatic brain metastases in metastatic colorectal cancer. *Clin Colorectal Cancer* 2020;19(4):263–9.
284. Hammoud MA, McCutcheon IE, Elsouki R, et al. Colorectal carcinoma and brain metastasis: Distribution, treatment, and survival. *Ann Surg Oncol* 1996;3(5):453–63.

285. Tokoto T, Okuno K, Hida J, et al. Prognostic factors for patients with advanced colorectal cancer and symptomatic brain metastases. *Clin Colorectal Cancer* 2014;13(4):226–31.

286. Quan J-C, Guan X, Ma C-X, et al. Prognostic scoring system for synchronous brain metastasis at diagnosis of colorectal cancer: A population-based study. *World J Gastrointest Oncol* 2020;12(2):195–204.

287. Chang Y, Wong C-E, Lee P-H, et al. Survival outcome of surgical resection vs. radiotherapy in brain metastasis from colorectal cancer: A meta-analysis. *Front Med* 2022;9:768896.

288. Cardinal T, Pangal D, Strickland BA, et al. Anatomical and topographical variations in the distribution of brain metastases based on primary cancer origin and molecular subtypes: A systematic review. *Neurooncol Adv* 2021;4(1):vdab170.

289. Naxerova K, Reiter JG, Bachtel E, et al. Origins of lymphatic and distant metastases in human colorectal cancer. *Science* 2017;357(6346):55–60.

290. Roussille P, Tachon G, Villalva C, et al. Pathological and molecular characteristics of colorectal cancer with brain metastases. *Cancers* 2018;10(12):504.

291. Dell'Aquila E, Rossini D, Fulgenzi CAM, et al. Bone metastases are associated with worse prognosis in patients affected by metastatic colorectal cancer treated with doublet or triplet chemotherapy plus bevacizumab: A subanalysis of the TRIBE and TRIBE2 trials. *ESMO Open* 2022;7(6):100606.

292. Hugen N, Verhoeven RH, Lemmens VE, et al. Colorectal signet-ring cell carcinoma: Benefit from adjuvant chemotherapy but a poor prognostic factor. *Int J Cancer* 2015;136(2):333–9.

293. van Zwam PH, Vink-Borger EM, Bronkhorst CM, et al. Prognosis of mucinous colon cancer is determined by histological biomarkers rather than microsatellite instability. *Histopathol* 2023;82:314–23.

294. Patel C, Behring M, Al Diffalha S, et al. Immunophenotypic profiles and prognosis for colorectal mucinous adenocarcinomas are dependent on anatomic location. *Cancer Med* 2023;12(8):9637–43.

295. O'Connell E, Reynolds IS, Salvucci M, et al. Mucinous and non-mucinous colorectal cancers show differential expression of chemotherapy metabolism and resistance genes. *Pharmacogenom J* 2021;21:510–9.

296. Philips RK, Hittinger R, Blesovsky L, et al. Large bowel cancer: Surgical pathology and its relationship to survival. *Br J Surg* 1984;71(8):604–10.

297. Chapuis PH, Dent OF, Fisher R, et al. A multivariate analysis of clinical and pathological variables in prognosis after resection of large bowel cancer. *Br J Surg* 1985;72(9):698–702.

298. Jass JR, Atkin WS, Cuzick J, et al. The grading of rectal cancer: Historical perspectives and a multivariate analysis of 447 cases. *Histopathol* 1986;10(5):437–59.

299. Newland RC, Dent OF, Lyttle MN, et al. Pathologic determinants of survival associated with colorectal cancer with lymph node metastases. A multivariate analysis of 579 patients. *Cancer* 1994;73(8):2076–82.

300. Fonseca GM, de Mello ES, Faraj SF, et al. Prognostic significance of poorly differentiated clusters and tumor budding in colorectal liver metastases. *J Surg Oncol* 2018;117(7):1364–75.

301. Galon J, Costes A, Sanchez-Cabo F, et al. Type, density, and location of immune cells within human colorectal tumors predict clinical outcome. *Science* 2006;313(5795):1960–4.

302. Mlecnik B, Van den Eynde M, Bindea G, et al. Comprehensive intrametastatic immune quantification and major impact of immunoscore on survival. *J Natl Cancer Inst* 2018;110(1):djx123.

303. Mlecnik B, Bindea G, Angell HK, et al. Integrative analyses of colorectal cancer show immunoscore is a stronger predictor of patient survival than microsatellite instability. *Immunity* 2016;44(3):698–711.

304. Minsky B, Mies C. The clinical significance of vascular invasion in colorectal cancer. *Dis Colon Rectum* 1989;32(9):794–803.

305. Mlecnik B, Bindea G, Angell HK, et al. Functional network pipeline reveals genetic determinants associated with in situ lymphocyte proliferation and survival of cancer patients. *Sci Transl Med* 2014;6(228):228ra237.

306. Fridman WH, Pages F, Sautes-Fridman C, Galon J. The immune contexture in human tumours: Impact on clinical outcome. *Nat Rev Cancer* 2012;12(4):298–306.

307. Halama N, Michel S, Kloor M, et al. Localization and density of immune cells in the invasive margin of human colorectal cancer liver metastases are prognostic for response to chemotherapy. *Cancer Res* 2011;71(17):5670–7.

308. Ahmed A, Halama N. Tertiary lymphoid structures in colorectal cancer liver metastases: Association with immunological and clinical parameters and chemotherapy response. *Anticancer Res* 2020;40:6367–73.

309. Dieu-Nosjean M-C, Giraldo NA, Kaplon H, et al. Tertiary lymphoid structures, drivers of the anti-tumor responses in human cancers. *Immunol Rev* 2016;271(1):260–5.

310. Sautes-Fridman C, Lawand M, Giraldo NA, et al. Tertiary lymphoid structures in cancers: Prognostic value, regulation, and manipulation for therapeutic intervention. *Front Immunol* 2016;7:407.

311. de Chaisemartin L, Goc J, Damotte D, et al. Characterization of chemokines and adhesion molecules associated with T cell presence in tertiary lymphoid structures in human lung cancer. *Cancer Res* 2011;71(20):6391–9.

312. Tanis E, Julié C, Emile J-F, et al. Prognostic impact of immune response in resectable colorectal liver metastases treated by surgery alone or surgery with perioperative FOLFOX in the randomised EORTC study 40983. *Eur J Cancer* 2015;51(17):2708–17.

313. Halama N, Michel S, Kloor M, et al. The localization and density of immune cells in primary tumors of human metastatic colorectal cancer shows an association with response to chemotherapy. *Cancer Immun* 2009;9:1.

314. van Dam P-J, van der Stok EP, Teuwen L-A, et al. International consensus guidelines for scoring the histopathological growth patterns of liver metastasis. *Br J Cancer* 2017;117(10):1427–41.

315. Latacz E, Hoppener D, Bohlok A, et al. Histopathological growth patterns of liver metastasis: Updated consensus guidelines for pattern scoring, perspectives and recent mechanistic insights. *Br J Cancer* 2022;127(6):988–1033.

316. Wu J-B, Lopez Sarmiento A, Fiset P-O, et al. Histologic features and genomic alterations of primary colorectal adenocarcinoma predict growth patterns of liver metastasis. *World J Gastroenterol* 2019;25(26):3408–25.

317. Van den Eynden GG, Bird NC, Majeed AW, et al. The histological growth pattern of colorectal cancer liver metastases has prognostic value. *Clin Exp Metastasis* 2012;29(6):541–9.

318. Nielsen K, Rolff HC, Eefsen RL, Vainer B. The morphological growth patterns of colorectal liver metastases are prognostic for overall survival. *Mod Pathol* 2014;27(12):1641–8.

319. Frentzas S, Simoneau E, Bridgeman VL, et al. Vessel co-option mediates resistance to anti-angiogenic therapy in liver metastases. *Nat Med* 2016;22(11):1294–302.

320. Stremitzer S, Vermeulen P, Graver S, et al. Immune phenotype and histopathological growth pattern in patients with colorectal liver metastases. *Br J Cancer* 2020;122(10):518–24.

321. Liang J-Y, Xi S-Y, Shao Q, et al. Histopathological growth patterns correlate with the immunoscore in colorectal cancer liver metastasis patients after hepatectomy. *Cancer Immunol Immunother* 2020;69(12):2623–34.

322. Uhlig J, Cecchini M, Sheth A, et al. Microsatellite instability and KRAS mutation in stage IV colorectal cancer: Prevalence, geographic discrepancies, and outcomes from the National Cancer Database. *J Natl Compr Canc Netw* 2021;19(3):307–18.

323. Andrè T, Shiu K-K, Kim TW, et al. Pembrolizumab in microsatellite-instability-high advanced colorectal cancer. *N Engl J Med* 2020;383:2207–18.

324. Bae JM, Kim MJ, Kim JH, et al. Differential clinicopathological features in microsatellite instability-positive colorectal cancers depending on CIMP status. *Virchow Arch* 2011;459(1):55–63.

325. Schirripa M, Biason P, Lonardi S, et al. Class 1, 2 and 3 BRAF-mutated metastatic colorectal cancer: A detailed clinical, pathologic, and molecular characterization. *Clin Cancer Res* 2019;25(13):3954–61.

326. Barras D, Missiaglia E, Wirapati P, et al. BRAF V600E mutant colorectal cancer subtypes based on gene expression. *Clin Cancer Res* 2017;23(1):104–15.

327. Seppala TT, Bohm JP, Friman M, et al. Combination of microsatellite instability and BRAF mutation status for subtyping colorectal cancer. *Br J Cancer* 2015;112:1966–75.

328. Guinney J, Dienstmann R, Wang X, et al. The consensus molecular subtypes of colorectal cancer. *Nat Med* 2015;21(11):1350–6.

329. Lenz H-J, Ou F-S, Venook AP, et al. Impact of Consensus Molecular Subtype on survival in patients with metastatic colorectal cancer: Results from CALGB/SWOG 80405 (Alliance). *J Clin Oncol* 2019;37:1876–85.

330. Eide PW, Moosavi SH, Eilertsen IA, et al. Metastatic heterogeneity of the consensus molecular subtypes of colorectal cancer. *Genom Med* 2021;6:59.

331. Kamal Y, Schmit SL, Hoehn HJ, et al. Transcriptomic differences between primary colorectal adenocarcinomas and distant metastases reveal metastatic colorectal cancer subtypes. *Cancer Res* 2019;79(16):4227–41.

332. Bramsen JB, Rasmussen MH, Ongen H, et al. Molecular-subtype-specific biomarkers improve prediction of prognosis in colorectal cancer. *Cell Reports* 2017;19:1268–80.

333. Pitroda SP, Khodarev NN, Huang L, et al. Integrated molecular subtyping defines a curable oligometastatic state in colorectal liver metastasis. *Nat Commun* 2018;9(1):1793.

334. ten Hoorn S, Sommeijer DW, Elliott F, et al. Molecular subtype-specific efficacy of anti-EGFR therapy in colorectal cancer is dependent on the chemotherapy backbone. *Br J Cancer* 2021;125:1080–8.

335. Okita A, Takahashi S, Ouchi K, et al. Consensus molecular subtypes classification of colorectal cancer as a predictive factor for chemotherapeutic efficacy against metastatic colorectal cancer. *Oncotarget* 2018;9(27):18698–711.

336. Del Rio M, Mollevi C, Bibeau F, et al. Molecular subtypes of metastatic colorectal cancer are associated with patient response to irinotecan-based therapies. *Eur J Cancer* 2017;76:68–75.

337. Innocenti F, Ou F-S, Qu X, et al. Mutational analysis of patients with colorectal cancer in CALGB/SWOG 80405 identifies new roles of microsatellite instability and tumor mutational burden for patient outcome. *J Clin Oncol* 2019;37:1217–27.

338. Mooi JK, Wirapati P, Asher R, et al. The prognostic impact of consensus molecular subtypes (CMS) and its predictive effects for bevacizumab benefit in metastatic colorectal cancer: Molecular analysis of the AGITG MAX clinical trial. *Ann Oncol* 2018;29:2240–6.

339. Fennell L, Dumenil T, Wockner L, et al. Integrative genome-scale DNA methylation analysis of a large and unselected cohort reveals 5 distinct subtypes of colorectal adenocarcinomas. *Cell Molec Gastroenterol Hepatol* 2019;8(2):269–90.

340. Wang J, Deng Z, Lang X, et al. Meta-analysis of the prognostic and predictive role of the CpG island methylator phenotype in colorectal cancer. *Dis Markers* 2022;2022:4254862.

341. Modest DP, Ricard I, Heinemann V, et al. Outcome according to KRAS-, NRAS- and BRAF-mutation as well as KRAS mutation variants: Pooled analysis of five randomized trials in metastatic colorectal cancer by the AIO colorectal cancer study group. *Ann Oncol* 2016;27:1746–53.

342. Tarantino I, Warschkow R, Worni M, et al. Prognostic relevance of palliative primary tumor removal in 37,793 metastatic colorectal cancer patients. A population-based, propensity score-adjusted trend analysis. *Ann Surg* 2015;262:112–20.

343. Hu C-Y, Bailey CE, You YN, et al. Time trend analysis of primary tumor resection for stage IV colorectal cancer: Less surgery, improved survival. *JAMA Surg* 2015;150(3):245–51.

344. Kanemitsu Y, Shitara K, Mizusawa J, et al. Primary tumor resection plus chemotherapy versus chemotherapy alone for colorectal cancer patients with asymptomatic, synchronous unresectable metastases (JCOG1007; iPACS): A randomized clinical trial. *J Clin Oncol* 2021;39(10):1098–107.

345. Park EJ, Baek J-H, Choi G-S, et al. The role of primary tumor resection in colorectal cancer patients with asymptomatic, synchronous, unresectable metastasis: A multicenter randomized controlled trial. *Cancers* 2020;12(8):2306.

346. Karoui M, Roudot-Thoraval F, Mesli F, et al. Primary colectomy in patients with stage IV colon cancer and unresectable distant metastases improves overall survival: Results of a multicentric study. *Dis Colon Rectum* 2011;54(8):930–8.

347. Colloca GA, Venturino A, Guarneri D. Primary tumor resection in patients with unresectable colorectal cancer with synchronous metastases could improve the activity of poly-chemotherapy: A trial-level meta-analysis. *Surg Oncol* 2022;44:101820.

348. Slesser AAP, Khan F, Chau I, et al. The effect of a primary tumour resection on the progression of synchronous colorectal liver metastases: An exploratory study. *Eur J Surg Oncol* 2015;41(4):484–92.

349. Faron M, Pignon J-P, Malka D, et al. Is primary tumour resection associated with survival improvement in patients with colorectal cancer and unresectable synchronous metastases? A pooled analysis of individual data from four randomised trials. *Eur J Cancer* 2015;51(2):166–76.

350. Wang Z, Liang L, Yu Y, et al. Primary tumour resection could improve the survival of unresectable metastatic colorectal cancer patients receiving bevacizumab-containing chemotherapy. *Cell Physiol Biochem* 2016;39(3):1239–46.

351. Cao G, Zhou W, Chen E, et al. A novel scoring system predicting survival benefits of palliative primary tumor resection for patients with unresectable metastatic colorectal cancer: A retrospective cohort study protocol. *Medicine* 2019;98(37):e17178.

352. Korkmaz L, Coskun HS, Dane F, et al. Kras-mutation influences outcomes for palliative primary tumor resection in advanced colorectal cancer-a Turkish Oncology Group study. *Surg Oncol* 2018;27(3):485–9.

353. Boselli C, Renzi C, Gemini A, et al. Surgery in asymptomatic patients with colorectal cancer and unresectable liver metastases: The authors' experience. *OncoTarg Ther* 2013;6:267–72.

354. Cetin B, Kaplan MA, Berk V, et al. Bevacizumab-containing chemotherapy is safe in patients with unresectable metastatic colorectal cancer and a synchronous asymptomatic primary tumor. *Jpn J Clin Oncol* 2013;43(1):28–32.

355. Kodaz H, Erdogan B, Hacibekiroglu I, et al. Impact of bevacizumab on survival outcomes in primary tumor resected metastatic colorectal cancer. *Med Oncol* 2015;32(1):441.

356. Liang L, Tian J, Yu Y, et al. An analysis of relationship between RAS mutations and prognosis of primary tumour resection for metastatic colorectal cancer patients. *Cell Physiol Biochem* 2018;50(2):768–82.

357. Shida D, Yoshida T, Tanabe T, et al. Prognostic impact of R0 resection and targeted therapy for colorectal cancer with synchronous peritoneal metastasis. *Ann Surg Oncol* 2018;25(6):1646–53.

358. Lim C, Doussot A, Osseis M, et al. Bevacizumab improves survival in patients with synchronous colorectal liver metastases provided the primary tumor is resected first. *Clin Transl Oncol* 2018;20(10):1274–9.

359. Cabart M, Frenel J-S, Campion L, et al. Bevacizumab efficacy is influenced by primary tumor resection in first-line treatment of metastatic colorectal cancer in a retrospective multicenter study. *Clin Colorectal Cancer* 2016;15(4):e165–74.

360. Ahmed S, Leis A, Chandra-Kanthan S, et al. Regional lymph nodes status and ratio of metastatic to examined lymph nodes correlate with survival in stage IV colorectal cancer. *Ann Surg Oncol* 2016;23(7):2287–94.

361. Ling J, Zhang J, Cai Y, et al. Primary tumor resection related to better outcome in Chinese metastatic colorectal cancer patients using bevacizumab. *Acta Chir Austriaca* 2015;47:S71–2.

362. Ghiringhelli F, Bichard D, Limat S, et al. Bevacizumab efficacy in metastatic colorectal cancer is dependent on primary tumor resection. *Ann Surg Oncol* 2014;21(5):1632–40.

363. de Mestiers L, Neuzillet C, Pozet A, et al. Is primary tumor resection associated with a longer survival in colon cancer and unresectable synchronous metastases? A 4-year multicentre experience. *Eur J Surg Oncol* 2014;40(6):685–91.

364. Lee B, Wong H-L, Tacey M, et al. The impact of bevacizumab in metastatic colorectal cancer with an intact primary tumor: Results from a large prospective cohort study. *Asia Pac J Clin Oncol* 2017;13(4):314–21.

365. Colloca GA, Venturino A, Guarneri D. Neutrophil-related variables have different prognostic effect based on primary tumor location in patients with metastatic colorectal cancer receiving chemotherapy. *Clin Colorectal Cancer* 2019;18(4):e343–8.

366. Colloca GA, Venturino A, Guarneri D. Leukocyte kinetics during the first cycle of chemotherapy predicts the outcome of patients with metastatic colorectal cancer and previous resection of the primary tumor. *Int J Colorectal Dis* 2021;36(4):847–55.

367. Turner N, Tran B, Tran PV, et al. Primary tumor resection in patients with metastatic colorectal cancer is associated with reversal of systemic inflammation and improved survival. *Clin Colorectal Cancer* 2015;14(3):185–91.

368. He W-Z, Rong Y-M, Jiang C, et al. Palliative primary tumor resection provides survival benefits for the patients with metastatic colorectal cancer and low circulating levels of dehydrogenase and carcinoembryonic antigen. *Chin J Cancer* 2016;35:58.

369. Chang Y-T, Tsai H-L, Chen Y-C, et al. Clinicopathological features and oncological outcomes of early and late recurrence in stage III colorectal cancer patients after adjuvant oxaliplatin-based therapy. *J Oncol* 2023:2439128.

370. Zok J, Bienkowski M, Radecka B, et al. Impact of relative dose intensity of oxaliplatin in adjuvant therapy among stage III colon cancer patients on early recurrence: A retrospective cohort study. *BMC Cancer* 2021;21(1):529.

371. O'Connell MJ, Campbell ME, Goldberg RM, et al. Survival following recurrence in stage II and III colon cancer: Findings from the ACCENT data set. *J Clin Oncol* 2008;26(14):2336–41.

372. Chu X, Xue P, Zhu S. Management of chemotherapy dose intensity for metastatic colorectal cancer. *Oncol Lett* 2022;23:141.

373. Aspinall SL, Good CB, Zhao X, et al. Adjuvant chemotherapy for stage III colon cancer: Relative dose intensity and survival among veterans. *BMC Cancer* 2015;15(1):62.

374. Nordlinger B, Sorbye H, Glimelius B, et al. Perioperative FOLFOX4 chemotherapy and surgery versus surgery alone for resectable liver metastases from colorectal cancer (EORTC 40983): Long-term results of a randomised, controlled, phase 3 trial. *Lancet Oncol* 2013;14:1208–15.

375. Sorbye H, Mauer M, Gruenberger T, et al. Predictive factors for the benefit of perioperative FOLFOX for resectable liver metastasis in colorectal cancer patients (EORTC Intergroup Trial 40983). *Ann Surg* 2012;255:534–9.

376. Primrose J, Falk S, Finch-Jones M, et al. Systemic chemotherapy with or without cetuximab in patients with resectable colorectal liver metastasis: The New EPOC randomised controlled trial. *Lancet Oncol* 2014;15:601–11.

377. Fonck M, Perez J-T, Catena V, et al. Pulmonary thermal ablation enables long chemotherapy-free survival in metastatic colorectal cancer patients. *Cardiovasc Intervent Radiol* 2018;41(11):1727–34.

378. Evrard S, Poston G, Kissmeyer-Nielsen P, et al. Combined ablation and resection (CARe) as an effective parenchymal sparing treatment for extensive colorectal liver metastases. *PLoS ONE* 2014;9(12):e114404.

379. Stintzing S, Modest DP, Rossius L, et al. FOLFIRI plus cetuximab versus FOLFIRI plus bevacizumab for metastatic colorectal cancer (FIRE-3): A post-hoc analysis of tumour dynamics in the final RAS wild-type subgroup of this randomised open-label phase 3 trial. *Lancet Oncol* 2016;17:1426–34.

380. Modest DP, Denecke T, Pratschke J, et al. Surgical treatment options following chemotherapy plus cetuximab or bevacizumab in metastatic colorectal cancer – Central evaluation of FIRE-3. *Eur J Cancer* 2018;88:77–86.

381. Holch JW, Stintzing S, Held S, et al. Right-sided colorectal cancer (RC): Response to the first-line chemotherapy in FIRE-3 (AIO KRK-0306) with focus on early tumor shrinkage (ETS) and depth of response (DpR). *J Clin Oncol* 2017;35:abs 3586.

382. Ychou M, Rivoire M, Thezenas S, et al. A randomized phase II trial of three intensified chemotherapy regimens in first-line treatment of colorectal cancer patients with initially unresectable or not optimally resectable liver metastases. The METHEP trial. *Ann Surg Oncol* 2013;20:4289–97.

383. Wong R, Cunningham D, Barbachano Y, et al. A multicentre study of capecitabine, oxaliplatin plus bevacizumab as perioperative treatment of patients with poor-risk colorectal liver-only metastases not selected for upfront resection. *Ann Oncol* 2011;22:2042–8.

384. Tang W, Ren L, Liu T, et al. Bevacizumab plus mFOLFOX6 versus mFOLFOX6 alone as first-line treatment for RAS mutant unresectable colorectal liver-limited metastases: The BECOME randomized controlled trial. *J Clin Oncol* 2020;38:3175–84.

385. Cremolini C, Loupakis F, Antoniotti C, et al. Early tumor shrinkage and depth of response predict long-term outcome in metastatic colorectal cancer patients treated with first-line chemotherapy plus bevacizumab: Results from phase III TRIBE trial by the Gruppo Oncologico del Nord Ovest. *Ann Oncol* 2015;26:1188–94.

386. Cremolini C, Casagrande M, Loupakis F, et al. Efficacy of FOLFOXIRI plus bevacizumab in liver-limited metastatic colorectal cancer: A pooled analysis of clinical studies by Gruppo Oncologico del Nord Ovest. *Eur J Cancer* 2017;73:74–84.

387. Ruers T, Punt C, Van Coevorden F, et al. Radiofrequency ablation combined with systemic treatment versus systemic treatment alone in patients with non-resectable colorectal liver metastases: A randomized EORTC Intergroup phase II study. *Ann Oncol* 2012;23:2619–26.

388. Binkley MS, Trakul N, Jacobs LR, et al. Colorectal histology is associated with an increased risk of local failure in lung metastases treated with stereotactic ablative radiation therapy. *Int J Radiat Oncol Biol Phys* 2015;92(5):1044–52.

389. Ahmed KA, Caudell JJ, El-Haddad G, et al. Radiosensitivity differences between liver metastases based on primary histology suggest implications for clinical outcomes after stereotactic body radiation therapy. *Int J Radiat Oncol Biol Phys* 2016;95(5):1399–404.

390. Najafi A, de Baere T, Purenne E, et al. Risk factors for local tumor progression after RFA of pulmonary metastases: A matched case-control study. *Eur Radiol* 2021;31:5361–9.

391. Kanemitsu Y. Reply to B. Bozkurt Duman et al. *J Clin Oncol* 2021;39:2970.

392. van der Kruijssen DEW, Elias SG, Vink GR, et al. Sixty-day mortality of patients with metastatic colorectal cancer randomized to systemic treatment vs primary tumor resection followed by systemic treatment. The CAIRO4 phase 3 randomized clinical trial. *JAMA Surg* 2021;156(12):1093–101.

393. Cremolini C, Antoniotti C, Stein A, et al. Individual patient data meta-analysis of FOLFOXIRI plus bevacizumab versus doublets plus bevacizumab as initial therapy of unresectable metastatic colorectal cancer. *J Clin Oncol* 2020;38:3314–24.

394. Bomze D, Mutti L, Goldman A, et al. Crossing survival curves of KEYNOTE-177 illustrate the rationale behind combining immune checkpoint inhibition with chemotherapy. *Lancet Oncol* 2022;23:e245.

395. Diaz LA, Shiu K-K, Kim T-W, et al. Pembrolizumab versus chemotherapy for microsatellite instability-high or mismatch repair-deficient metastatic colorectal cancer (KEYNOTE-177): Final analysis of a randomised, open-label, phase 3 study. *Lancet Oncol* 2022;23:659–70.

396. Tejpar S, Stintzing S, Ciardiello F, et al. Prognostic and predictive relevance of primary tumor location in patients with RAS wild-type metastatic colorectal cancer. Retrospective analyses of the CRYSTAL and FIRE-3 trials. *JAMA Oncol* 2017;3(2):194–201.

397. Maughan TS, Adams RA, Smith CG, et al. Addition of cetuximab to oxaliplatin-based first-line combination chemotherapy for treatment of advanced colorectal cancer: Results of the randomised phase 3 MRC COIN trial. *Lancet* 2011;377:2103–14.

398. Qin S, Li J, Wang L, et al. Efficacy and tolerability of first-line cetuximab plus leucovorin, fluorouracil, and oxaliplatin (FOLFOX-4) versus FOLFOX-4 in patients with RAS wild-type metastatic colorectal cancer: The open-label, randomized, phase III TAILOR trial. *J Clin Oncol* 2018;36:3031–9.

399. Venook AP, Niedzwiecki D, Lenz H-J, et al. Effect of first-line chemotherapy combined with cetuximab or bevacizumab on overall survival in patients with KRAS wild-type advanced or metastatic colorectal cancer. A randomized clinical trial. *JAMA* 2017;317(23):2392–401.

400. Holch JW, Ricard I, Stintzing S, et al. Relevance of baseline carcinoembryonic antigen for first-line treatment against metastatic colorectal cancer with FOLFIRI plus cetuximab or bevacizumab (FIRE-3 trial). *Eur J Cancer* 2019;106:115–25.
401. Rossini D, Antoniotti C, Lonardi S, et al. Upfront modified fluorouracil, leucovorin, oxaliplatin, and irinotecan plus panitumumab versus fluorouracil, leucovorin, and oxaliplatin plus panitumumab for patients with RAS/BRAF wild-type metastatic colorectal cancer: The phase III TRIPLETE study by GONO. *J Clin Oncol* 2022;40:2878–88.
402. Peeters M, Price T, Taieb J, et al. Relationships between tumour response and primary tumour location, and predictors of long-term survival, in patients with RAS wild-type metastatic colorectal cancer receiving first-line panitumumab therapy: Retrospective analyses of the PRIME and PEAK clinical trials. *Br J Cancer* 2018;119:303–12.
403. Holch JW, Stintzing S, Held S, et al. Right-sided colorectal cancer (RC): Response to first-line chemotherapy in FIRE-3 (AIO KRK-0306) with focus on early tumor shrinkage (ETS) and depth of response (DpR). *J Clin Oncol* 2017;35(suppl 15):3586.
404. Ince WL, Jubb AM, Holden SN, et al. Association of k-ras, b-raf, and p53 status with the treatment effect of bevacizumab. *J Natl Cancer Inst* 2005;97:981–9.
405. Hurwitz HI, Yi J, Ince W, et al. The clinical benefit of bevacizumab in metastatic colorectal cancer is independent of K-ras mutation status: Analysis of a phase III study of bevacizumab with chemotherapy in previously untreated metastatic colorectal cancer. *Oncologist* 2009;14:22–8.
406. Passardi A, Nanni O, Tassinari D, et al. Effectiveness of bevacizumab added to standard chemotherapy in metastatic colorectal cancer: Final results for first-line treatment from the ITACa randomised clinical trial. *Ann Oncol* 2015;26:1201–7.
407. Modest DP, Fischer von Weikersthal L, Decker T, et al. Sequential versus combination therapy of metastatic colorectal cancer using fluoropyrimidines, irinotecan, and bevacizumab: A randomized, controlled study – XELAVIRI (AIO KRK0110). *J Clin Oncol* 2019;37:22–32.
408. Cremolini C, Antoniotti C, Rossini D, et al. Upfront FOLFOXIRI plus bevacizumab and reintroduction after progression versus mFOLFOX6 plus bevacizumab followed by FOLFIRI plus bevacizumab in the treatment of patients with metastatic colorectal cancer (TRIBE2): A multicentre, open-label, phase 3, randomised, controlled trial. *Lancet Oncol* 2020;21:497–507.
409. Aranda E, Viéitez JM, Gòmez-Espana A, et al. FOLFOXIRI plus bevacizumab versus FOLFOX plus bevacizumab for patients with metastatic colorectal cancer and ≥3 circulating tumor cells: The randomised phase III VISNU-1 trial. *ESMO Open* 2020;5:e000944.
410. Yamada Y, Takahari D, Matsumoto H, et al. Leucovorin, fluorouracil, and oxaliplatin plus bevacizumab versus S-1 and oxaliplatin plus bevacizumab in patients with metastatic colorectal cancer (SOFT): An open-label, non-inferiority, randomised phase 3 trial. *Lancet Oncol* 2013;14:1278–86.
411. Yamazaki K, Nagase N, Tamagawa H, et al. Randomized phase III study of bevacizumab plus FOLFIRI and bevacizumab plus mFOLFOX6 as first-line treatment for patients with metastatic colorectal cancer (WJOG4407G). *Ann Oncol* 2016;27:1539–46.
412. Cunningham D, Lang I, Marcuello E, et al. Bevacizumab plus capecitabine versus capecitabine alone in elderly patients with previously untreated metastatic colorectal cancer (AVEX): An open-label, randomised phase 3 trial. *Lancet Oncol* 2013;14:1077–85.
413. Van Cutsem E, Danielewicz I, Saunders MP, et al. Trifluridine/tipiracil plus bevacizumab in patients with untreated metastatic colorectal cancer ineligible for intensive therapy: The randomized TASCO1 study. *Ann Oncol* 2020;31:1160–8.
414. Wasan HS, Gibbs P, Sharma NK, et al. First-line selective internal radiotherapy plus chemotherapy versus chemotherapy alone in patients with liver metastases from colorectal cancer (FOXFIRE, SIRFLOX, and FOXFIRE-Global): A combined analysis of three multicentre, randomised, phase 3 trials. *Lancet Oncol* 2017;18:1159–71.
415. Gibbs P, Heinemann V, Sharma NK, et al. Effect of primary tumor side on survival outcomes in untreated patients with metastatic colorectal cancer when selective internal radiation therapy is added to chemotherapy: Combined analysis of two randomized controlled studies. *Clin Colorectal Cancer* 2018;17(4):e617–29.
416. Chibaudel B, Maindrault-Goebel F, Lledo G, et al. Can chemotherapy be discontinued in unresectable metastatic colorectal cancer? The GERCOR OPTIMOX2 study. *J Clin Oncol* 2009;27:5727–33.
417. Adams RA, Meade AM, Seymour MT, et al. Intermittent versus continuous oxaliplatin and fluoropyrimidine combination chemotherapy for first-line treatment of advanced colorectal cancer: Results of the randomised phase 3 MRC COIN trial. *Lancet Oncol* 2011;12:642–53.

418. Luo HY, Li YH, Wang W, et al. Single-agent capecitabine as maintenance therapy after induction of XELOX (or FOLFOX) in first-line treatment of metastatic colorectal cancer: Randomized clinical trial of efficacy and safety. *Ann Oncol* 2016;27:1074–81.
419. Diaz-Rubio E, Gomez-Espana A, Massutì B, et al. First-line XELOX plus bevacizumab followed by XELOX plus bevacizumab or single-agent bevacizumab as manteinance therapy in patients with metastatic colorectal cancer: The phase III MACRO TTD study. *Oncologist* 2012;17:15–25.
420. Hegewisch-Becker S, Graeven U, Lerchenmuller CA, et al. Maintenance strategies after first-line oxaliplatin plus fluoropyrimidine plus bevacizumab for patients with metastatic colorectal cancer (AIO 0207): A randomised, non-inferiority, open-label, phase 3 trial. *Lancet Oncol* 2015;16:1355–69.
421. Aparicio T, Ghiringhelli F, Boige V, et al. Bevacizumab maintenance versus no maintenance during chemotherapy-free intervals in metastatic colorectal cancer: A randomized phase III trial (PRODIGE 9). *J Clin Oncol* 2018;36:674–81.
422. Pinto C, Orlandi A, Normanno N, et al. Phase III study with FOLFIRI/cetuximab versus FOLFIRI/cetuximab followed by cetuximab (Cet) alone in first-line therapy of RAS and BRAF wild-type (wt) metastatic colorectal cancer (mCRC) patients: The ERMES study. *Ann Oncol* 2022;33(7):LBA22.
423. Wasan H, Meade AM, Adams R, et al. Intermittent chemotherapy plus either intermittent or continuous cetuximab for first-line treatment of patients with KRAS wild-type advanced colorectal cancer (COIN-B): A randomised phase 2 trial. *Lancet Oncol* 2014;15:631–9.
424. Boige V, Blons H, Francois E, et al. Maintenance therapy with cetuximab after FOLFIRI plus cetuximab for RAS wild-type metastatic colorectal cancer. A phase 2 randomized clinical trial. *JAMA Network Open* 2023;6(9):e2333533.
425. Pietrantonio F, Morano F, Corallo S, et al. Maintenance therapy with panitumumab alone vs panitumumab plus fluorouracil-leucovorin in patients with RAS wild-type metastatic colorectal cancer. A phase 2 randomized clinical trial. *JAMA Oncol* 2019;5(9):1268–75.
426. Modest DP, Karthaus M, Fruehauf S, et al. Panitumumab plus fluorouracil and folinic acid versus fluorouracil and folinic acid alone as maintenance therapy in RAS wild-type metastatic colorectal cancer: The randomized PANAMA trial (AIO KRK 0212). *J Clin Oncol* 2022;40:72–82.
427. Raimondi A, Nichetti F, Stahler A, et al. Optimal maintenance strategy following FOLFOX plus anti-EGFR induction therapy in patients with RAS wild type metastatic colorectal cancer: An individual patient data pooled analysis of randomised clinical trials. *Eur J Cancer* 2023;190:112945.
428. Kopetz S, Grothey A, Yaeger R, et al. Encorafenib, binimetinib, and cetuximab in BRAF V600E-mutated colorectal cancer. *N Engl J Med* 2019;381:1632–43.
429. Bennouna J, Sastre J, Arnold D, et al. Continuation of bevacizumab after first progression in metastatic colorectal cancer (ML18147): A randomised phase 3 trial. *Lancet Oncol* 2013;14:29–37.
430. Van Cutsem E, Tabernero J, Lakomy R, et al. Addition of aflibercept to fluorouracil, leucovorin, and irinotecan improves survival in a phase III randomized trial in patients with metastatic colorectal cancer previously treated with an oxaliplatin-based regimen. *J Clin Oncol* 2012;30:3499–506.
431. Tabernero J, Yoshino T, Lee Cohn A, et al. Ramucirumab versus placebo in combination with second-line FOLFIRI in patients with metastatic colorectal carcinoma that progressed during or after first-line therapy with bevacizumab, oxaliplatin, and a fluoropyrimidine (RAISE): A randomised, double-blind, multicentre, phase 3 study. *Lancet Oncol* 2015;16:499–508.
432. Mulcahy MF, Mahvash A, Pracht M, et al. Radioembolization with chemotherapy for colorectal liver metastases: A randomized, open-label, international, multicenter, phase III trial. *J Clin Oncol* 2021;39:3897–907.
433. Cremolini C, Rossini D, Dell'Aquila E, et al. Rechallenge for patients with RAS and BRAF wild-type metastatic colorectal cancer with acquired resistance to first-line cetuximab and irinotecan. A phase 2 single-arm clinical trial. *JAMA Oncol* 2019;5(3):343–50.
434. Sartore-Bianchi A, Pietrantonio F, Lonardi S, et al. Circulating tumor DNA to guide rechallenge with panitumumab in metastatic colorectal cancer: The phase 2 CHRONOS trial. *Nat Med* 2022;28:1612–8.
435. Martinelli E, Martini G, Famiglietti V, et al. Cetuximab rechallenge plus avelumab in pretreated patients with RAS wild-type metastatic colorectal cancer. The phase 2 single-arm clinical CAVE trial. *JAMA Oncol* 2021;7(10):1529–35.
436. Tsuji A, Nakamura M, Watanabe T, et al. Phase II study of third-line panitumumab rechallenge in patients with metastatic wild-type KRAS colorectal cancer who obtained clinical benefit from first-line panitumumab-based chemotherapy: JACCRO CC-09. *Target Oncol* 2021;16(6):753–60.
437. Masuishi T, Tsuji A, Kotaka M, et al. Phase 2 study of irinotecan plus cetuximab rechallenge as third-line treatment in KRAS wild-type metastatic colorectal cancer: JACCRO CC-08. *Br J Cancer* 2020;123:1490–5.

438. Kato T, Kagawa Y, Kuboki Y, et al. Safety and efficacy of panitumumab in combination with trifluridine/tipiracil for pre-treated patients with unresectable, metastatic colorectal cancer with wild-type RAS: The phase 1/2 APOLLON study. *Int J Clin Oncol* 2021;26:1238–47.

439. Sartore-Bianchi A, Trusolino L, Martino C, et al. Dual-targeted therapy with trastuzumab and lapatinib in treatment-refractory , KRAS codon 12/13 wild-type, HER2-positive metastatic colorectal cancer (HERACLES): A proof-of-concept, multicentre, open-label, phase 2 trial. *Lancet Oncol* 2016;17:738–46.

440. Siena S, Di Bartolomeo M, Raghav K, et al. Trastuzumab deruxtecan (DS-8201) in patients with HER2-expressing metastatic colorectal cancer (DESTINY-CRC01): A multicentre, open-label, phase 2 trial. *Lancet Oncol* 2021;22:779–89.

441. Chang J, Xu M, Wang C, et al. Dual HER2 targeted therapy with pyrotinib and trastuzumab in refractory HER2 positive metastatic colorectal cancer: A result from HER2-FUSCC-G study. *Clin Colorectal Cancer* 2022;21(4):347–53.

442. Sartore-Bianchi A, Lonardi S, Martino C, et al. Pertuzumab and trastuzumab emtasine in patients with HER2-amplified metastatic colorectal cancer: Tha phase II HERACLES-B trial. *ESMO Open* 2020;5:e000911.

443. Brulè SY, Jonker DJ, Karapetis CS, et al. Location of colon cancer (right-sided versus left-sided) as a prognostic factor and a predictor of benefit from cetuximab in NCIC CO.17. *Eur J Cancer* 2015;51:1405–14.

444. Grothey A, Van Cutsem E, Sobrero A, et al. Regorafenib monotherapy for previously treated metastatic colorectal cancer (CORRECT): An international, multicentre, randomised, placebo-controlled, phase 3 trial. *Lancet* 2013;381:303–12.

445. Li J, Qin S, Xu R, et al. Regorafenib plus best supportive care versus placebo plus best supportive care in Asian patients with previously treated metastatic colorectal cancer (CONCUR): A randomised, double-blind, placebo-controlled, phase 3 trial. *Lancet Oncol* 2015;16:619–29.

446. Li J, Qin S, Xu R-H, et al. Effect of fruquitinib vs placebo on overall survival in patients with previously treated metastatic colorectal cancer. The FRESCO randomized clinical trial. *JAMA* 2018;319(24):2486–96.

447. Dasari A, Lonardi S, Garcia-Carbonero R, et al. Fruquintinib versus placebo in patients with refractory metastatic colorectal cancer (FRESCO-2): An international, multicentre, randommised, double-blind, phase 3 study. *Lancet* 2023;402:41–53.

448. Bekaii-Saab TS, Ou S-F, Ahn DH, et al. Regorafenib dose-optimisation in patients with refractory metastatic colorectal cancer (ReDOS): A randomised, multicentre, open-label, phase 2 study. *Lancet Oncol* 2019;20:1070–82.

449. Mayer RJ, Van Cutsem E, Falcone A, et al. Randomized trial of TAS-102 for refractory metastatic colorectal cancer. *N Engl J Med* 2015;372:1909–19.

450. Xu J, Kim TW, Shen L, et al. Results of a randomized, double-blind, placebo-controlled, phase III trial of trifluridine/tipiracil (TAS-102) monotherapy in Asian patients with previously treated metastatic colorectal cancer: The TERRA study. *J Clin Oncol* 2018;36:350–8.

451. Pfeiffer P, Yilmaz M, Moller S, et al. TAS-102 with or without bevacizumab in patients with chemorefractory metastatic colorectal cancer: An investigator-initiated, open-label, randomised, phase 2 trial. *Lancet Oncol* 2020;21:412–20.

452. Fiorentini G, Aliberti C, Tilli M, et al. Intra-arterial infusion of irinotecan-loaded drug-eluting beads (DEBIRI) versus intravenous therapy (FOLFIRI) for hepatic metastases from colorectal cancer: Final results of a phase III study. *Anticancer Res* 2012;32:1387–96.

453. Martin RCG, Scoggins CR, Schreeder M, et al. Randomized controlled trial of irinotecan drug-eluting beads with simultaneous FOLFOX and bevacizumab for patients with unresectable colorectal liver-limited metastasis. *Cancer* 2015;121:3649–58.

10 Anal cancer

10.1 INTRODUCTION

10.1.1 EPIDEMIOLOGY

A GLOBOCAN analysis estimated 30,416 cases of anal cancer (AC) for 2020, of which 19,792 in women and 10,624 in men, respectively 65% and 53% in countries with a very high human development index [1]. In the US in 2024 are expected 10,540 new cases and 2,190 deaths [2]. AC remains a rare tumor, representing only 2% of the gastrointestinal tract malignancies. The incidence age-adjusted standardized rate (ASR) for AC in Europe in 2022 was 2.2/100,000, with 9,901 new cases, and mortality ASR of 0.7/100,000 with 2,968 cancer deaths. The tumor was more prevalent among females with an incidence ASR of 2.3 vs. 1.9/100,000, and a mortality ASR of 0.6 vs. 0.6/100,000 [3].

In the US, an increase of incidence of 2.7% per year from 2001 to 2015 was registered [4], and similar findings were documented in Europe and Australia [5]. In particular, in Europe, the estimated incidence by the year 2040 is increasing by an additional 18.39% [3]. However, among 8,032 human papillomavirus (HPV) vaccine-eligible individuals in the US, a reduction in the incidence of in situ and invasive AC was reported [6].

10.1.2 STAGING OF METASTATIC DISEASE

For diagnosis, clinical examination of inguinal lymph nodes and digital rectal examination are essential. Anoscopy/proctoscopy completes the local evaluation, and sometimes is useful to obtain a confirmatory biopsy, which is mandatory.

For staging, multiparametric high-resolution T2-weighted MRI of the pelvis, chest-abdomen CT, and gynecological examination are required. Sometimes, FDG-PET/CT can be considered for its high sensitivity for nodal and distant metastases, modifying the stage in 41% and treatment plan in 28% [7, 8]. In addition, some parameters related to MRI or FDG-PET could predict recurrence [9, 10].

HIV testing and p16/HPV evaluation could be useful for treatment plans and follow-up.

TNM staging system of the American Joint Committee on Cancer (AJCC), 9th edition is the currently recommended stage classification [11].

10.1.3 PROGNOSIS OF METASTATIC DISEASE

From 1980 to 2010 5-year survival rates of AC patients increased from 64% to 75% [12]. Unresectable relapsed or metastatic anal cancer (mAC) patients report 5-year survival rates of 35% [13], and only 10–20% have metastases at diagnosis with another 10–20% experiencing a recurrence after a curative treatment [14, 15]. In recent prospective trials, the median overall survival (OS) ranges between 12–20 months [16]. A monoinstitutional mAC series demonstrated that a multimodal treatment, including regional treatment of primary tumor or metastasis, can improve OS (53 vs. 22 months) and progression-free survival (PFS) [17]. Further analyses of the National Cancer Database (NCDB) confirmed these findings [18–20]. Given the rarity of mAC, a prospective trial is unlikely, then regional treatments in the context of a palliative strategy should be considered, and represent an additional reason to better evaluate prognostic variables (PFs) in the individual patient.

10.2 ANALYSIS OF PROGNOSTIC VARIABLES IN EARLY METASTATIC DISEASE

A systematic review of 13 studies, 6 prospective phase II trials and 7 retrospectives, that investigated upfront therapies in mAC patients, resulted in the selection of one prospective trial, which however was excluded from the selection because the PFs analysis was performed considering PFS as the outcome [21]. Due to the low number of studies enrolling mAC patients, three retrospective studies that analyzed the relationship of PFs with OS were included in the analysis [22–24] (Table S1).

10.3 PATIENT-RELATED PROGNOSTIC FACTORS

10.3.1 PERFORMANCE STATUS

In a prospective trial enrolling mAC patients receiving three-drug first-line chemotherapy, only patients with ECOG performance status (PS) 0–1 were included, and the comparison of patients with PS 1 vs. PS 0 did not document any PFS differences [21].

TABLE S1
Prognostic factors analysed in the three selected retrospective studies of patients with unresectable or metastatic anal cancer receiving upfront treatment

Variable	No. trials	Prognostic relationship	No prognostic relationship
Patient-related			
Performance status	1	0	1
Demographic			
Age	3	0	3
Sex	3	0	3
Anthropometric			
Clinic			
Lab			
Hemoglobin	1	0	1
Neutrophil-to-lymphocyte ratio	1	1	0
Albumin	1	0	1
Lactic dehydrogenase	1	0	1
Tumor-related			
Tumor burden			
Disease status	1	0	1
No. sites metastases	2	0	2
Location			
Timing metastasis			
Synchronous vs. metachronous	2	0	2
Site of metastasis			
Liver metastases	2	1	1
Nodal metastases	1	1	0
Pathology			
Histologic grade	1	0	1
Previous treatments			
Multimodal treatment	1	1	0
CDDP vs. MMC-based CRT	1	0	1

10.3.1.1 Selected studies

A Danish retrospective study from the Danish Hospital registers of patients treated with paclitaxel and capecitabine for mAC, detected a trend for poor OS of both comparisons, PS 1 vs. PS 0 (HR 1.93 0.98–3.83) and PS 2 vs. PS 0 (HR 2.06 0.86–4.93) [24].

10.3.2 DEMOGRAPHIC

10.3.2.1 Age

Population databases agree on the prognostic role of age. Three NCDB analyses of mAC patients reported shorter OS for >70 [18, 20, 25], but another report from the same database [23] and a study of patients receiving salvage surgery [26] did not find any prognostic effect of age.

10.3.2.2 Sex

A reduced OS of males compared to females was reported by four studies on different cohorts of mAC of the NCDB [18–20, 25] but was not confirmed by a retrospective study [26].

10.3.2.3 Other demographic variables

Different regions of the US [25] or urban vs. rural areas [20] did not affect the prognosis of mAC patients.

Two NCDB studies excluded a relationship between race and the outcome of mAC patients [18, 19].

10.3.2.4 Selected studies

Two studies assessed age around a cut-off of 65 [23, 24], and one around 60 [22], but none documented a prognostic effect.

Although the trend was unfavorable for males, this was not associated with a significant difference in OS (HR 1.41, 0.80–2.48) [27], while no prognostic relationships for sex were reported in the other two studies.

10.3.3 ANTHROPOMETRIC

Body mass index (BMI) can influence anal microbiome composition [27], and obesity in heterosexual males may favor HPV16 persistence [28]. Conversely, sarcopenia was associated with some characteristics, such as anemia and deterioration of the PS, but did not affect the outcome [29].

10.3.4 CLINIC

Local symptoms correlate with more advanced T-stage, in particular, perianal pain, painful defecation, and weight loss [30].

Two of three NCDB reports suggest an unfavorable prognostic role for the increasing values of the Charlson-Deyo comorbidity score [18–20].

Some viral diseases, in addition to having a relationship with the incidence, could affect prognosis. CDC estimated that 97% of all AC arise from HPV infection [31], but few data are available on the prognostic role of serum HPV positivity and viral load, as well as unknown is the role of HPV subtypes other than HPV16, that is responsible for mono-infection of 80% of AC patients [32].

Many HIV-associated malignancies are linked to oncogenic viruses, such as HPV in the AC [33], but only 21% of AC in males and 3% in females occur in HIV-positive, with ASR of 0.07 and 0.02 [1]. However, considering the results of HAART on HIV, an increasing AC incidence in HIV-positive subjects is expected [34].

Still, among AC patients the risk of second primary tumors is increased, and only among females it was related to radiotherapy [35].

10.3.5 Laboratory

10.3.5.1 Hematology

Anemia has been associated with higher rates of distant metastases [36] and poor OS [37]. However, among mAC patients hemoglobin concentrations <10 g/dL did not influence OS [21].

Data about mAC patients remain very limited, and in a prospective study of patients receiving palliative chemotherapy, no differences in OS were reported for the lymphocyte count with a cut-off of 1,000 [21].

10.3.5.2 Tumor markers

HPV circulating tumor DNA (ctDNA) is the most promising marker of mAC [38] and is measurable in 91% of mAC patients [39]. An evaluation of 59 mAC patients from the Epitopes-HPV02 study documented that baseline HPV ctDNA levels <7,148 copies/mL were associated with longer PFS [40], and a similar effect on OS was suggested by a meta-analysis of 16 studies [41].

Although CEA kinetics have shown a longitudinal behavior similar to mAC during treatment, CEA is expressed by only a third of mACs [42].

10.3.5.3 Selected studies

The Danish population-based analysis evaluated the relationship between hemoglobin and OS. Despite the better prognosis for increased hemoglobin, OS prolongation was not significant, while in the same study neutrophil-to-lymphocyte ratio (NLR) >4 was associated with a poor prognosis (HR 2.22, CI: 1.18–4.17) [24]

No significant relationships with OS were evident for lactic dehydrogenase (LDH) >245 U/L and albumin >35 g/L [24].

10.4 TUMOR-RELATED PROGNOSTIC FACTORS

10.4.1 Tumor burden

Although many variables are ultimately attributable to tumor burden (TB), none of them was standardized.

Population-based studies did not report an effect of the primary tumor size [20], whereas a more extended T-stage, namely T3–T4 vs. T2 [25] or T3–T4 vs. T1 [19] and N3 vs. N0 stage [19], have been associated with poor survival of mAC patients. Similarly, no prognostic role was reported for the size of relapsing/persistent disease [26].

Few data are available about the comparison of metastatic vs. loco-regional spread, and a retrospective study did not find any OS difference [26].

Multiple sites of metastasis vs. single site conferred poor prognosis to mAC patients [20], and having more than three metastatic sites correlated with a trend for shorter PFS [21].

10.4.1.1 Selected studies

Only one retrospective study analyzed the relationship of disease status (metastatic vs. locally advanced) with OS, but the relationship was not significant [24].

Similarly, the number of metastatic sites was not associated with OS [23, 24].

10.4.2 Primary tumor location

Anal malignancies are mostly those of the anal canal, a region extending from the anorectal junction to the skin of the anal margin, including the dentate line, which begins about 1 cm inferior to the rectal epithelium, and which separates the glandular mucosa from the squamous epithelium. Formally, all tumors arising in the skin 5 cm around the anal canal are also AC (anal margin), but their clinical evolution and treatment are similar to skin cancer. The distinction is often not simple, especially when both areas are involved, so it is common to formulate a diagnosis of primary tumors of the anal canal whenever it is involved. Consequently, it is rare to find studies that define different sites of origin for AC, since involvement of the anal canal indicates a rather homogeneous behavior of the disease.

10.4.3 TIMING OF METASTASIS

The timing of metastases has been poorly evaluated. Only 10% of AC at diagnosis have metastases and another 10–20% will have a recurrence. As with other malignancies, patients with synchronous metastases appear to have more aggressive disease, as suggested by shorter PFS of mAC patients receiving chemotherapy [21].

A retrospective study analyzed a surgical series of relapsing/persistent AC patients after chemoradiation and did not find different outcomes by the timing of relapse [26].

10.4.3.1 Selected studies

One study calculated the time-to-metastasis >12 months and verified that it was not associated with OS differences [23], while another study evaluated the OS of the synchronous and metachronous metastasis groups, that were identical, around 20 months [22].

10.4.4 SITE OF METASTASIS

The most frequent sites of metastasis are para-aortic nodes and liver, then lungs, peritoneum, and skin. Bone localizations occur in 1% [43], and brain metastases have rarely been described.

NCDB data evidentiated that only multiple sites of metastasis were associated with poor prognosis, while 5-year survival rates were increasing from bone metastases (14.8%) to liver (20.4%) and lung (21.3%) [20]. Another evaluation from the same database reported a better outcome for patients with non-regional lymph node metastases compared to other sites of metastases [19], a finding that was confirmed after immunotherapy [44]. On the other hand, a lymph node involvement associated with recurrence, after salvage surgery, correlated with poor prognosis [26].

10.4.4.1 Selected studies

The presence of liver metastases was associated with poor OS in one study [23], while it had no influence on prognosis in another [24]. A comparison of lymph node metastases vs. visceral was instead reported in the other retrospective analysis and documented a relationship between the visceral site of metastases and reduced OS (36 vs. 17 months) [22].

10.4.5 PATHOLOGY

10.4.5.1 Histology

Squamous cell carcinoma of the anus (SCCA) is the more frequent histotype, while other histologies are rare. The patterns of SCCA, such as basaloid, transitional, spheroidal or cloacogenic, have not demonstrated any impact on prognosis, as with the keratinizing aspect, even though an NCDB report suggested a poor prognosis of cloacogenic AC and no effect from keratinizing [20].

10.4.5.2 Other pathological variables

The degree of differentiation did not influence mAC outcome [20].

HPV status and p16 are PFs. While HPV determination is generally not necessary in the pathology report, it predicts better prognosis and sensitivity to treatments [32, 45]. Although associated with HPV–DNA expression, p16 expression has an independent prognostic role [32], with a better outcome for HPV+/p16+ mACs [46].

The massive occurrence of tumor-infiltrating lymphocytes (TILs) was related to improved survival, regardless of AC stage [47]. Some studies documented that high TIL infiltration prevailed among HPV-positive ACs, for which the role of TILs during response to chemoradiation is the most relevant feature [48]. Indeed, E6 and E7 viral proteins, in addition to oncogenic transformation, induce host response and TIL recruitment. As in other HPV-related tumors, a better understanding of the TME is needed. HPV persistence supports local inflammation, which facilitates AC development [49].

HIV-positivity does not affect the composition of the TME, in terms of immune cells and PD-L1 expression, suggesting that such patients should not be excluded from immunotherapy trials [50].

10.4.5.3 Molecular biology

In AC patients, HPV-positive tumors are the vast majority, and among these some genomic analyses have detected mutations activating the PI3K/mTOR signaling pathway [32, 51], among which PIK3CA mutations occur in 88% of mAC patients [82]. PIK3CA mutations were associated with an increased risk of recurrence [52] and with poor outcomes after salvage surgery [53]. Similarly, TP53 mutations were more frequent in recurrences [53].

HPV-negative AC patients are often associated with an unfavorable trend of OS, they are more likely to be nonwhite and to have a strong tobacco exposure [54], express more frequently actionable mutations (TP53, CDNK2A [51], BRAF [55]). TP53 mutations in HPV-negative AC are associated with poor prognosis [45, 46]. High tumor mutation burden (TMB-high) is rare in AC [56, 57] like microsatellite instability-high (MSI-H) status, and they never occur in the same patients [55], nor TMB predicts the efficacy of immunotherapy [58, 59].

10.4.5.4 Selected studies

One study compared patients with moderately vs. poorly differentiated AC, without detecting any relationship with OS [23].

10.4.6 Previous treatments

In AC with metachronous metastases, previous therapy affects OS. The analysis of 1,160 mAC patients from the NCDB documented that regional treatment, even in the presence of metastases, improved OS [20]. Other authors reported a similar retrospective favorable effect from adding radiation therapy to chemotherapy in mAC [18, 19].

Additionally, several studies have reported poor OS for patients receiving incomplete radiation [60, 61] or long-lasting chemoradiation [62]. The analysis included 1,125 patients who underwent definitive chemoradiation and identified factors associated with treatment interruptions leading to OS reduction. Elderly patients (>70 years) and those with at least one co-morbidity were less likely to complete the chemoradiation program [63].

10.4.6.1 Selected studies

If previous cisplatin-based vs. mitomycin-based therapy did not affect OS [22], prior multimodal therapy was associated with a better prognosis (22 vs. 13 months) [22].

10.5 PROGNOSTIC FACTORS IN DECISION-MAKING

For patients with poor general conditions (ECOG PS >2) antineoplastic treatment is not indicated. Some recommendations about PFs can be reported (Table 10.1).

10.5.1 Upfront treatment

The recommended standard of care is a platinum-based chemotherapy, preferring a platinum and taxane-based regimen [64], and considering a platinum-fluoropyrimidine doublet in the presence of a contraindication to paclitaxel [65, 66].

TABLE 10.1

Prognostic and predictive variables in clinical decision-making in metastatic anal cancer

A. Upfront systemic treatment

1	Tumor burden	
	• Low: multimodal treatment favored (primary tumor, metastases)	
	• High: platinum-based chemotherapy favored	
2	Site of metastases	
	• Nodal metastases (or para-aortic only): multimodal treatment favored	
	• Liver-limited disease and OMD: aggressive regional approach favored	
3	Co-morbidities	
	• Low number: consider aggressive multimodal approach	

B. Treatment of refractory disease

1	Progression-free survival	
	• Longer than 12 months: alternative drugs favored (not received as upfront)	
2	Performance status	
	• Good: alternative drugs favored (not received as upfront)	
3	Immune activation	
	• PD-L1 positive (CPS>1–20): consider immunotherapy (clinical trials)	
	• high CD8 infiltration: consider immunotherapy (clinical trials)	
	• positive tumor-inflammation signature: consider immunotherapy (clinical trials)	

Legend: CPS, combined positive score. OMD, oligometastatic disease. PD-L1, programmed death ligand 1.

However, some studies, mostly retrospective, support a more aggressive approach in the setting of liver-limited [67] or oligometastatic disease [17], frequently proposing articulated treatment plans including radiation treatment of the primary tumor [18, 19, 22] and/or locoregional therapies of metastases [22]. These approaches are more justified in the presence of low TB or disease confined to para-aortic nodes [68] or only lymph node metastases [20], early onset AC [17], low number of comorbidities [69].

10.5.2 TREATMENT OF REFRACTORY DISEASE

Patients with good PS progressing after more than 12 months from the conclusion of the upfront treatment are ideal candidates for a second-line regimen with alternative cytotoxic drugs, such as paclitaxel [70] or fluoropyrimidines.

To date, it is not clear the subgroup of mAC patients, who could benefit from immunotherapy, around 10–20%, so immunotherapy should preferably be proposed in the context of clinical trials [71, 72]. However, the recommendation for immunotherapy could be stronger in the subgroup with PD-L1 positive CPS>1–20 [73], high CD8 T-cell infiltration [72], or a positive tumor-inflammation signature [58].

10.6 CONCLUSION

Within the limited evidence on PFs in mAC, a central role continues to be played by primary tumor stage, both T-stage and N-stage, and chemoradiation on the primary tumor, as reported in Table 10.2. Less solid is the evidence in favor of the negative role of the number of metastatic sites and the site of metastasis, visceral vs. lymph node. On the other hand, HPV is too frequently involved to expect it to improve prognosis assessment in the future.

In contrast, TILs infiltration and its change after chemoradiation should be better characterized in mAC, especially their relationship to systemic inflammation and its kinetics.

TABLE 10.2

Prognostic factors evaluated in prospective trials of upfront treatment in patients with unresectable or metastatic anal cancer

Suggested	Not suggested	Needing study
-	HIV	Performance status
		Age
		Sex
		HPV, HPV ctDNA
		Hemoglobin
		Neutrophil count, NLR
T-stage	Primary tumor location	T diameter
N-stage	Disease status	Timing metastases
Multiple sites of metastases		
Nodal metastases only		
TILs infiltration		
Multimodal therapy		
Complete RT/CRT		

Legend: CRT, chemo-radiation therapy. HIV, Human Immunodeficiency Virus. HPV, Human Papilloma Virus. HPV ctDNA, Human papilloma virus circulating tumor DNA. N, nodes. NLR, neutrophil-to-lymphocyte ratio. RT, radiation therapy. T, tumor. TILs, tumor-infiltrating lymphocyte.

REFERENCES

1. Deshmukh AA, Damgacioglu H, Georges D, et al. Global burden of HPV-attributable squamous cell carcinoma of the anus in 2020, according to sex and HIV status: A worldwide analysis. *Int J Cancer* 2023;152(3):417–28.
2. American Cancer Society. Anal cancer: Key statistics, available at: https://www.cancer.org/cancer/types/anal-cancer/about/what-is-key-statistics.html, accessed January 9, 2024.
3. ECIS – European Cancer Information System, available at: https://ecis.jrc.ec.europa.eu, accessed October 31, 2023.
4. National Cancer Institute 2020, available at: https://www.cancer.gov/news-events/cancer-currents-blog/2019/anal-cancer-incidence-mortality-rise, accessed October 31, 2023.
5. Islami F, Ferlay J, Lortet-Tieulent J, et al. International trends in anal cancer incidence rates. *Int J Epidemiol* 2017;46(3):924–38.
6. Berenson AB, Guo F, Chang M. Association of human papillomavirus vaccination with the incidence of squamous cell carcinomas of the anus in the US. *JAMA Oncol* 2022;8(4):639–41.
7. Jones M, Hruby G, Stanwell P, et al. Multiparametric MRI as an outcome predictor for anal canal cancer managed with chemoradiotherapy. *Ann Surg Oncol* 2015;22:3574–81.
8. Mahmud A, Poon R, Jonker D. PET imaging in anal canal cancer: A systematic review and meta-analysis. *Br J Radiol* 2017;90(1080):20170370.
9. Owkzarczyk K, Prezzi D, Cascino M, et al. MRI heterogeneity analysis for prediction of recurrence and disease free survival in anal cancer. *Radioth Oncol* 2019;134:119–26.
10. Jones MP, Hruby G, Metser U, et al. FDG-PET parameters predict for recurrence in anal cancer – Results from a prospective, multicentre clinical trial. *Radiation Oncol* 2019;14:140.
11. Janczewski LM, Faski J, Nelson H, et al. Survival outcomes used to generate version 9 American Joint Committee on Cancer staging system for anal cancer. *CA Cancer J Clin* 2023;73:516–23.
12. Sekhar H, Zwahlen M, Trelle S, et al. Nodal stage migration and prognosis in anal cancer: A systematic review, meta-regression, and simulation study. *Lancet Oncol* 2017;18(10):1348–59.
13. NCI SEER 2023, available at: https://seer.cancer.gov/statfacts/html/anus.html, accessed October 31, 2023.

14. No authors. Epidermoid anal cancer: Results from the UKCCCR randomised trial of radiotherapy alone versus radiotherapy, 5-fluorouracil, and mitomycin. UKCCCR Anal Cancer Trial Working Party. UK Coordinating Committee on Cancer Research. *Lancet* 1996;348(9034):1049–54.
15. Horner MJ, Ries LAG, Krapcho M, et al. SEER Cancer Statistics Review, 1975-2006. Bethesda, MD; National Cancer Institute, available at: https://seer.cancer.gov/csr/1975_2006/, based on November 2008 SEER data submission, posted to the SEER web site, 2009.
16. Rao S, Sclafani F, Eng C, et al. International rare cancers initiative multicenter randomized phase II trial of cisplatin and fluorouracil versus carboplatin and paclitaxel in advanced anal cancer: InterAAct. *J Clin Oncol* 2020;38:2510–8.
17. Eng C, Chang GJ, You YN, et al. The role of systemic chemotherapy and multidisciplinary management in improving the overall survival of patients with metastatic squamous cell carcinoma of the anal canal. *Oncotarget* 2014;5:11133–42.
18. Abdelazim YA, Rushing CN, Palta M, et al. Role of pelvic chemoradiation therapy in patients with initially metastatic anal canal cancer: A National Cancer Database Review. *Cancer* 2019;125:2115–22.
19. Wang Y, Yu X, Zhao N, et al. Definitive pelvic radiotherapy and survival of patients with newly diagnosed metastatic anal cancer. *J Natl Compr Canc Netw* 2019;17(1):29–37.
20. Atallah RP, Zhang Y, Zakka K, et al. Role of local therapy in the management of patients with metastatic anal squamous cell carcinoma: A National Cancer Database study. *J Gastrointest Oncol* 2022;13(5):2306–21.
21. Kim S, Francois E, André T, et al. Docetaxel, cisplatin, and fluorouracil chemotherapy for metastatic or unresectable locally recurrent anal squamous cell carcinoma (Epitopes-HPV02): A multicentre, single-arm, phase 2 study. *Lancet Oncol* 2018;19:1094–106.
22. Evesque L, Benezery K, Follana P, et al. Multimodal therapy of squamous cell carcinoma of the anus with distant metastasis: A single-institution experience. *Dis Colon Rectum* 2017;60:785–91.
23. Sclafani F, Morano F, Cunningham D, et al. Platinum-fluoropyrimidine and paclitaxel-based chemotherapy in the treatment of advanced anal cancer patients. *Oncologist* 2017;22:402–8.
24. Truelsen CG, Serup-Hansen E, Smedegaard Storm K, et al. Nonplatinum-based therapy with paclitaxel and capecitabine for advanced squamous cell carcinomas of the anal canal: A population-based Danish anal cancer group study. *Cancer Med* 2021;10:3224–30.
25. Repka MC, Aghdam N, Karlin AW, et al. Social determinants of stage IV anal cancer and the impact of pelvic radiotherapy in the metastatic setting. *Cancer Med* 2017;8:2497–506.
26. Hagemans JAW, Blinde SE, Nuyttens JJ, et al. Salvage abdominoperineal resection for squamous cell anal cancer: A 30-year single-institution experience. *Ann Surg Oncol* 2018;25:1970–9.
27. Wells J, Bai J, Tsementzi D, et al. Exploring the anal microbiome in HIV positive and high-risk HIV negative women. *AIDS Res Hum Retroviruses* 2022;38(3):228–36.
28. Nyitray AG, Peng F, Day RS, et al. The association between body mass index and anal canal human papillomavirus prevalence and persistence: The HIM study. *Hum Vacc Immunother* 2019;15(7–8):1911–9.
29. Martin D, von der Grun J, Rodel C, et al. Sarcopenia is associated with hematologic toxicity during chemoradiotherapy in patients with anal carcinoma. *Front Oncol* 2020;10:1576.
30. Sauter M, Keilholz G, Kranzbuhler H, et al. Presenting symptoms predict local staging of anal cancer: A retrospective analysis of 86 patients. *BMC Gastroenterol* 2016;16:46.
31. Centers for Disease Control and Prevention (CDC). Human papillomavirus-associated cancers – United States, 2004–2008. *Morb Mortal Wkly Rep* 2012;61:258–61.
32. Serup-Hansen E, Linnemann D, Skovrider-Ruminski W, et al. Human papillomavirus genotyping and p16 expression as prognostic factors for patients with American Joint Committee on Cancer stages I to III carcinoma of the anal canal. *J Clin Oncol* 2014;32(17):1812–7.
33. Grulich AE, van Leeuwen MT, Falster MO, et al. Incidence of cancers in people with HIV/AIDS compared with immunosuppressed transplant recipients: A meta-analysis. *Lancet* 2007;370(9581):59–67.
34. Sumner L, Kamitani E, Chase S, et al. A systematic review and meta-analysis of mortality in anal cancer patients by HIV status. *Cancer Epidemiol* 2022;76:102069.
35. Jani KS, Lu S-E, Murphy JD, et al. Malignancies diagnosed before and after anal squamous cell carcinomas: A SEER registry analysis. *Cancer Med* 2021;10:3575–83.
36. Kapacee ZA, Susnerwala S, Wise M, et al. Chemoradiotherapy for squamous cell anal carcinoma: A review of prognostic factors. *Colorectal Dis* 2016;18:1080–6.
37. Banerjee R, Roxin G, Eliasziw M, et al. The prognostic significance of pretreatment leukocytosis in patients with anal cancer treated with radical chemioradiotherapy or radiotherapy. *Dis Colon Rectum* 2013;56(9):1036–42.

38. Cabel L, Jeannot E, Bieche I, et al. Prognostic impact of residual HPV ctDNA detection after chemora-diotherapy for anal squamous cell carcinoma. *Clin Cancer Res* 2018;24(22):5767–71.

39. Bernard-Tessier A, Jeannot E, Guenat D, et al. Clinical validity of HPV circulating tumor DNA in advanced anal carcinoma: An ancillary study to the Epitopes-HPV02 trial. *Clin Cancer Res* 2019;25(7):2109–15.

40. Bernard-Tessier A, Jeannot E, Guenat D, et al. HPV circulating tumor DNA as predictive biomarker of sus-tained response to chemotherapy in advanced anal carcinoma. *Ann Oncol* 2018;26(suppl_8):viii14–viii57.

41. Urbute A, Rasmussen CL, Belmonte F, et al. Prognostic significance of HPV DNA and p16INK4a in anal cancer: A systematic review and meta-analysis. *Cancer Epidemiol Biomarkers Prev* 2020;29:703–10.

42. Hester R, Advani S, Rashid A, et al. CEA as blood-based biomarker in anal cancer. *Oncotarget* 2021;12(11):1037–45.

43. Huang J-F, Shen J, Li X, et al. Incidence of patients with bone metastases at diagnosis of solid tumors in adults: A large population-based study. *Ann Transl Med* 2020;8(7):482.

44. Peddireddy AS, Johnson B, Wolff RA, et al. Survival benefit to immunotherapy according to site of organ involvement in metastatic anal cancer. *J Clin Oncol* 2023;41(suppl2):3.

45. Meulendijks D, Tomasoa NB, Dewit L, et al. HPV-negative squamous cell carcinoma of the anal canal is unresponsive to standard treatment and frequently carries disruptive mutations in TP53. *Br J Cancer* 2015;112(8):1358–66.

46. Parwaiz I, MacCabe TA, Thomas MG, et al. A systematic review and meta-analysis of prognostic biomarkers in anal squamous cell carcinoma treated with primary chemoradiotherapy. *Clin Oncol* 2019;31(12):e1–e13.

47. Rubio CA, Nilsson PJ, Petersson F, et al. The clinical significance of massive intratumoral lymphocyto-sis in squamous cell carcinoma of the anus. *Int J Clin Exp Pathol* 2008;1:376–80.

48. Gilbert DC, Serup-Hansen E, Linnemann D, et al. Tumour-infiltrating lymphocyte scores effec-tively stratify outcomes over and above p16 post chemo-radiotherapy in anal cancer. *Br J Cancer* 2016;114(2):134–7.

49. Smola S. Immunopathogenesis of HPV-associated cancers and prospects for immunotherapy. *Viruses* 2017;9(9):254.

50. Yanik EL, Kaunitz GJ, Cottrell TR, et al. Association of HIV status with local immune response to anal squamous cell carcinoma. Implications for immunotherapy. *JAMA Oncol* 2017;3(7):974–8.

51. Chung JH, Sanford E, Johnson A, et al. Comprehensive genomic profiling of anal squamous cell carci-noma reveals distinct genomically defined classes. *Ann Oncol* 2016;27:1336–41.

52. Morris V, Rao X, Pickering C, et al. Comprehensive genomic profiling of metastatic squamous cell carcinoma of the anal canal. *Mol Cancer Res* 2017;15(11):1542–50.

53. Cacheux W, Rouleau E, Briaux A, et al. Mutational analysis of anal cancers demonstrates frequent PIK3CA mutations associated with poor outcome after salvage abdominoperineal resection. *Br J Cancer* 2016;114(12):1387–95.

54. Morris VK, Rashid A, Rodriguez-Bigas M, et al. Clinicopathologic features associated with human papillomavirus/p16 in patients with metastatic squamous cell carcinoma of the anal canal. *Oncologist* 2015;20:1247–52.

55. Armstrong SA, Malley R, Wang H, et al. Molecular characterization of squamous cell carcinoma of the anal canal. *J Gastrointest Oncol* 2021;12(5):2423–37.

56. Cacheux W, Dangles-Marie V, Rouleau E, et al. Exome sequencing reveals aberrant signalling pathways as hallmark of treatment-naive anal squamous cell carcinoma. *Oncotarget* 2017;9(1):464–76.

57. Salem ME, Puccini A, Grothey A, et al. Landscape of tumor mutation load, mismatch repair defi-ciency, and PD-L1 expression in a large patient cohort of gastrointestinal cancers. *Mol Cancer Res* 2018;16(5):805–12.

58. Rao S, Anandappa G, Capdevila J, et al. A phase II study of retifanlimab (INCMGA00012) in patients with squamous carcinoma of the anal canal who have progressed following platinum-based chemo-therapy (PODIUM-202). *ESMO Open* 2022;7(4):100529.

59. Marabelle A, Fakih M, Lopez J, et al. Association of tumour mutational burden with outcomes in patients with advanced solid tumours treated with pembrolizumab: Prospective biomarker analysis of the multicohort, open-label, phase 2 KEYNOTE-158 study. *Lancet Oncol* 2020;21(10):1353–65.

60. Shakir R, Adams R, Cooper R, et al. Patterns and predictors of relapse following radical chemoradiation therapy delivered using intensity modulated radiation therapy with a simultaneous integrated boost in anal squamous cell carcinoma. *Int J Radiat Oncol* 2020;106:329–39.

61. Rouard N, Peiffert D, Rio E, et al. Intensity-modulated radiation therapy of anal squamous cell carcinoma: Relationship between delineation quality and regional recurrence. *Radiother Oncol* 2019;131:93–100.

62. Schernberg A, Escande A, Del Campo ER, et al. Leukocytosis and neutrophilia predicts outcome in anal cancer. *Radiother Oncol* 2017;122(1):137–45.
63. Raphael MJ, Ko G, Booth CM, et al. Factors associated with chemoradiation therapy interruption and noncompletion among patients with squamous cell anal carcinoma. *JAMA Oncol* 2020;6(6):881–7.
64. Rao S, Sclafani F, Eng C, et al. International rare cancers initiative multicenter randomized phase II trial of cisplatin and fluorouracil versus carboplatin and paclitaxel in advanced anal cancer: InterAAct. *J Clin Oncol* 2020;38(22): 2510–8.
65. Faivre C, Rougier P, Ducreux M, et al. 5-fluorouracile and cisplatinum combination chemotherapy for metastatic squamous-cell anal cancer. *Bull Cancer* 1999;86(10): 861–5.
66. Eng C, Pathak P. Treatment options in metastatic squamous cell carcinoma of the anal canal. *Curr Treat Options Oncol* 2008;9:400–7.
67. Pawlik TM, Gleisner AL, Bauer TW, et al. Liver-directed surgery for metastatic squamous cell carcinoma to the liver: Results of a multi-center analysis. *Ann Surg Oncol* 2007;14(10):2807–16.
68. Holliday EB, Lester SC, Harmsen WS, et al. Extended-field chemoradiation therapy for definitive treatment of anal cancer squamous cell carcinoma involving the para-aortic lymph nodes. *Int J Radiat Oncol Biol Phys* 2018;102(1):102–8.
69. Bilimoria KY, Bentrem DJ, Rock CE, et al. Outcomes and prognostic factors for squamous-cell carcinoma of the anal canal: Analysis of patients from the National Cancer Data Base. *Dis Colon Rectum* 2009;52(4):624–31.
70. Abbas A, Nehme E, Fakih M. Single-agent paclitaxel in advanced anal cancer after failure of cisplatin and 5-fluorouracil chemotherapy. *Anticancer Res* 2011;31(12): 4637–40.
71. Ott PA, Elez E, Hiret S, et al. Pembrolizumab in patients with extensive-stage small-cell lung cancer: Results from the phase Ib KEYNOTE-028 study. *J Clin Oncol* 2017;35(34):3823–9.
72. Morris VK, Salem ME, Nimeiri H, et al. Nivolumab for previously treated unresectable metastatic anal cancer (NCI9673): A multicentre, single-arm, phase 2 study. *Lancet Oncol* 2017;18(4):446–53.
73. Burtness B, Harrington KJ, Greil R, et al. Pembrolizumab alone or with chemotherapy versus cetuximab with chemotherapy for recurrent or metastatic squamous cell carcinoma of the head and neck (KEYNOTE-048): A randomised, open-label, phase 3 study. *Lancet* 2019;394(10212):1915–28.

Index

Printed in the United States
by Baker & Taylor Publisher Services